INTRODUCTION TO MATERNAL AND CHILD HEALTH

Zwannda Kwinda

ALLIED HEALTH PRESS

Introduction to Maternal and Child Health

Author: **Zwannda Kwinda**

Allied Health Press
4164 Lakeshore Road
Burlington ON L7L 1A4
Canada
www.alliedhealthpress.com
Email: orders@arclereducation.com

ISBN: 978-1-77956-254-8

ABOUT THE AUTHOR

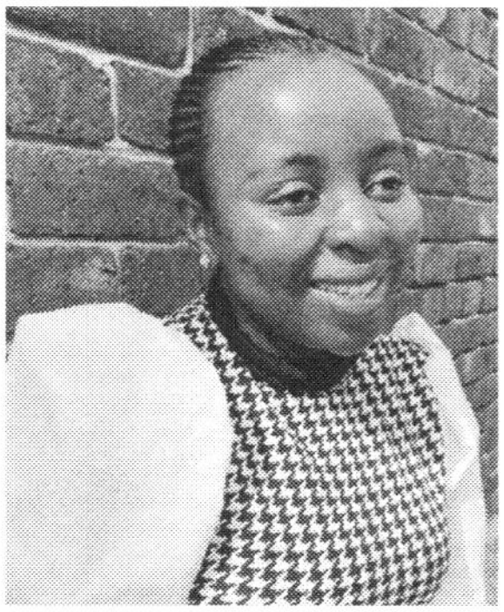

Zwannda Kwinda is a passionate public health professional with a strong background in epidemiology, HIV research, and maternal and child health. Currently serving as an Associate at the Clinton Health Access Initiative (CHAI) in South Africa. She supports the National Paediatric and Adolescent HIV program, focusing on improving health outcomes for children and adolescents living with HIV. Her role involves contributing to key national initiatives, including the path to elimination of vertical transmission of HIV and the implementation of the South African chapter of Global Alliance to end AIDS in children by 2030.

Word Roots, Prefixes, and Suffixes by Chapter

Chapter 1 Introduction to Maternal and Child Health

able (capable of, able) inflammable, notable, reliable

ac (pertaining to) hypochondriac, maniac

acean (class or order) crustacean, cetacean

aceous (of the nature of) herbaceous, sebaceous

acious (tending toward) gracious, rapacious, spacious

Chapter 2 Anatomy and Physiology of Pregnancy

fet/o: fetus, unborn offspring

gravid/o: pregnancy

lact/o: milk

nat/o: birth

omphal/o: umbilicus, navel

puerper/o: childbirth

Chapter 3 Prenatal Care

-aemia related to blood Bacteraemia

-algia pain Hyperalgia

angio- vessel Angiogram

ante- before Antenatal

anti- attacks, treats condition Antibacterial

arthro- related to a joint Artherosclerosis

-ase an enzyme Lipase

Chapter 4 Childbirth and Postpartum Care

a/an Without or none anemia

ectomy to cut out or remove appendectomy, tonsillectomy

gram the image (X-ray) mammogram

Chapter 5 Newborn Care

Cardi(o)- Cardiology

Gastr(o)- Gastroenteritis

-ase an enzyme Lipase

baro- pressure Baroreceptor

Chapter 6 Child Health and Development

astro star astronaut

aud hear audio

auto self automobile

dict say dictator

meter measure centimeter

micro small microorganism

Chapter 7 Promoting Children's Health

Brady - Slow

De - Away from, down

Hyper - Excessive, above normal

Hypo - Below normal, deficient

Inter - Between, among

Chapter 8 Community Health

-oma - Tumor, mass

-pathy - Disease, suffering

-rrhea - Flow, discharge

-scopy - Visual examination

Chapter 9 Child Maltreatment

Dys - Abnormal, difficult, painful

Endo - Within, inner

Epi - Upon, over, above

Intro - Within, inside

Macro - Large, great

Chapter 10 Immunization, Infectious Diseases, and Managing Illness

-aemia related to blood Bacteraemia

-algia pain Hyperalgia

angio- vessel Angiogram

ante- before Antenatal

anti- attacks, treats condition Antibacterial

Table of Contents

List of Figures *xiii*
List of Tables *xv*
Preface *xvii*

1 Introduction to Maternal and Child Health 1

Unit Introduction 2
1.1. Overview of Maternal and Child Health 4
1.1.1. Historical Perspectives on Maternal and Child Health 4
1.1.2. Contribution to Maternal and Child Health 7
1.2. Concept Maternal and Child Healthcare 7
1.2.1. Definition of Maternal and Neonatal 8
1.3. Philosophy of Maternal and Neonatal Health 10
1.4. Family Concepts and Types of Family 12
1.4.1. Family Types 12
1.4.2. The Communal Family 14
1.4.3. Family-Centered Care 14
1.4.4. Family Centered Maternity Care (FCMC) 15
1.5. Standards of Maternal and Child Health Practice 16
1.5.1. Ethics and Standards of Practice Issues 16
1.5.2. Theory 19
1.6. Major Health Issues for Women 21
1.6.1. Maternal and Child Health Today 22
1.6.2. National Health Goals 22
1.6.3. Trends in the Maternal and Child Health Population 22
1.6.4. Trends in Healthcare Environment 34
Summary 44
References 44

2 Anatomy and Physiology of Pregnancy 47

Unit Introduction 48
2.1. Gravidity and Parity 50
2.2. Pregnancy Tests 51
2.3. Adaptations to Pregnancy 52
2.3.1. Signs of Pregnancy 52
2.3.2. Reproductive System and Breasts 54
2.3.3. General Body Systems 60
Summary 77
References 77

3 Prenatal Care 79

Unit Introduction 79
3.1. An Overview of Antenatal Care 81
3.1.1. Early Registration 82
3.1.2. Detection of Pregnancy 83
3.1.3. Number and Timing of Visits 83
3.1.4. Seek Help for Early Registration and Antenatal Check-Up 84

3.1.5. Estimate the Number of Pregnancies in Your Area 84
3.1.6. Keep a Track of All Pregnant Women by Name 84
3.1.7. Record Keeping 85
3.1.8. Antenatal Check-Up 85
3.2. Nutrition During Pregnancy 86
3.2.1. Dietary and Caloric Recommendations 86
3.2.2. Fluid Intake During Pregnancy 86
3.2.3. Ideal Foods to Eat During Pregnancy 86
3.2.4. Foods to Avoid During Pregnancy 87
3.2.5. Guidelines for Safe Food Handling 87
3.2.6. Prenatal Vitamin and Mineral Supplements 87
3.3. Common Health Problems During Pregnancy 88
3.3.1. High Blood Pressure 88
3.3.2. Gestational Diabetes 89
3.3.3. Infections 89
3.3.4. Preeclampsia 90
3.3.5. Preterm Labor 91
3.3.6. Depression and Anxiety 91
3.3.7. Pregnancy Loss/Miscarriage 91
3.3.8. Stillbirth 92
3.3.9. Other Complications 92
3.4. Psychological Changes in Pregnancy 92
3.5. Planned Intervention for the Alleviation of Psychological Difficulties During the Perinatal Period 94
3.5.1. Antenatal Classes 94
3.5.2. The Effectiveness of Antenatal Classes 95
3.5.3. Controlled Trials of Explicit Social and Psychological Support in the Perinatal Period 97
3.6. Psychosocial Effects of the Actual Provision of Prenatal Care 99
3.7. Routine Screening and Diagnostic Tests 100
3.7.1. Tests to Confirm Pregnancy 101
3.7.2. Prenatal Tests to Monitor the Health of the Mother and the Baby 102
3.7.3. Tests for Specific Medical Conditions in Pregnancy 102
3.7.4. Screening Tests and Diagnostic Tests in Pregnancy 102
3.7.5. Making Decisions About Diagnostic Testing in Pregnancy 104
3.7.6. Immunizations in Pregnancy 104
3.7.7. Best Practice for Health Professionals Talking to Families About Screening and Test Results 104
3.8. Fetal Assessment 105
3.8.1. Prenatal Diagnosis 105
3.8.2. Antepartum Tests of Fetal Well-Being 109
3.8.3. Intrapartum Tests of Fetal Well-Being 111
3.8.4. Tests of Fetal Lung Maturity 114
Summary 118
References 118

4 Childbirth and Postpartum Care 121

Unit Introduction 122
4.1. Overview of Childbirth 124
4.1.1. Signs and Symptoms 124
4.2. Vaginal Birth 125
4.2.1. Onset of Labor 126
4.2.2. Stages of Labor 127
4.2.3. Early Skin-to-Skin Contact 130
4.2.4. Discharge 130
4.3. Labor Induction and Caesarean Section 131
4.3.1. Labor Induction 131
4.3.2. Cesarean Section 132
4.4. Management 132
4.4.1. Preparation 132
4.4.2. Forceps or Vacuum Assisted Delivery 133
4.4.3. Pain Management During Childbirth 133
4.4.4. Augmentation 135
4.4.5. Episiotomy 135
4.4.6. Multiple Births 135
4.4.7. Fetal Monitoring 135
4.5. Complications 136
4.5.1. Maternal Mortality and Adverse Health Consequences 136
4.5.2. Infant Mortality 137
4.5.3. Labor and Delivery Complications 137
4.5.4. Maternal Complications 137

4.5.5. Fetal Complications 139
4.6. Postpartum Care 141
4.6.1. Adjusting to Motherhood 141
4.6.2. Baby Blues vs. Postpartum Depression 142
4.6.3. Function 142
4.6.4. Issues of Concern 144
4.6.5. Clinical Significance 144
4.6.6. Other Issues 145
Summary 147
References 147

5 Newborn Care 149

Unit Introduction 150
5.1. Newborn Assessment and Care 152
5.1.1. Apgar Scoring 152
5.1.2. Birthweight 152
5.1.3. Measurements 152
5.1.4. Physical Examination 153
5.1.5. Care of the Newborn 154
5.2. Common Newborn Health Problems 155
5.2.1. Abdominal Distension 155
5.2.2. Birth Injuries 155
5.2.3. Bluish Skin 155
5.2.4. Coughing 156
5.2.5. Jaundice 156
5.2.6. Respiratory Distress 156
5.2.7. Vomiting 156
5.2.8. Fever 157
5.2.9. Colic 157
5.2.10. Skin Problems 157
5.2.11. Cold and Flu 157
5.2.12. Ear Infections 157
5.2.13. Oral Thrush 158
5.2.14. Diarrhea 158
5.2.15. Constipation 158
5.3. Neonatal Resuscitation 158
5.3.1. Apgar Score 159
5.3.2. Resuscitation 161
5.3.3. Initial Measures 162
5.3.4. Ventilation and Oxygenation 163
5.3.5. Intubation and Chest Compression 164
5.3.6. Failure to Respond to Resuscitation 165
5.3.7. No Resuscitation 166
5.4. Screening and Diagnostic Tests for Newborns 166
5.4.1. The Screening Procedures 168
Summary 172
References 172

6 Child Health and Development 173

Unit Introduction 174
6.1. Growth and Development Milestones 176
6.1.1. Physical Development Milestones 176
6.1.2. Cognitive Development Milestones 176
6.1.3. Emotional Development Milestones 177
6.1.4. Parental Role in Supporting Child Development 178
6.1.5. Cultural Differences in Child Development Milestones 178
6.1.6. Supporting Children with Developmental Disabilities 179
6.2. Health and Nutrition of Children 180
6.2.1. The Importance of Nutrition for Children 181
6.2.2. Nutrition and Health in Pre-School- and School-Age Children 182
6.2.3. Nutrition and Health in Adolescents 183
6.2.4. Dietary Guidelines for Children and Adolescents 183
6.2.5. Childhood Obesity and Its Impact on Health 184
6.2.6. Food Safety for Children 185
6.3. Basic Nutrition for Children 188
6.3.1. Choosing Foods for Children 188
6.3.2. How to Encourage Healthy Eating Habits? 189
6.3.3. Vegetarian Diets for Children 189
6.3.4. What Nutrients Do Children Need? 189
6.4. Common Childhood Illnesses 193
6.4.1. The Integrated Management of Childhood Illness 195
6.4.2. Daily Health Check 196
6.4.3. Recommendations for Exclusion 197

6.4.4. Preparing for Managing Illness 197
6.4.5. Key Criteria for Exclusion of Children Who Are Ill 198
6.5. Child Abuse and Neglect 199
6.5.1. The Types of Child Abuse and Neglect 199
6.5.2. The Effects of Child Abuse and Neglect 200
6.5.3. The Risk Factors for Child Abuse and Neglect 201
6.5.4. Recognizing and Reporting Child Abuse and Neglect 201
6.5.5. Prevention of Child Abuse and Neglect 202
6.5.6. The Legal and Ethical Issues Related to Child Abuse and Neglect 203
6.5.7. The Role of Trauma-Informed Care in Addressing Child Abuse and Neglect 204
Summary 206
References 207

7 Promoting Children's Health 209

Unit Introduction 210
7.1. Concept of Promoting Children's Health 212
7.1.1. Promoting Healthy Mental and Intellectual Development 212
7.1.2. Components of Health Promotion/Health Maintenance Visits 213
7.1.3. Mental and Spiritual Health 214
7.1.4. Disease Prevention Strategies 214
7.1.5. Promoting Optimal Health and Development of Children 215
7.2. Public Health Issues Related to Maternal and Child Health 217
7.2.1. Epidemiology and Disease Control 219
7.2.2. Disaster Management and Emergency Preparedness 220
7.2.3. Healthcare Systems and Policies 221
7.3. Relationship Between Diet and Health in Children and Adolescents 222
7.3.1. Primary Changes Occurring in Children and Adolescents as They Grow 223
7.3.2. Relationship Between Diet and Chronic Diseases in Children 226
7.4. Healthy Diet for Child 228
7.4.1. Setting a Good Example 228
7.4.2. Using Vegetables and Fruit as Snacks 229
7.4.3. Making Vegetables and Fruits More Appealin229
7.4.4. How to Feed Your Child a Balanced Diet? 230
7.4.5. How to Keep Your Child Healthy? 234
Summary 240
References 240

8 Community Health 241

Unit Introduction 241
8.1. Overview of Community Health 244
8.1.1. Common Responsibilities of a Community Health 245
8.1.2. Public Health Issues Related to Maternal and Child Health 246
8.1.3. Impact 246
8.1.4. Global Goals 247
8.1.5. U.S. Government Efforts 248
8.1.6. Organization 248
8.1.7. Key Issues for the U.S. 251
8.2. Epidemiology and Disease Control 251
8.2.1. Chain of Infection 253
8.2.2. Epidemiologic Methods 257
8.2.3. Epidemic Investigation 259
8.3. Disaster Management and Emergency Preparedness 260
8.3.1. Gender Differences in the Aftermath 262
8.3.2. Effect of Disasters on Women 262
8.4. Healthcare Systems and Policies 268
8.4.1. Healthcare Needs of Women, Children, and Adolescents 269
8.4.2. Healthcare Benefits for Women and Children 271
8.4.3. Coordinated Healthcare Services for Women and Children 273
Summary 280
References 280

9 Child Maltreatment 283

Unit Introduction 284
9.1. Abuse and Neglect: Scope of the Problem 286
9.1.1. Consequences of Maltreatment 287

9.1.2. Risk Factors 287
9.1.3. Child 287
9.1.4. Parent or Caregiver 288
9.1.5. Relationship 288
9.1.6. Community and Societal Factors 288
9.1.7. Prevention 288
9.1.8. WHO Response 289
9.2. Classification of Child Maltreatment 289
9.2.1. Physical Abuse 290
9.2.2. Sexual Abuse 290
9.2.3. Emotional Abuse 290
9.2.4. Neglect 291
9.2.5. Special Considerations 291
9.2.6. Etiology of Child Maltreatment 291
9.3. Symptoms and Signs of Child Maltreatment 292
9.3.1. Physical Abuse 292
9.3.2. Sexual Abuse 293
9.3.3. Diagnosis of Child Maltreatment 294
9.4. Treatment of Child Maltreatment 296
9.4.1. Immediate Safety 296
9.4.2. Follow-Up 297
9.4.3. Removal From the Home 298
9.5. Prevention of Child Maltreatment 298
9.5.1. Child Maltreatment: A Public Health and Prevention Considerations 299
9.5.2. Risk and Protective Factors Related to Child Maltreatment 303
9.5.3. Considerations for Nurses 304
9.5.4. The Importance of Prevention in Child Maltreatment 305
Summary 309
References 309

10 Immunization, Infectious Diseases, and Managing Illness 313

Unit Introduction 314
10.1. Importance of Childhood Immunization 316
10.1.1. Common Childhood Infectious Diseases 317
10.1.2. Vaccination Schedules and Coverage 318
10.2 Integrated Management of New-born and Childhood Illness (IMNCI) 319
10.2.1 The IMNCI Strategy 320
10.2.2 Importance and Objectives of the IMNCI Strategy 321
10.2.3 The IMNCI Assessment 322
10.3. Childhood Illnesses 322
10.4. Nutritional Management 323
10.4.1. Supporting Breastfeeding 323
10.4.2. Assessing a Breastfeed 323
10.4.3. Overcoming Difficulties 323
10.4.4. Nutritional Management of Sick Children 327
10.4.5. Fluid Management 327
10.4.6. Management of Fever 329
10.4.7. Pain Control 329
10.4.8. Management of Anemia 330
10.5. Care for a Sick Child 333
10.5.1. Making a Sick Child Comfortable 333
10.5.2. Feeding a Sick Child 335
10.5.3. Treating a Sick Child at Home 335
10.5.4. Seeing a Doctor 336
10.5.5. Reducing the Spread of Illness in Childcare 337
10.5.6. Measures to Promote Good Hygiene in Childcare 338
Summary 341
References 341

Index 343

LIST OF FIGURES

Figure 1.1. Maternal and child health includes care of the pregnant woman, child, and family

Figure 1.2. Data on average ages

Figure 1.3. Maternal mortality rates in India

Figure 1.4. Infant mortality rates in 2017

Figure 1.5. Parenthood

Figure 1.6. A nurse prepares an infant transport incubator to move a premature infant to a regional hospital. Helping with safe movement of pregnant women and ill newborns to regional centers is an important responsibility

Figure 2.1. Changes in pregnancy

Figure 2.2. Gestation

Figure 2.3. Displacement of internal abdominal structures and diaphragm by the enlarging uterus at 4, 6, and 9 months of gestation

Figure 2.4. Hegar sign. Bimanual examination for assessing compressibility and softening of the isthmus (lower uterine segment) while the cervix is still firm

Figure 2.5. Internal ballottement (18 weeks)

Figure 2.6. Cervix during pregnancy

Figure 2.7. (A) Pelvic floor in nonpregnant woman. (B) Pelvic floor at end of pregnancy. Note marked hypertrophy and hyperplasia below dotted line joining tip of coccyx and inferior margin of symphysis. Note elongation of bladder and urethra as a result of compression. Fat deposits are increased

Figure 2.8. Changes in position of heart, lungs, and thoracic cage in pregnancy. Broken line, nonpregnant; solid line, change that occurs in pregnancy

Figure 2.9. Hemorrhoids

Figure 2.10. Linea nigra

Figure 2.11. Postural changes during pregnancy

Figure 2.12. Possible change in rectus abdominis muscles during pregnancy. (A) Normal position in nonpregnant woman. (B) Diastasis recti abdominis in pregnant woman

Figure 2.13. Change in position of appendix in pregnancy. Note McBurney's point

Figure 3.1. Nutrition in pregnancy

Figure 3.2. Gestational hypertension

Figure 3.3. Schematic illustration with the assumption of the compensatory carry-over action model (CCAM) for changes in pregnancy

Figure 3.4. Non-invasive prenatal test (NIPT) analysis. [CNVs: copy number variations, SNPs: single

nucleotide polymorphisms]
Figure 3.5. Examples of fetal heart rate monitoring
Figure 4.1. The core stages associated with labor
Figure 4.2. Non-pharmacological pain management in labor
Figure 4.3. Preterm births
Figure 5.1. Blue skin
Figure 5.2. Infant care
Figure 5.3. Resuscitation of neonates
Figure 5.4. Mask position
Figure 5.5. Manual ventilation
Figure 6.1. Food safety in children
Figure 6.2. Child abuse is serious
Figure 7.1. Issues of maternal and child health
Figure 7.2. School meal planning-points
Figure 7.3. Tobacco addiction in children
Figure 7.4. Recommended screen time for children of different age groups in minutes
Figure 8.1. The sustainable development goals
Figure 8.2. Summary of important aspects involved in the chain of any infection
Figure 8.3. An example of a disease showing a seasonal trend. The seasonality of several human infectious disease pathogens in England and Wales
Figure 8.4. Natural disasters (1971–2001)
Figure 9.1. Prevalence of subtypes of maltreatment by age group between 2011 and 2020
Figure 9.2. Preventing child abuse
Figure 9.3. Findings from a study on child abuse and child protection in Australia
Figure 9.4. Addressing maltreatment
Figure 10.1. Breastfeeding is an important aspect of motherhood
Figure 10.2. Caring for sick children: This toy consists of a cord, hooks, and various materials with holes, such as rings made from glittering tapes of different colors and bells, threaded onto the cord. For children in bed, the cord is hooked at the bedrail, and rings are slid toward the opposite side at a signal from HPS, such as "Here they go! Choo!," so that they enjoy the movements and sounds of rings that move while rotating and changes of color

LIST OF TABLES

Table 1.1. Collaborative networks and practices contributing to social sustainability in healthcare context

Table 1.2. Quality indicators and definitions

Table 1.3. Infant mortality and poverty level in the southeastern US from 2005–2009

Table 1.4. Differences in infant mortality by the month of prenatal care began in the southeastern US from 2005 to 2009

Table 2.1. Effect of pregnancy on endocrine function tests [5]

Table 2.2. Signs of pregnancy

Table 2.3. Laboratory values for pregnant and nonpregnant women

Table 2.4. Cardiovascular changes in pregnancy

Table 2.5. Respiratory changes in pregnancy

Table 5.1. Resuscitation at birth-the terms

Table 5.2. Neonatal deaths and addressing them

Table 5.3. Neonatal oxygen saturation targets

Table 8.1. The SDGs, assessed variables, and sources of data

Table 8.2. Emerging and re-emerging zoonotic viruses

Table 8.3. Examples of contraception-based studies

Table 8.4. STI pathogens

Table 9.1. Allegations of maltreatment types published in a study

Table 10.1. Complementary feeding practices

PREFACE

Maternal healthcare represents a foundational pillar for not just safeguarding the lives and well-being of mothers and their infants, but it also holds profound significance for the overarching health and prosperity of societies globally. Within the domain of maternal healthcare, clinicians stand at the forefront, endowed with the pivotal opportunity to mitigate the myriad challenges that mothers encounter in seeking and obtaining quality healthcare services. Their roles are instrumental in guiding mothers through the labyrinth of healthcare systems toward leading healthier and more fulfilled lives.

Maternal health encompasses the comprehensive care of women throughout the continuum of pregnancy, childbirth, and the ensuing postnatal period. Each phase in this continuum is crucial and should be characterized by nurturing and positive experiences that aspire not just towards survival but towards maximizing the health and well-being potential of both mother and child. The journey through pregnancy and childbirth is one of profound transformation and growth, meriting an environment that fosters safety, respect, and dignity.

This book provides readers with a comprehensive understanding of the key principles, practices, and challenges associated with maternal and child healthcare. The book endeavors to blend theoretical knowledge with practical insights, offering a foundational overview of maternal and child health from a global perspective. It covers a broad spectrum of topics, including prenatal care, childbirth, postnatal care, and the early years of child development, emphasizing the importance of healthcare access, quality, and equity in ensuring the health and well-being of mothers and children.

This book is designed to cater to a wide audience, making it an invaluable resource for students pursuing degrees in public health, nursing, and medicine. Additionally, it serves as a critical reference for healthcare professionals, including nurses, midwives, and public health practitioners, who are directly involved in the delivery of maternal and child health services. By integrating evidence-based research findings with real-world case studies, the book aims to equip its readers with the knowledge and skills necessary to contribute effectively to the improvement of maternal and child health outcomes in various healthcare settings and socio-economic contexts.

Chapter

INTRODUCTION TO MATERNAL AND CHILD HEALTH

1

Contents

Unit Introduction 2
1.1. Overview of Maternal and Child Health 4
1.2. Concept Maternal and Child Healthcare 7
1.3. Philosophy of Maternal and Neonatal Health 10
1.4. Family Concepts and Types of Family 12
1.5. Standards of Maternal and Child Health Practice 16
1.6. Major Health Issues for Women 21
Summary 44
References 44

Unit Introduction

Maternal and child health, which includes the development and health of infants, children, and adolescents, as well as the well-being of women during pregnancy, childbirth, and the postnatal period, is an essential part of public health.

To ensure that moms and their newborns reach their maximum potential for health and wellbeing, each stage of the pregnancy, childbirth, and postpartum process should be a positive experience for women. This is known as maternal health. Child health pertains to the well-being of children under five years old, and safeguarding and enhancing the health of these individuals is crucial. In the framework of the family, maternal and child health focuses on giving the client evidence-based, case-managed care. To provide cost-effective, outcome-focused, and quality-oriented care continuity, an interdisciplinary plan must be implemented collaboratively. In addition to working together with other fields like education, social work, and justice, maternity and neonatal clinicians plan for discharge and offer care in the community.

Maternal and child health and wellbeing demands a multifaceted approach that takes into account social, medical, cultural, and economic factors. It takes access to high-quality medical care to support the health of mothers and their children. This covers immunizations, preventative health services, skilled attendance at birth, postnatal care for moms and babies, and prenatal care. Comprehensive healthcare services should also take into account the unique requirements of women and children, including those related to family planning, nutrition, mental health, and reproductive health. Through the provision of knowledge and skills that enable women to make informed decisions regarding their own and their children's health, educational interventions are essential in promoting maternal and child health practices. Information on healthy eating, breastfeeding, personal hygiene, and child care are all included in this. Encouraging positive health behaviors and dispelling myths about the significance of maternal and child health can be achieved through educating communities.

Maternal and child health outcomes can be significantly impacted by socioeconomic factors like poverty, substandard housing, and limited access to opportunities for education and employment. Improving access to healthcare services, lowering disparities, and advancing health equity all depend on addressing these socioeconomic determinants of health. Maternal and child health can be significantly impacted by initiatives to reduce poverty, increase access to education, and give women more economic power.

Additionally, cultural factors influence the health outcomes for mothers and children. Cultural customs and beliefs may affect how people perceive illness, how they seek medical attention, and how they make decisions about having children and giving birth. Respecting cultural diversity and advocating for evidence-based methods that put mothers' and kids' health and wellbeing first are both crucial.

Orientation and Directional Terms

Term	Definition	Illustration
Childbirth	Childbirth is the completion of pregnancy where one or more babies exits the internal environment of the mother via vaginal delivery or caesarean section.	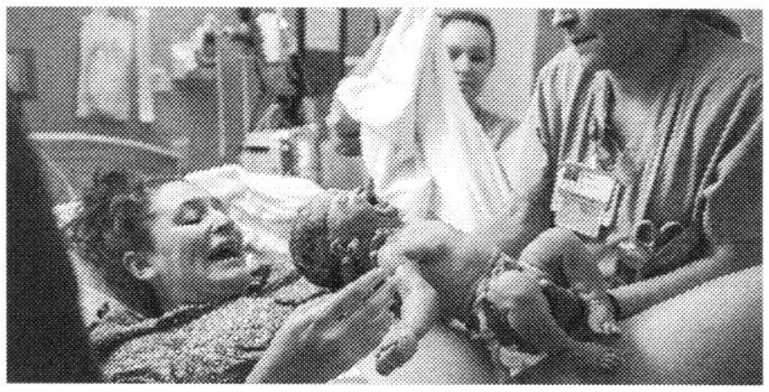
Postpartum	Postpartum (or postnatal) refers to the period after childbirth.	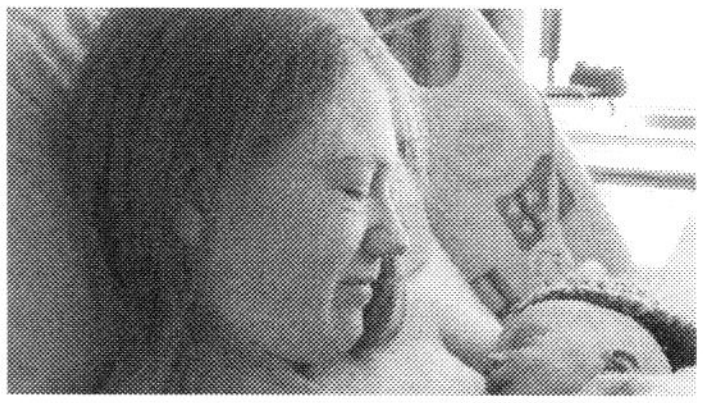
Antibiotic	An antibiotic is a type of antimicrobial substance active against bacteria	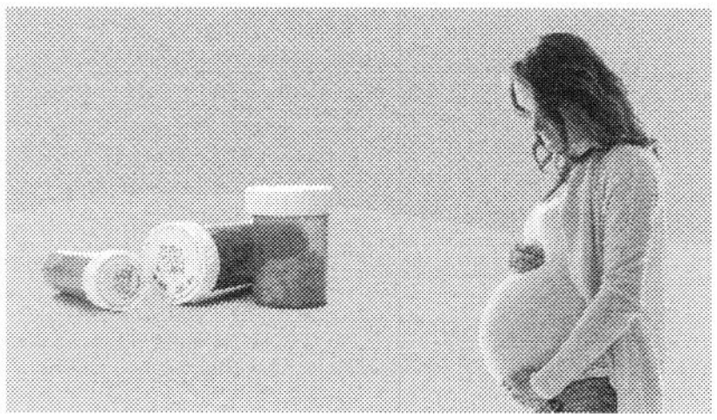
Postnatal Care	Postnatal care is the care given to a mother and newborn after birth.	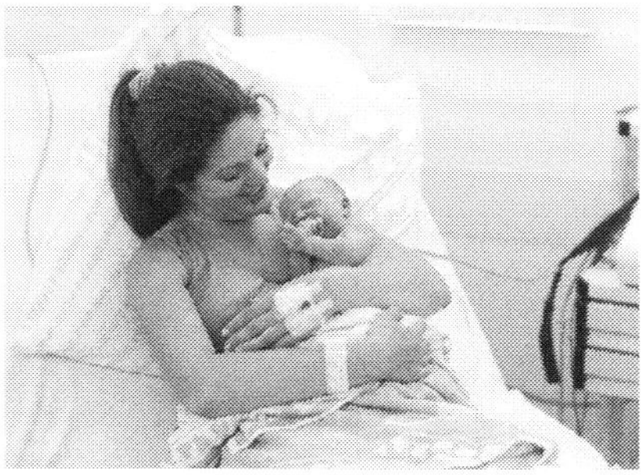
Neonatal	Neonatal means newborn or the first 28 days of a child's life. The neonatal period is a time of rapid change for a child, and is considered the most vulnerable time for a child's survival.	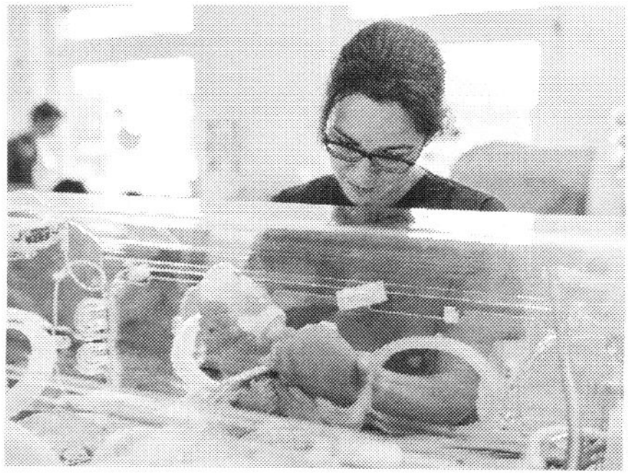

1.1. Overview of Maternal and Child Health

Maternal and child health (MCH) is one of the most important public health services and has been a global priority for many years. MCH is an important public health issue which provides an opportunity to end preventable death for mother and child. A global maternal mortality rate of less than 70 per 100,000 live births is the target set by the Sustainable Development Goals (SDGs) for 2030, but in many nations, poor maternal and child health is still a major problem. A study conducted in 2017 by the United Nations Interagency Group estimated that 295,000 maternal deaths occurred annually, and in 2018, there were 18 neonatal deaths for every 1000 live births worldwide. Approximately 86% of maternal deaths reported globally are reported from Sub-Saharan Africa and Southern Asia. (Hutchins VL. et al. 1994)

1.1.1. Historical Perspectives on Maternal and Child Health

Over the course of human history, societies have developed a variety of practices and interventions to ensure the health and well-being of mothers and children. However, due to influences from science, society, culture, and the economy, historical viewpoints on mother and child health have changed dramatically over time.

Maternal and child health practices were primitive in ancient Egypt, Mesopotamia, and ancient Indian civilizations. These societies valued childbirth and raising children, frequently attributing their significance to supernatural forces. Important roles in pregnancy, childbirth, and postnatal care were played by midwives, herbal remedies, and religious rituals. Yet, there was still a lack of knowledge in the medical field, and the death rates for mothers and children were still high. In Europe throughout the Middle Ages, superstitions and religious beliefs persisted in having an impact on mother and child health. Midwives attended childbirth and were frequently community women with little formal training. Still, giving birth was dangerous, and the rate of maternal death was high. Infectious diseases, poor hygiene, and malnutrition all contributed to the high infant death rate.

Maternal and child health saw some improvements during the Renaissance due to advances in medical knowledge and practices. But real advancements didn't come about until the 19th century. The rate of maternal and infant mortality in Western societies has decreased as a result of advancements in science, better sanitation, and public health initiatives. Obstetrics and public health were revolutionized by pioneers such as Louis Pasteur, who developed germ theory, and Ignaz Semmelweis, who promoted handwashing as a preventative measure against childbed fever.

Organizations and programs for maternal and child health were established in the late 19th and early 20th centuries to lower the death rates of mothers and children. Governments, nonprofits, and philanthropists contributed to projects like immunization campaigns, clean water supplies, prenatal care, and mother education. Maternal and child health was advanced by the work of individuals like Florence Nightingale, who highlighted the value of cleanliness and nursing care, and Margaret Sanger, who promoted birth control and reproductive rights.

Significant strides in maternal and child health were made in the middle of the 20th century as a result of scientific discoveries, technical developments, and public health campaigns. In many regions of the world, the introduction of vaccinations, antibiotics, and better obstetric procedures resulted in additional drops in the rates of mother and child mortality. Through international campaigns and initiatives, governments and organizations like UNICEF and the World Health Organization (WHO) have been instrumental in promoting maternal and child health.

To improve mother and child health outcomes, there has been a growing recognition in recent decades of the significance of addressing social determinants of health, such as poverty, education, and gender inequality. Maternal and child health initiatives now take a comprehensive approach that incorporates social, economic, and cultural aspects with medical interventions. Furthermore, a growing focus is being placed on the rights of mothers and children, empowering them, and ensuring equity in healthcare delivery and access.

Throughout history, the understanding of maternal and child health has undergone significant changes, influenced by advancements in medical science, societal beliefs, and public health focus. Despite notable improvements, obstacles still exist, especially in communities with limited resources where maternal and child mortality rates are alarmingly high. To address these challenges, it is crucial to continue building upon past successes and implement holistic, research-based strategies to enhance the health and prosperity of mothers and children globally.

1.1.1.1. The Past

1. **Obstetrics:** The skills related to obstetrics have evolved over centuries. The earliest concerning childbirth are in the Egyptian (circa 1550 BC). Soranus, a Greek physician who practiced in Rome in the 2nd century and who is known as the father of obstetrics, made later advances. He instituted the practice of the pediatric version, a procedure used to rotate a fetus to a breech or feet-first, position. Podalic version is important in the vaginal delivery of the second infant in a set of twins. In this procedure, the physician reaches into the uterus and grasps one or both of the infant's feet to facilitate delivery. Planned cesarean birth is used today, as it is safer than the pediatric version.

With the decline of the Roman Empire and the ensuing Dark Ages, scientific exploration and associated medical improvement came to a halt. During the 19th century, however, Karl Crede (1819–1892) and Ignaz Semmelweis (1818–1865) made contributions that improved the safety and the health of mother and child during and after childbirth. In 1884 Crede recommended instilling 2% silver nitrate into the eyes of newborns to prevent blindness caused by gonorrhea. Crede's innovation has saved the eyesight of incalculable numbers of babies.

Semmelwels' story is a classic in the history of maternity care. In the 1840s, he worked as an assistant professor in the maternity ward of the Vienna General Hospital. There he discovered a relationship between the incidence of puerperal fever (or "childbed fever"), which caused many deaths among women in lying-in wards, and the examination of new mothers by student doctors who had just returned from dissecting cadavers. Semmelweis deduced that puerperal fever was septic, contagious and transmitted by the unwashed hands of physicians and medical students.

Louis Pasteur (1822–1895), a French chemist, confirmed that puerperal fever was caused by bacteria and could be spread by improper hand washing and control with contaminated objects. The simple, but highly effective, procedure of hand washing continues to be one of the most important means of preventing the spread of infection in the hospital and the home today.

Joseph Lister (1827–1912), a British surgeon influenced by Pasteur, experimented with chemical means of preventing infection. He revolutionized surgical practice by introducing antiseptic surgery.

2. **Pediatrics:** Methods of child care have varied throughout history. The culture of a society has a strong influence on standards of child care. Many primitive tribes were nomads. Strong children survived, whereas the weak were left to die. This practice of infanticide (French and Latin infans, "infant" and caedere, "to kill") helped to ensure the safety of the group. As tribes became settled, more attention was given to children, but they were still frequently valued only for their productivity. Certain cultures, such as the Egyptians and the Greeks, were advanced in their attitudes. The Greek physician Hippocrates (460–370 BC) wrote about illnesses peculiar to children.

In the Middle Ages, the concept of childhood did not exist. Infancy lasted until about age seven years at which time the child was assimilated into the adult world. The art of the time depicts children wearing adult clothes and wigs. In the early 17th century, Saint Vincent de Paul founded several children's asylums. Many of these eventually became hospitals, although their original concern was for abandoned children. The first children's hospital was founded in Paris in 1802. In the United States, the Children's Aid Society, founded in New York City 1853, cared for numerous homeless children. In 1855, the first pediatric hospital in the United States, Children's Hospital of Philadelphia, was founded.

Abraham Jacobi (1830–1919) is known as the father of pediatrics because of his many contributions to the field. The establishment of pediatrics as a specialty paralleled the establishment of departments of pediatrics in medical schools, the founding of the children's hospitals, and the development of separate units for children in foundling homes and general hospitals. By the 1960s separate pediatric units were also common in hospitals. Parents were restricted by rigid visiting hours that allowed parent-infant contact for only a few hours each day, when medically indicated, mothers were allowed to enter the pediatric unit for 1 hour at a time to breastfeeds their infants.

1.1.1.2. The Present

In a family-centric approach to childbirth, the family is viewed as a distinct system where every member is impacted by the arrival of a new child. Therefore, involving the family during pregnancy and birth is considered essential for bonding and support. To meet the needs of families, alternative birthing centers, birthing rooms, and mother-infant coupling programs have been created. These alternatives replace the traditional practice of separating labor and delivery areas, which often required moving the mother between different rooms and interrupting her care.

The maternity unit's three distinct departments—labor and delivery, postpartum, and newborn nursery—have combined. All of the action could happen in a single set of labor, delivery, and recovery (LDR) rooms. The patient is cared for during labor and delivery in a single room, and she stays there to recuperate and tend to her newborn instead of being transferred to a different location. These spaces are frequently furnished to look cozy.

Low-risk maternity patients are drawn to freestanding birthing centers that are not part of the traditional hospital environment. Comprehensive care is offered by these birthing centers, including antepartum, labor and delivery, postpartum, mother's education, lactation education, and family planning follow-up. Because hiring midwives for home births is not currently common, there is a lack of emergency equipment in case of unforeseen complications and high costs associated with malpractice insurance.

1.1.1.3. The Future

The struggle between quality of care and cost containment is central to the healthcare revolution. Cost containment and managed care emerged as the healthcare sector turned into a lucrative business. Care that is managed can lead to higher quality because it evaluates provided care in an open and ongoing manner. The routine management of patients is being looked into by the quality assurance committee, particularly with regard to testing and preventive care.

In an effort to lower healthcare costs and increase accessibility for all Americans, the federal government passed healthcare reform laws in 2010 and 2017. The community's resource availability affects access to care as well. The provision of healthcare has benefited greatly from health insurance. Because the insurance company frequently needs to approve (or deny) the expenditure before a test or treatment is provided, having health insurance does not guarantee access to care. In the past, families without health insurance frequently forewent receiving preventive medical care, including well-baby checkups, infant vaccinations, and prenatal care. Prior to the ACA of 2010, access to healthcare for follow-up and preventive care was restricted. While Somalia spends $33 per person on healthcare annually, the United States spends thousands of dollars per person on healthcare. However, some argue that waste and inefficiencies impede efforts to reduce costs and improve access to therapeutic and preventive care for everyone. Proposals for future changes and restructuring of the US healthcare system are still being made. In the fight for healthcare reform, clinicians take on the role of patient advocates to guarantee high-quality care.

1.1.2. Contribution to Maternal and Child Health

For any society to be healthy and prosperous, it is essential to protect the health of mothers and children. Maternal and child health is influenced by a wide range of factors, including socioeconomic status, cultural norms, and access to healthcare services. As a result, dealing with these complex problems calls for an all-encompassing strategy that incorporates community involvement, policy changes, education, and healthcare interventions. The involvement in maternity and child health encompasses multiple areas, all with the goal of enhancing results and creating a supportive atmosphere for both moms and their offspring.

1.2. Concept Maternal and Child Healthcare

Maternal and child healthcare (MCH) encompasses a range of services aimed at improving the health and well-being of mothers and their children. The primary goal is to ensure safe pregnancies, healthy childbirth, and optimal development during infancy and early childhood. Key components include:

- *Prenatal Care:* Regular check-ups during pregnancy to monitor the health of both mother and fetus, identify potential complications, and provide education on nutrition and healthy behaviors.
- *Skilled Birth Attendance*: Ensuring that childbirth is attended by trained healthcare professionals to manage labor and delivery safely, minimizing risks to both mother and child.

- *Postnatal Care*: Follow-up care for mothers and newborns shortly after birth to address recovery, breastfeeding support, and newborn health assessments.
- *Child Health Services*: Routine immunizations, growth monitoring, and education on child development to promote healthy growth in infants and young children.
- *Family Planning and Reproductive Health*: Providing education and resources to help families make informed decisions about spacing and planning pregnancies.
- *Mental Health Support*: Addressing the psychological well-being of mothers, recognizing that mental health is crucial for effective caregiving and overall family health.
- *Community Engagement*: Involving families and communities in MCH initiatives to enhance awareness, accessibility, and support for healthcare services.

By integrating these components, maternal and child healthcare aims to reduce mortality and morbidity rates, enhance health outcomes, and promote the overall development of future generations.

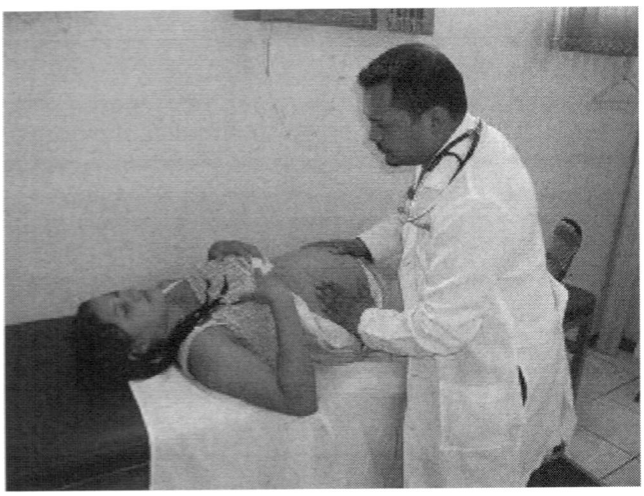

Figure 1.1. *Maternal and child health includes care of the pregnant woman, child, and family.*

Source: *By This image is a work of a United States Agency for International Development employee, taken or made as part of that person's official duties. As a work of the U.S. federal government, the image is in the public domain in the United States. See also: The USAID privacy policy and the USAID Office of Inspector General "Disclaimers & Notices" page, Public Domain, https://commons.wikimedia.org/w/index.php?curid=1046.*

1.2.1. Definition of Maternal and Neonatal

Neonatal includes instruction in perinatal and newborn health assessment, stabilization, and care; pathophysiology of pregnancy, fetuses, and the newborn; clinical management of high-risk pregnancies and newborns; perinatal and neonatal technology and clinical procedures; and patient education. Is a program that prepares registered clinicians to provide prenatal care to pregnant women and to mothers and their newborn infants

1. Objectives of Maternal and Child Health Programs:

- Provide basic healthcare to all mothers and children;
- Prevent communicable diseases;
- Promoting reproductive health; Regulate fertility so that desired and healthy children can be born when desired;
- Ensure the birth of a healthy child;
- Encourage healthy growth and development.

2. Components of Maternal and Child Health:

- Maternal health;
- Child health;
- Family planning;
- School health;
- Handicapped children;
- Care of children in special setting such as day care.

3. Factors Affecting Maternal and Child Health:

- Education level; Knowledge of one's own right;
- Sociocultural practices;
    - Cultural taboos;
    - Early marriage and pregnancy;
    - Women's internalization of patriarchal values;
    - Gender-based violence;
    - Social services;
- Provision of clean water and sanitation; Water, food and sanitation; Unbalanced diet;
- Healthcare access and utilization; Lack of accessibility to family planning services.
- Healthcare quality;
- Income/employment;
- Economic status;
- Family health; Poor health status of family members;

4. Importance of Maternal and Child Health:

- It ensures a healthy pregnancy and good healthcare;
- It aids in the delivery of a healthy baby by providing immunization services, guaranteeing a balanced diet, and maintaining sanitation;
- It safeguards reproductive rights and promotes a happy life;
- It ensures the health of both mother and child;
- It helps to reduce the preventable deaths among women and children.

5. Common Health Problems of Mother and Child:

i. **Infection:** Maternal infection can cause:

- Growth retardation;
- Abortion;
- Low birth weight;
- Puerperal sepsis.

Infection among children can cause:

- Diarrhea;
- Respiratory tract infection;
- Chronic infections like malaria, tuberculosis (TB).

ii. **Uncontrolled Fertility:** Consequences of uncontrolled fertility:

- Increase prevalence of LBW;
- Anemia;
- Abortion;
- Malnutrition.

6. Challenges in Ensuring Maternal and Child Health:

- Universalization of services;
- Existing rural-urban differentiation;
- Political and administrative will in this sector;
- Socio-cultural and attitudes.

7. Emerging Issues in Maternal and Child Health:

- Issues like the emergence of new viruses like the Zika virus, Coronavirus as pandemics can result in an overall decrease in coverage across all maternal and child health interventions like the number of institutional deliveries, antenatal care services, immunization services.
- Increase in infertility due to various reasons can potentially affect various aspects of women's quality of life such as physical health, mental health, social health and the total quality of life significantly.
- Consumption of junk food is on trend among younger children. This has certain short and long-term consequences like lethargy, bloating, indigestion, obesity, dental problems, etc. in children as well as adults.

1.3. Philosophy of Maternal and Neonatal Health

The core tenet of maternal and neonatal health philosophy is that all expectant mothers and their babies have the right to safe, humane care throughout their pregnancies, deliveries, and postpartum periods. It includes a holistic strategy that puts the physical, mental, and social health of the mother and child first. The understanding that pregnancy and childbirth are normal, life-changing experiences that call for individualized, evidence-based care catered to each person's particular needs is fundamental to this philosophy. The philosophy of maternal and neonatal health is based on the idea that autonomy and informed decision-making are crucial. Women ought to have the freedom to actively engage in all facets of their care, including interventions, pain management techniques, and delivery options. Ensuring that care is provided in a sensitive, compassionate, and culturally competent manner requires respect for women's rights, preferences, and cultural beliefs.

Another fundamental tenet of the philosophy of maternal and newborn health is safety. It is imperative to make every effort to guarantee a low-risk and safe childbirth experience for both mother and child. This means having trained birth attendants on hand, giving women access to emergency obstetric care, and performing the necessary medical interventions. All women should have equal access to high-quality healthcare services, irrespective of their socioeconomic background, place of residence, or other demographic characteristics.

Furthermore, continuity of care throughout the pregnancy and delivery journey is emphasized by the philosophy of maternal and neonatal health. This entails fostering open communication, building trusting relationships between women and their healthcare providers, and making sure that transitions between various levels of care are seamless. Better health outcomes, greater satisfaction with the birthing process, and enhanced mother-infant bonding are all encouraged by continuity of care. The concept of maternal and newborn health also includes preventative care and health promotion as essential components. This entails offering thorough prenatal education, doing risk factor and complication screenings, and encouraging healthy lifestyle choices. We can prevent maternal and neonatal morbidity and mortality and promote optimal health for both mother and child by enabling women to make educated decisions and adopt healthy habits.

Respect, safety, continuity of care, and health promotion are the cornerstones of the philosophy of maternal and newborn health. We can work to improve maternal and newborn health outcomes for every person by adhering to these principles and making sure that care is woman-centered, evidence-based, and culturally sensitive. In their collaborative efforts to enhance maternal and newborn health across the globe, communities, legislators, and healthcare professionals can all find guidance in this philosophy.

Maternal and child health is family-centered; assessment must include both family and individual assessment data:

- Maternal and child health is community-centered; the health of families depends on and influences the health of communities.
- Maternal and child health is evidence-based, because this is the means whereby critical knowledge increases.
- A maternal and child health nurse serves as an advocate to protect the rights of all family members, including the fetus.
- Maternal and child health includes a high degree of independent functions because teaching and counseling are major interventions.
- Promoting health and disease prevention are important roles because these protect the health of the next generation.
- Maternal and child health clinicians serve as important resources for families during childbearing and childrearing as these can be extremely stressful times in a life cycle.
- Personal, cultural, and religious attitudes and beliefs influence the meaning and impact of childbearing and childrearing on families.
- Circumstances such as illness or pregnancy are meaningful only in the context of a total life.
- Maternal and child health is a challenging role for clinicians and a major factor in keeping families well and optimally functioning.

The promotion and maintenance of optimal family health to ensure cycles of optimal childbearing and childrearing can be summed up as the main objective of maternity and child healthcare. The broad scope of practice in maternal and child healthcare necessitates broad goals.

The range of services and care provided by a nurse based on state requirements includes:

- Preconceptual healthcare.
- Care of women during three trimesters of pregnancy and the puerperium (the 6 weeks after childbirth, sometimes termed the fourth trimester of pregnancy).
- Care of children during the perinatal period (6 weeks before conception to 6 weeks after birth).
- Care of children from birth through adolescence.
- Care in settings as varied as the birthing room, the pediatric intensive care unit, and the home.

Maintaining the family at the center of care delivery is a crucial objective in all settings and forms of care. Family is the primary unit of care in maternal and child health, and this is always the case. Individual health status is influenced by the functioning level of one's families because low functioning levels can negatively impact members of the family's potential and their emotional, physical, and social well-being. On the other hand, a healthy family creates a setting that supports development and behaviors that promote health and help family members get through difficult times. In a similar vein, a person's health and capacity for function have a significant impact on the health of their family members and the general functioning of the family. These factors make it possible for clinicians to provide more comprehensive care by helping them to better understand each patient.

1.4. Family Concepts and Types of Family

The family is an essential social institution that shapes people's identities, relationships, and values. It provides a sense of security and belonging and is the main hub for emotional support, socialization, and caregiving. A group of people who are connected by blood, marriage, or adoption and who share emotional ties and responsibilities are generally referred to as a family, though the definition of family can differ among cultures and societies. Families come in a variety of forms, each with special dynamics and structure. Within many societies, the most prevalent family type is the nuclear family, which consists of the parents and their biological or adopted children. This family structure is frequently linked to ideas of stability and continuity and typically highlights the relationship between parents and children.

Conversely, extended families consist of a larger network of relatives that go beyond the traditional nuclear family. Grandparents, aunts, uncles, cousins, and other relatives who live together or close by may fall under this category. In addition to offering financial support, childcare, and emotional support, extended families frequently play a vital role in promoting intergenerational solidarity and ties. Apart from traditional nuclear and extended families, there exist non-traditional family structures that defy accepted standards and beliefs. For instance, blended families consist of parents who have remarried and might include children from past relationships in the new family. Families with only one parent raise one or more children; this is frequently the result of a spouse passing away, divorcing, or being separated from one another. These various family configurations demonstrate the variety of family structures and the tenacity of familial ties in the face of shifting social norms.

Furthermore, another type of family is represented by chosen families, which are made up of people who are not related by blood but who develop strong bonds through friendship, support, and caregiving. Members of marginalized communities, roommates, or close friends who band together to create alternative sources of support and belonging are examples of chosen families. All things considered, the idea of a family is fluid and changing, mirroring the various ways that people connect, form bonds with one another, and establish support systems. Family, in all its forms, continues to be the foundation of society, offering people of all ages a vital source of resilience, love, and belonging.

Understanding various family structures can aid in concentrating on family-centered care or creating a setting that is family-friendly for receiving medical care. "A group of people related by blood, marriage, or adoption living together" is the definition of a family. Some families consist of unrelated couples, and not all family members may live together at different times in life. An alternative definition of a family is "two or more people who live in the same household share a common emotional bond, and perform certain interrelated social tasks." This definition is far more expansive."

1.4.1. Family Types

Many types or structures of families exist, and family structures change over time as they are affected by birth, work, death, divorce, and the growth of family members. To assess families in maternal and child health, two basic family types can be described:

- Family of orientation (the family one is born into; or oneself, mother, father, and siblings); and
- Family of procreation (a family one establishes; or oneself, spouse or significant other, and children).

Specific descriptions of family types vary greatly depending on family roles, generational issues, means of family support, and sociocultural influences.

1.4.1.1. The Dyad Family

A dyad family is made up of two single adults without children who live together, typically a woman and a man. For instance, recentlyweds are dyad families. Although dyad families are typically thought of as transient situations, they can also be considered lifetime arrangements if the couple decides to live childfree.

1.4.1.2. The Cohabitation Family

Cohabitation families are made up of heterosexual couples who live together but are not married, as well as possibly some children. Cohabitation is often chosen by couples who want to get to know a potential life partner better before getting married, as it is thought to strengthen the bond between them. Similar to marriage, a successful cohabitation agreement provides both financial stability and psychological comfort. These kinds of long-term cohabitation partnerships are becoming more common. The rising number of people living together and maintaining monogamous relationships may help lower the rate of STDs and lessen the financial strain on cohabiting partners.

1.4.1.3. The Nuclear Family

A nuclear family is made up of a husband, wife, and kids. Nonetheless, the proportion of nuclear families has decreased to roughly 49% of all families. The rise in divorce rates, the growing acceptance of single parenthood, and the growing acceptance of alternative lifestyles are the causes of this. Because of its small size, a nuclear family has the advantage of being able to support other family members since everyone gets to know one another well and can truly feel affection for one another. It can be a big responsibility to assist nuclear families in finding and reaching out to people in need of support during a crisis.

1.4.1.4. The Polygamous Family

In the world, polygamy—a marriage in which one man has multiple wives—is a common practice. Polygyny is the condition in which women are undervalued for their unique talents or have a low social status. Because it allows for sexual variety, it may appeal to men. Given that wives are expensive, it can be a sign of a wealthy man. The likelihood that a marriage will result in a male heir also rises when multiple wives bear children. One benefit for women in polygyny marriages is that their chances of dying in childbirth are reduced because they can have fewer children than they would if they were a single wife. Women who experience significant income disparities might choose polygyny over marrying a poor man. Envy and rivalry between spouses due to perceived favoritism can be problematic.

1.4.1.5. The Single-Parent Family

Health issues in a single-parent household can be especially challenging. When the parent is sick, there is no one else to provide childcare. And if the child gets sick, there may not be anyone to offer support or a second opinion on their well-being. Single-parent families, usually headed by women, also often face financial struggles. Single fathers may find it difficult to manage household tasks or care for their children if they were not previously accustomed to those responsibilities.

1.4.1.6. Blended Family

The blended family, also known as a reconstituted or widowed family, is formed when a parent who has children gets married to another parent who also has children. Having resources for the new family and more security are benefits of blended families. Children of blended families also benefit from exposure to diverse customs and cultures, which may help them become more situationally adaptive. Rivalry among the kids for a parent's attention can lead to parenting issues in this kind of household. Youngsters may not accept a stepparent for a variety of reasons, including unresolved feelings regarding the biological parents' separation (via divorce or death), the stepparent's possible differences from the biological parent, especially in terms of parenting and discipline, or the possibility that the stepparent poses a threat to their bond. They might also be biased against their new parent when they join the new family because they have heard so many stories about bad stepparents. When they witness their other biological parent move into a new residence and take on the role of stepparent to other kids, they could get very upset. Even though blended families typically experience less financial hardship, resources can still be extremely tight, particularly if one or both parents must support the children of their current marriage while also being responsible for paying child support for children from a previous marriage.

1.4.2. The Communal Family

Groups of people who decide to live together as an extended family form communes. Rather than being bonded by blood, their relationship is driven by social or religious ideals. Members of a commune might value freedom and autonomy more than members of a traditional family. It may be difficult for residents of a commune to adhere to conventional medical protocols; instead, they may choose to use complementary or alternative therapies.

1.4.2.1. The Gay or Lesbian Family

Individuals of the same sex who live together as partners for companionship, financial security, and sexual fulfillment are known as homosexual unions. A relationship of this kind provides crisis support on par with that of a nuclear or cohabitation family. Children from prior heterosexual marriages, adoptions, surrogate motherhood, and artificial insemination are all common among lesbian and gay families.

1.4.2.2. The Foster Family

A child protection agency may place a child in a foster home or substitute home if their parents are unable to care for them. Foster parents could be parents of their own children or not. They get paid for looking after the foster child. Foster homes are meant to be temporary placements for kids until they are able to go back to their biological parents. Unfortunately, children may grow up in foster care until they are adults if return is not possible or is not imminent. These kids may be insecure almost all the time, worrying that they'll have to move again soon.

1.4.2.3. The Adoptive Family

Nowadays, a wide range of families—including nuclear, extended, cohabitational, single-parent, homosexual, and lesbian—adopt children. Regardless of the makeup of the family, adopting presents a number of difficulties for the child, the adopting parents, and any other children in the home.

1.4.3. Family-Centered Care

The cooperative relationship between the patient, family, and caregivers to set objectives, exchange information, provide support, and create healthcare plans is known as family-centered care. It is commonly understood to be a methodology that views patients and their families as essential partners in the decision-making and provision of healthcare.

Informational support is intended to give the family understanding communication about their member's condition, treatment, growth, and care; as well as about their needs and behavioral and emotional reactions. It also aims to prepare the family for future developments related to their member's condition.

When a family member is ill, emotional support encompasses listening, showing compassion, and showing concern in a way that supports the family in managing the illness and its effects on other aspects of their lives. The idea behind appraisal support, also known as esteem support, is to strengthen, uphold, and promote the family role. Family-centered care acknowledges the family as the constant, with each member's functional abilities and overall health influencing the client's and the family's overall health. Family-centered care is based on the fundamental principles of treating clients and their families with dignity and respect, collaborating with them and their families to deliver care, and providing meaningful and accurate health information. It also encourages clients and their families to participate in decisions about their care.

From preventive care to long-term care, family-centered care is effective across the board in the medical field. Family-centered care helps people feel more confident about their abilities and helps them get ready to take charge of their own healthcare needs. The nurse must determine the level of knowledge the client's family already possesses regarding their health or illness.

Positive results include reduced anxiety, better pain management, quicker recovery times, and increased confidence and problem-solving abilities when a family-centered approach is used. Better communication between the family and the medical team also results in higher satisfaction for the families, who are the healthcare consumers, as well as the medical staff. To build trust and keep lines of communication open with all family members, clinicians must act impartially toward everything they see and hear.

1.4.4. Family Centered Maternity Care (FCMC)

Since ICEA's founding in 1960, family-centered maternity care, or FCMC, has been a defining feature. "Family-centered" at the time meant involving the father in both the actual delivery and classes for expectant parents. Over time, technology became more and more integrated into the birthing process, even though family members were still welcome to attend. In response to this, Celeste Phillips wrote the textbook entitled "Family-Centered Maternity Care" in the mid-1970s. A decade later, McMaster University published a definition of FCMC that was then adopted by ICEA (ICEA, n.d.). In 1996, the Coalition for Maternity Services published the Mother Friendly Childbirth Initiative which was endorsed by many professional and consumer organizations. In 2000, Canada's Public Health Agency published national guidelines for family-centered care. Following the Institute of Medicine's release of "Crossing the Quality Chasm," a number of professional associations have released declarations regarding "patient-centered care" or "family entered care." On "woman-centered care," the Royal College of Midwives has released position papers. It also sets standards for women who enter care in its position paper on high-quality midwifery care. Most recently, an initiative outlining the best care for the mother-baby dyad was developed by the International Mother Baby Childbirth Organization.

Family centered care is an attitude, not simply a list of protocols. In an atmosphere of FCMC, a woman will:

1. Choose the caregiver and place of birth that is most beneficial.
2. Work in collaboration with healthcare providers and other advisers.
3. Have the support of people she desires present whenever she wishes.
4. Move around and use whatever position she feels is beneficial during labor.
5. Refuse routine procedures that are not evidence-based.
6. Practice uninterrupted skin-to-skin contact and breastfeeding immediately after birth.
7. Have access to a variety of support groups including those for breastfeeding, postpartum emotional health, and parenting.

Facilities that promote FCMC will provide education for their staff that includes:

1. Information and training in communication skills;
2. Labor support;
3. Non-pharmacologic forms of pain relief;
4. Breastfeeding support;
5. Perinatal mood disorders.

1.5. Standards of Maternal and Child Health Practice

The American clinicians Association's Division of Maternal-Child Health Practice, in partnership with the Society of Pediatric Nurses, has created standards in the field of maternal-child health.

The Association of Women's Health, Obstetric, and Neonatal clinicians (AWHONN) has developed similar standards for the care of women and newborns.

These standards include:

- Access to skilled birth attendants: Every woman and child should have access to a skilled birth attendant and support staff at all times.
- Competent staff: Skilled birth attendants and support staff should have the right skills and competence for labor, childbirth, and the early postnatal period.
- Leadership: Health facilities should have leadership that develops and implements policies and supports quality improvement.
- Physical environment: Health facilities should have the right physical environment, including water, sanitation, energy, medicines, supplies, and equipment.

1.5.1. Ethics and Standards of Practice Issues

Some of the most difficult ethical quandaries in healthcare today are those that involve children and their families. Are:

- Conception issues, especially those related to in vitro fertilization, embryo transfer, ownership of frozen oocytes or sperm, cloning, and stem cell research.
- Abortion, particularly partial-birth abortions.
- Fetal rights versus rights of the mother.
- Use of fetal tissue for research.
- Resuscitation (for how long should it be continued?).
- Number of procedures or degree of pain that a child should be asked to endure to achieve a degree of better health.
- Balance between modern technology

and quality of life, Legal and ethical aspects of issues are often intertwined, which makes the decision-making process complex.

It is common for a patient's values and those of a healthcare provider to diverge. For instance, if a woman becomes seriously ill during her pregnancy, the family will have to decide whether to end the pregnancy and forfeit the child or to continue the pregnancy and help the mother get through this difficult time. Making the decision may be simpler if the fetus is also at risk for the illness; however, most cases involve complex circumstances and difficult choices. Practice will inevitably bring up these and other problems.

Nurses can help clients who are facing such difficult decisions by providing factual information and supportive listening and helping the family clarify their values.

The legal implications pertinent to maternal and child health are:

- Informed consent is rarely needed as children are unable to understand this.
- All adolescents over age 14 are able to sign consent for their own healthcare.
- Children who feel they have been wronged can sue years into the future.
- Pregnant women are not legally mandated to protect the health of their fetus.

Table 1.1. *Collaborative Networks and Practices Contributing to Social Sustainability in Healthcare Context*

Collaborative Networks	**Collaborative Practices**	**References**
Patients-professionals	Communication, sharing information, shared decision making.	[17, 28, 67, 69]
Inter-professionals	Shared responsibility, joint decision making, communication, shared knowledge and experience, cooperative work, conflict management and shared problem solving.	[30, 56, 70, 71, 73]
Scientists–scientists	Sharing knowledge and view.	[74, 75]
Managers-policy makers-professionals	Sharing knowledge, view, power and responsibility, and joint decision making.	[62, 77, 80, 81]
Inter-organizational	Sharing resources and sharing knowledge.	[58, 82]
Professionals-scientists-supplier of healthcare products	Sharing knowledge, communication, cooperative work.	[83, 84, 85]

Source: Maghsoudi, T., Cascón-Pereira, R., & Beatriz, H. L. A., (2020). The role of collaborative healthcare in improving social sustainability: A conceptual framework. Sustainability, 12(8), 3195. https://doi.org/10.3390/su12083195.

To guarantee consistency and quality of care, the best kind of care is planned and carried out meticulously utilizing a structured set of procedures. The method is a tried-and-true approach to problem solving grounded in the scientific method; it forms the foundation for all aspects of healthcare management, including diagnosis, planning, organizing, and evaluation. The fact that the procedure works in every medical setting—from the pediatric intensive care unit to the prenatal clinic—demonstrates how comprehensive the approach is to act as the foundation for all medical care.

Multidisciplinary Care Maps are included throughout the text to illustrate the application of the process for specific clients, offer examples of critical thinking, and clarify care for particular client needs, as clinicians rarely work in isolation but rather as members of a healthcare team or unit. Rather than care plans, multidisciplinary care maps are displayed because they highlight the growing significance of the nurse's role as a client care coordinator in addition to illustrating the procedure.

In evidence-based practice, clinical knowledge is combined with research or controlled investigation of an issue to serve as a basis for action. Professionals in that field plan and conduct research, which results in the growth and expansion of bodies of knowledge. Research, which is the methodical examination of issues that have practical applications, offers practice-relevant evidence, which serves as the cornerstone for practice's development. Furthermore, the implementation of activities for outcome achievement is justified by evidence-based practice, which ultimately leads to better and more affordable patient care.

The application of Rubin's (1963) research on a mother's approach to her newborn is a classic example of how research findings can impact practice. Before the release of this study, clinicians believed that a mother was "cold" or heartless if she did not hold and cuddle her newborn right away. Rubin concluded that attachment typically starts with simple fingertip touching after witnessing a large number of new mothers. After learning about Rubin's research and applying it to their work, clinicians were better equipped to distinguish between bonding behaviors that were healthy and unhealthy in postpartum mothers and their babies. Women who adhered to this methodical attachment pattern were accepted as normal and no longer seen as emotionless. clinicians can identify women who do not follow this pattern by recording these normal parameters. Based on this information, interventions can be planned and implemented to help these mothers develop a stronger attachment to their newborns. The significance of this initial investigation has been further supported by additional research in this field.

Evidence-based practice requires ongoing research to substantiate current actions as well as to provide guidelines for future actions.

- What is the most effective stimulus to encourage women to come for prenatal care or parents to bring children for health maintenance care?
- How can clinicians be instrumental in fostering diversity in care?
- What are the special needs of women who are discharged from a hospital or birthing center within a short time after childbirth? Of children, after ambulatory surgery?
- How much self-care should young children be expected (or encouraged) to provide during an illness?
- What is the effect of market-driven healthcare on the quality of care?
- What active measures can clinicians take to reduce the incidence of child or intimate partner abuse?
- How can clinicians best help families cope with the stress of long-term healthcare?
- What are the long-term effects of violence on families, and how can clinicians help modify these effects?

- How can clinicians be active in helping prevent violence in communities?
- What do maternal-child health clinicians need to know about alternative therapies such as herbal remedies to keep their practices current?

1.5.2. Theory

A prerequisite for a profession is that the body of knowledge within a discipline originates from well-established theory, along with other crucial factors like member-set standards, practice quality monitoring, and research involvement. Theorists provide useful perspectives on clients so that activities can best meet the needs of the client. For instance, they suggest viewing pregnant women as dynamic forces with significant psychosocial needs rather than just physical forms, or they suggest viewing children as both independent beings and extensions of their families. Clinicians are only able to recognize the profound impact that a child's illness or the addition of a new family member has on the family when they have this wide theoretical perspective.

The objectives of care and how clinicians should be perceived are other topics that most theorists touch on. The purpose of care could have once been defined as "giving sick and injured people comfort and care." Since most clinicians nowadays are qualified to provide preventive care as well, they would likely view this as a narrow perspective. The focus on maternity and child health has shifted significantly as maintaining the health of parents and children—also known as health promotion—has taken precedence. The activities of care are a third topic that nurse theorists address: as goals expand, so do the activities. For instance, actions were restricted to bathing, feeding, and comforting sick individuals when it was thought that caring for them was the main objective. Currently, advocating, teaching, counseling, and support are common roles, with one of the main goals being health promotion. Additionally, clinicians are providing care for patients who are sicker than ever thanks to new technologies. Maternal-child health clinicians perform these expanded roles to a unique and special degree because caring for women during pregnancy and for children during their formative years helps protect not only the health of the present generation but also the health of the future one.

Table 1.2 outlines the basic ideas of several popular theorists and offers examples of how they might be used in the case of a single child to improve maternal-child healthcare. The table's third column, "Emphasis of Care," illustrates that while the theoretical underpinnings of these care approaches vary, each one leads to the provision of a higher caliber of care. These different theories, therefore, do not contradict but rather complement each other in the planning and implementation of holistic care.

Table 1.2. Summary of Theories

Theorist	Major Concepts of Theory	Emphasis of Care
Patricia Benner	Patricia Benner is a caring relationship. Clinicians grow from novice to expert as they practice in clinical settings.	Assess Terry as a whole. An expert nurse is able to do this intuitively from knowledge gained from practice.
Dorothy Johnson	A person comprises subsystems that must remain in balance for optimal functioning. Any actual or potential threat to this system balance is a concern.	Assess the effect of lack of arm function on Terry as a whole; modify care to maintain function to all systems, not just musculoskeletal.

Imogene King	is a process of action, reaction, interaction, and transaction; needs are identified based on client's social system, perceptions, and health; the role of the nurse is to help the client achieve goal attainment.	Discuss with Terry the way she views herself and illness. She views herself as a well-child, active in Girl Scouts and school; structure care to help her meet these perceptions.
Madeleine Leininger	The essence of is care. To provide transcultural care, the nurse focuses on the study and analysis of different cultures with respect to caring behavior.	Assess Terry's family for beliefs about healing. Incorporate these into care.
Florence Nightingale	The role of the nurse is viewed as changing or structuring elements of the environment such as ventilation, temperature, odors, noise, and light to put the client into the best opportunity for recovery	Turn Terry's bed into the sunlight; provide adequate covers for warmth; leave her comfortable with electronic games to occupy her time.
Betty Neuman	A person is an open system that interacts with the environment; is aimed at reducing stressors through primary, secondary, and tertiary prevèntion.	Assess for stressors such as loss of self-esteem and derive ways to prevent further loss such as praising her for combing her own hair.
Dorothea Orem	The focus of is on the individual; clients are assessed in terms of ability to complete self-care. Care given may be wholly compensatory (client has no role); partly compensatory (client participates in care); or supportive-educational (client performs own care).	Arrange overbed table so Terry can feed herself; urge her to participate in care by doing as much for herself as she can.
Ida Jean Orlando	The focus of the nurse is interaction with the client; effectiveness of care depends on the client's behavior and the nurse's reaction to that behavior. The client should define his or her own needs.	Ask Terry what she feels is her main need. Terry says that returning to school is what she wants most. Stress activities that allow her to maintain contact with school, such as doing homework or telephoning friends.
Rosemarie Rizzo Parse	Is a human science. Health is a lived experience. Man-living-health as a single unit guides practice.	Ask Terry what being sick means to her. Allow her to participate in care decisions based on her response.
Hildegard Peplau	The promotion of health is viewed as the forward movement of the personality; this is accomplished through an interpersonal process that includes orientation, identification, exploitation, and resolution.	Plan care together with Terry. Encourage her to speak of school and accomplishments in Girl Scouts to retain self-esteem.
Martha Rogers	The purpose of is to move the client toward optimal health; the nurse should view the client as whole and constantly changing and help people to interact in the best way possible with the environment.	Help Terry to make use of her left side as much as possible so that she returns to school and to her previous level of functioning as soon as possible.

Sister Callista Roy	The role of the nurse is to aid clients to adapt to the change caused by illness; levels of adaptation depend on the degree of environmental change and state of coping ability; full adaptation includes physiologic interdependence.	Assess Terry's ability to use her left hand to replace her right-hand functions, which are now lost; direct care toward replacing deficit with other factors, self-concept, role function, and skills.

1.6. Major Health Issues for Women

Women's Health Issues (WHI) is committed to enhancing women's overall health and access to healthcare across a range of communities and life stages.

Here are 9 of the main issues regarding women's health that keep me awake at night:

1. **Reproductive Health:** Sexual and reproductive health problems are responsible for one-third of health issues for women between the ages of 15 and 44 years.
2. **Maternal Health:** Many women are now benefitting from massive improvements in care during pregnancy and childbirth introduced in the last century. The women died from complications in pregnancy and childbirth. Most of these deaths could have been prevented, had access to family planning and to some quite basic services been in place.
3. **HIV:** Three decades into the AIDS epidemic, it is young women who bear the brunt of new HIV infections. Too many young women still struggle to protect themselves against sexual transmission of HIV and to get the treatment they require.
4. **Sexually Transmitted Infections:** The importance of protecting against HIV and human papillomavirus (HPV) infection (the world's most common STI) is known. But it is also vital to do a better job of preventing and treating diseases like gonorrhea, chlamydia and syphilis.
5. **Violence Against Women:** Women can be subject to a range of different forms of violence, but physical and sexual violence – either by a partner or someone else – is particularly invidious. Violence affects their physical and mental health in the short and long-term.
6. **Mental Health:** Evidence suggests that women are more prone than men to experience anxiety, depression, and somatic complaints – physical symptoms that cannot be explained medically. Depression is the most common mental health problem for women and suicide is a leading cause of death for women under 60.
7. **Noncommunicable Diseases:** Some women died from Noncommunicable diseases before they reached the age of 70 —most of them in low- and middle-income countries. They died as a result of road traffic accidents, harmful use of tobacco, abuse of alcohol, drugs and substances, and obesity.
8. **Being Young:** Adolescent girls face several sexual and reproductive health challenges: STIs, HIV, and pregnancy. Adolescent girls (under 20) give birth every year. Complications from those pregnancies and childbirth are a leading cause of death for those young mothers. Many suffer the consequences of unsafe abortion.
9. **Getting Older:** Having often worked in the home, older women may have fewer pensions and benefits, and less access to healthcare and social services than their male counterparts. Combine the greater risk of poverty with other conditions of old age, like dementia, and older women also have a higher risk of abuse and generally, poor health.

1.6.1. Maternal and Child Health Today

At the beginning of the 20th century, the infant mortality rate in the United States (i.e., the number of infants per 1,000 births who die during the first year of life) was greater than 100 per 1,000. In response to efforts to lower this rate, healthcare shifted from a treatment focus to a preventive one, dramatically changing the scope of maternal and child health. Research on the benefits of early prenatal care led to the first major national effort to provide prenatal care to all pregnant women through prenatal services (home visits) and clinics. Today, thanks to these and other community health measures (such as efforts to encourage breast-feeding, increased immunization, and injury prevention), as well as many technological advances, the U.S. infant mortality rate has fallen to 6.9 per 1,000.

Numerous significant advancements in maternal and child health have been made possible by medical technology: vaccinations have nearly eliminated childhood diseases like measles and poliomyelitis; specific genes responsible for many inherited diseases have been identified; stem cell therapy may one day allow for the replacement of diseased cells with new growth cells; more couples than ever before can conceive thanks to new fertility drugs and techniques; and the capacity to postpone preterm birth and improve the lives of premature infants has increased dramatically. Furthermore, an increasing number of childbearing and childrearing families are actively involved in their own health monitoring and care due to a growing trend toward healthcare consumerism, or self-care. Additionally, as a result of healthcare consumerism, care is now provided in community settings rather than in hospitals, and surgery and overnight stays have replaced long-term hospital stays.

There is still much more to be done, even in light of these developments. The significance of maternal and child health to the general health of the community is still emphasized in the national healthcare goals for the year 2010 that were set in 2000. Even with the advancements in healthcare, not everyone has access to it. The provision of high-quality maternity and child healthcare has become a persistent challenge as a result of these and other social changes and trends, which have also broadened the roles of clinicians in this area.

1.6.2. National Health Goals

In 1979, the U.S. Public Health Service first initiated the formulation of healthcare objectives. Healthcare goals were reestablished in 2000, to be completed in 2010. Many of these objectives directly involve maternal and child healthcare, because improving the health of this young age group will have such long-term effects. National health goals are intended to help everyone more easily understand the importance of health promotion and disease prevention and to encourage wide participation in improving health in the next decade. Given their critical role in assisting the country in achieving these goals through practice and research, maternal and child health clinicians should be well-versed in these objectives. The goals also serve as the basis for grant funding and financing of evidence-based practice.

1.6.3. Trends in the Maternal and Child Health Population

Due to shifting patterns of illness, changes in family lifestyles, and shifts in social structures, the population of mothers and children is always changing. Table 1.2 lists some of the societal shifts that have taken place in the last 20 to 30 years and affected maternal and child health nurses' priorities for healthcare. Clinicians have responded to these shifts by taking on new roles, emphasizing health education more, adopting a cost-containment mindset, and advocating for clients.

Table 1.2. *Quality Indicators and Definitions*

Category	**Quality Indicators[1] or Definitions**	**Numerator**	**Denominator**
Onset of labor	Inductions of labor	Number of inductions of labor [2]	Total number of deliveries[2]
	Planned cesarean deliveries	Number of planned cesarean deliveries performed on or before the scheduled due date (surgical indication recorded ≥ 48 h before performance) [2]	Total number of cesarean deliveries[2]
	Planned cesareans ≥ 39 wk	Number of planned cesarean deliveries ≥ 39 wk performed on or before the scheduled due date (surgical indication recorded ≥ 48 h before performance)[2]	Total number of planned cesarean deliveries[2]
	Cesareans before labor	Number of cesarean deliveries before labor [2]	Total number of cesarean deliveries [2]
Delivery	Vaginal deliveries	Number of vaginal deliveries [2]	Total number of deliveries [2]
	Spontaneous vaginal deliveries (non-instrumental)	Number of non-instrumental spontaneous vaginal deliveries[2]	Total number of vaginal deliveries[2]
	Instrumental vaginal deliveries	Number of instrumental vaginal deliveries[2,3]	Total number of vaginal deliveries [2]
	Global cesarean deliveries	Number of cesareans[2]	Total number of deliveries[2]
	Global cesareans ≥ 37 wk with a singleton pregnancy in breech presentation.	Number of cesareans ≥ 37 wk with a singleton pregnancy in breech presentatio[n]2	Total number of deliveries ≥ 37 wk with a singleton pregnancy in breech presentatio[n]2
	Cesareans among nulliparas	Number of cesareans among nulliparas[2]	Total number of deliveries for nulliparas [2]
	Cesareans during labor	Number of cesareans during labor (among planned cesareans or planned vaginal deliveries) [2]	Total number of cesarean deliveries[2]

	Cesareans ≥ 37 wk for nulliparas with a singleton pregnancy in cephalic presentation.	Number of cesareans ≥ 37 wk for nulliparas with a singleton pregnancy in cephalic presentatio[n]2	Total number of deliveries ≥ 37 wk for nulliparas with a singleton pregnancy in cephalic presentatio[n]2
	Cesareans after one previous cesarean.	Number of cesareans after only one previous cesarean delivery[2]	Total number of deliveries with only one previous cesarean delivery[2]
	Cesareans in non-singleton pregnancy.	Number of cesareans in non-singleton pregnancy[2]	Total number of non-singleton deliveries[2]
	Planned cesareans ≥ 39 wk	Number of planned cesareans ≥ 39 wk[2]	Total number of cesarean deliveries [2]
	Unplanned cesareans after failure of induction.	Number of unplanned cesareans after induction of labor[2]	Total number of inductions of labor[2]
	Definition of low risk at the end of pregnancy.	Low-risk women at the end of pregnancy defined as initially at low risk at the beginning of pregnancy (1), and at low risk during pregnancy (2), without placenta previa or other obstacle for a vaginal delivery, with a fetus in cephalic presentation.	
		(1) Initially (at first consultation) at low risk: • Age: ≥18 years and <35 years. • No medical history negatively affecting the pregnancy. • No history of preterm birth, stillbirth, neonatal death. • Singleton pregnancy. • No previous cesarean or other uterine scar.	(2) Low-risk women during pregnancy: • Initially at low risk and no disorders of pregnancy. • No threatened premature delivery. • No hypertension. • No diabetes. • No amniotic fluid abnormality. • No uterine growth abnormality.
	Cesareans in women at low risk.	Number of cesareans in women at low risk[2,4]	Total number of deliveries in women at low risk[2]

	Cesarean sections according to Robson 10-group classification.	Number of cesareans[2] in: • Nulliparas, singleton cephalic fetus, ≥37 wk, in spontaneous labor. • Nulliparas, singleton cephalic fetus ≥37 wk, induction or cesarean before labor. • Multiparas (excluding previous cesarean), singleton cephalic fetus, ≥37 wk, in spontaneous labor. • Multiparas (excluding previous cesarean), singleton cephalic fetus, ≥37 wk, induction or cesarean before labor. • Previous cesarean, singleton cephalic fetus, ≥37 wk. • All nulliparas with fetus in breech presentation. • All multiparas with fetus in breech presentation (including previous cesarean). • All multiple pregnancies (including previous cesarean). • All abnormal lies (including previous cesarean). • All singleton cephalic fetuses, ≤36 wk (including previous cesarean).	Total number of deliveries[2] according to the description of each group (e.g., for group 1: total number of deliveries in nulliparas, with a singleton cephalic fetus, ≥37 wk, in spontaneous labor).
Pain management	General anesthesia for cesarean delivery.	Number of women receiving general anesthesia for cesareans[2]	Total number of cesarean deliveries [2]
	Epidural analgesia for vaginal delivery.	Number of women receiving epidural analgesia for vaginal delivery[2]	Total number of vaginal deliveries[2]
	Spinal analgesia for cesareans	Number of women receiving spinal analgesia for cesareans[2]	Total number of cesarean deliveries[2]

Neonatal morbidity and mortality	Apgar score < 7 at 5 min	Number of live-born infants with Apgar score < 7 at 5 min[2]	Total number of live-born infants (stillborn infants excluded) [2]
	Births ≥ 37 wk with Apgar score < 7 at 5 min	Number of live-born infants with a birth ≥ 37 wk and an Apgar score < 7 at 5 min[2]	Total number of live-born infants ≥ 37 wk (stillborn infants excluded)[2]
	Live-born preterm neonate.	Number of live-born infants before < 37 wk gestation[2]	Total number of live-born infants[2]
	Live-born infants before < 34 wk gestation	Number of live-born infants before < 34 wk gestation[2]	Total number of live-born infants[2]
	Live-born infants before < 32 wk gestation	Number of live-born infants before < 32 wk gestation[2]	Total number of live-born infants[2]
	Live-born infants before < 28 wk gestation.	Number of live-born infants before < 28 wk gestation [2]	Total number of live-born infants[2]
	Arterial pH < 7.10	Number of live-born infants with umbilical artery pH < 7.10[2]	Total number of live-born infants with umbilical artery pH measured[2]
	Arterial pH < 7.0	Number of live-born infants with umbilical artery pH < 7.0[2]	Total number of live-born infants with umbilical artery pH measured[2]
	Birth weights < 3rd percentile for gestational age.	Number of infants with a birth weight < 3rd percentile for gestational age[2]	Total number of newborns[2]
	Neonatal transfers to intensive care or neonatology unit.	Number of live-born infants transferred to an intensive care or neonatology unit[2]	Total number of live-born infants (admissions for congenital malformations and transfer to kangaroo care unit excluded)[2]
	Neonatal transfers to intensive care unit.	Number of live-born infants transferred to intensive care unit[2]	Total number of live-born infants (admissions for congenital malformations excluded)[2]
	Immediate transfers to any neonatal unit for infants born ≥ 37 wk.	Number of infants born ≥37 wk transferred to any neonatal unit[2]	Total number of live-born infants ≥ 37 wk (admissions for congenital malformations excluded)[2]
	Stillbirths	Number of fetal or immediate neonatal deaths (including fetal deaths in utero, medical terminations of pregnancy, and intrapartum deaths)2	Total number of births (live-born or stillborn infants) [2]

Maternal morbidity	Postpartum hemorrhages >500 mL for vaginal delivery.	Number of postpartum hemorrhages > 500 mL for vaginal delivery[2]	Total number of vaginal deliveries[2]
	Postpartum hemorrhages > 1000 mL (regardless of mode of delivery).	Number of postpartum hemorrhages > 1000 mL for delivery[2]	Total number of deliveries[2]
	Postpartum hemorrhage > 1000 mL for vaginal delivery.	Number of postpartum hemorrhages > 1000 mL for vaginal delivery[2]	Total number of vaginal deliveries[2]
	Postpartum hemorrhages > 1000 mL for cesarean deliveries.	Number of postpartum hemorrhages > 1000 mL for cesareans[2]	Total number of cesarean deliveries[2]
	Blood transfusions in delivery or operating room.	Number of blood transfusions in the delivery or operating room[2]	Total number of deliveries[2]
	Hemostatic hysterectomies	Number of hemostatic hysterectomies[2]	Total number of deliveries[2]
	Hemostatic surgery (other than hysterectomy).	Number of hemostatic surgeries other than hysterectomies[2]	Total number of deliveries[2]
	Uterine ruptures	Number of complete or subperitoneal uterine ruptures (dehiscences excluded)[2]	Total number of deliveries[2]
	Discharge from delivery unit by transfer to adult intensive care unit.	Number of women discharged from the delivery unit by a transfer to an intensive care unit[2]	Total number of deliveries[2]
	Intact perineum	Number of women with an intact perineum (without suture)[2]	Total number of deliveries[2]
	Episiotomies	Number of women with an episiotomy for vaginal delivery[2]	Total number of vaginal deliveries[2]
	Episiotomies in primiparas	Number of primiparas with an episiotomy in vaginal delivery[2]	Total number of vaginal deliveries in primiparas[2]
	Severe perineal tears	Number of women with 3rd- and 4th-degree perineal tears[5] in vaginal delivery[2]	Total number of vaginal deliveries[2]

	Severe perineal tears for instrumental vaginal delivery.	Number of women with 3rd- and 4th-degree perineal tears[5] for instrumental vaginal delivery[2]	Total number of instrumental vaginal deliveries (forceps, vacuum, spatula)[2]
	Severe perineal tears for non-instrumental vaginal delivery.	Number of women with 3rd- and 4th-degree perineal tears[5] in non-instrumental vaginal delivery[2]	Total number of non-instrumental vaginal deliveries[2]
	Severe perineal tears for forceps delivery.	Number of women with 3rd- and 4th-degree perineal tears[5] in instrumental vaginal delivery using forceps [2]	Total number of instrumental vaginal deliveries using forceps[2]
	International definition of perineal tears (first, second, third, and fourth degrees).	• 1st degree: tears affecting the skin or the vaginal mucosa. • 2nd degree: tears affecting the muscle of the perineum but not the sphincter. • 3rd degree: tears affecting the anal sphincter. • 4th degree: tears involving the anal sphincter and tears into the rectal mucosa.	

Note: Wk: Weeks of amenorrhea.

[1]Quality indicators are expressed as percentages.

[2]For births ≥ 22 wk or birth weight ≥ 500 g in the absence of a known pregnancy onset.

[3]Forceps, spatula, or vacuum extractor.

[4]According to the previously proposed definition during the Delphi process.

[5]Third-degree tears involve the anal sphincter, with either total or partial damage to the sphincter and fourth-degree tears involving the anal sphincter and tears into the rectal mucosa.

Source: *Guiguet-Auclair, C., Rivière, O., Gerbaud, L., & Vendittelli, F., (2023). Quality indicators during delivery, and the immediate postpartum period: A modified Delphi study.* ***Healthcare****, 11(6), 848. https://doi.org/10.3390/healthcare110608481.6.4. Measuring Maternal and Child Health.*

1.6.3.1. Birth Rate

The birth rate in the United States has gradually decreased over the past 10 years to 13.9 per 1,000 population at present (Figure 1.2). Currently, the average family in the United States has 1.2 children. Boys are born more often than girls, at a rate of 1,050 boys to every 1,000 girls.

Births to teenage mothers are steadily declining, and those to women older than 40 years of age are steadily increasing.

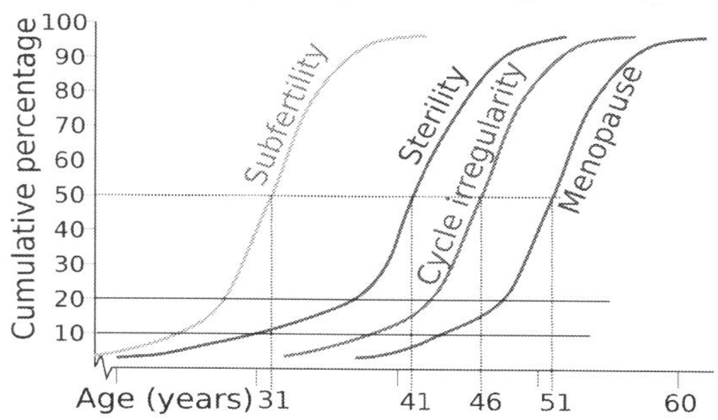

Figure 1.2. *Data on average ages.*

Source: *By Mikael Häggström, by work of Egbert, R. T. V., & Peter, L. P., (2002) – Own work, adapted from: The variability of female reproductive ageing. Human Reproduction Update, 8(2), 141–154. doi: 10.1093/humupd/8.2.141. ISSN 1355-4786. Sterility data further specified from: Leridon, Henri (2005). The biological obstacles to late childbearing and the limits of ART. Ined-Inserm, Paris. Archived from the original on 2016-04-19. Retrieved on 2012-08-26, CC0, https://commons.wikimedia.org/w/index.php?curid=47074986.*

1.6.3.2. Perinatal Death Rate

There are several ways to define the perinatal period. According to statistics, the period is defined as the period of time that starts at week 20 of pregnancy, or when the fetus weighs 500 grams, and ends four to six weeks after delivery. The total of the fetal and neonatal death rates is the perinatal death rate.

1.6.3.3. Fetal Death Rate

A fetus that weighs 500 grams or more—roughly the weight of a fetus that is 20 weeks or more gestation—is considered to have died in utero. It is possible for maternal factors (e.g., malnourishment, early cervical dilation, and maternal illness) or fetal factors (e.g., chromosomal abnormality, poor placental attachment, and fetal disease). Unknown causes are the cause of many fetal fatalities. Since it indicates the general standard of maternal health and prenatal care, the fetal death rate is a useful indicator of a country's health. The emphasis on both pre-conceptual and prenatal care has helped to reduce this rate from a number as high as 18% in 1950 to 6.4% at present.

1.6.3.4. Neonatal Death Rate

An infant is referred to as a neonate during the first 28 days of life, which is also known as the neonatal period. The quality of care provided to babies in their first month of life is also reflected in the neonatal death rate, in addition to the care that women receive during their pregnancies and deliveries. In the first four weeks of life, low birth weight (less than 2,500 g), congenital anomalies, and prematurity (early gestational age) are the main causes of infant mortality. Around 80% of newborns that pass away within 48 hours of delivery weigh less than 2,500 grams (5 pounds, five ounces). Approximately 7% of all births result in a low birth weight baby. Because of improved prenatal care, babies who would have died in utero (fetal death) are able to be born and survive, which causes this number to slightly increase annually.

1.6.3.5. Maternal Mortality Rate

The number of maternal deaths that result directly from reproduction per 100,000 live births is known as the maternal mortality rate. In the United States, this rate rose to 600 per 100,000 live births at the beginning of the 20th century. This dramatic decrease can be attributed to improved preconceptual, prenatal, labor and birth, and postpartum care, such as the following:

- Greater detection of disorders such as ectopic pregnancy or placenta previa and prevention of related complications through the use of ultrasound.
- Increased control of complications associated with hypertension during pregnancy.
- Decreased use of anesthesia with childbirth.

Uterine bleeding and infection were the main causes of death during pregnancy and childbirth for the majority of the 20th century. Due to the improved ability to stop or manage bleeding and infections, this has changed, and hypertensive disorders are now the main causes of maternal death. Particularly in older women, pregnancy-induced hypertension exacerbates preexisting hypertensive disorders. Pregnant and postpartum women's health is greatly protected by clinician who are knowledgeable about the warning signs and symptoms of hypertension (Figure 1.3).

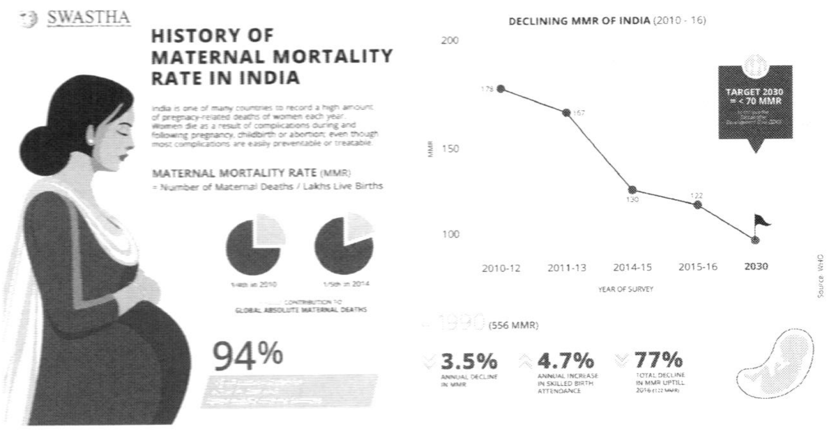

Figure 1.3. *Maternal mortality rates in India.*

Source: *https://upload.wikimedia.org/wikipedia/commons/2/2c/Maternal_Mortality_in_India_-_History_inforgraphic.jpg.*

1.6.3.6. Infant Mortality Rate

A nation's infant mortality rate serves as a gauge of its overall health since it considers both the infant's health and the quality of prenatal care, nutrition, and sanitation. This rate is the conventional benchmark for evaluating the current status of national healthcare in relation to past performance or other nations.

Thanks to healthcare advances and improvements in childcare, the infant mortality rate in the United States has been steadily declining in recent years. Unfortunately, infant mortality is not equal for all races. African-American infants, for example, have a mortality rate of almost 15%. This difference in African-American and white infant deaths is thought to be related to the higher proportion of births to young African-American mothers, unequal provision of healthcare, and the higher percentage of low-birth-weight babies born to African-American women: 12%, compared with approximately 5% for white and Asian women. Despite this negative trend, the overall steady drop in total infant mortality is encouraging (Figure 1.4).

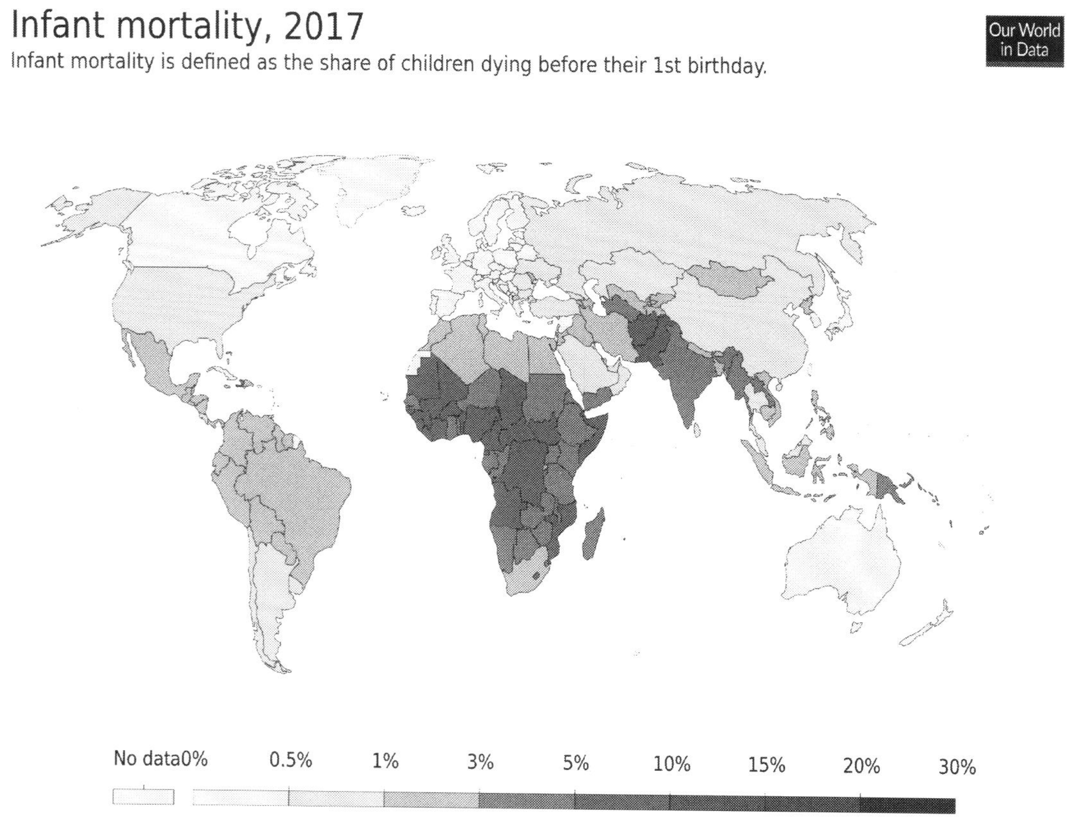

Figure 1.4. *Infant mortality rates in 2017.*

Source: *By Max Roser – https://ourworldindata.org/child-mortality, CC BY 4.0, https://commons.wikimedia.org/w/index.php?curid=83581872.*

State	Rate	State	Rate	State	Rate
Massachusetts	4.8	South Dakota	6.4	Missouri	7.7
New Hampshire	4.9	Wyoming	6.5	Ohio	7.7
Maine	5.1	Idaho	6.6	Illinois	7.8
Utah	5.3	Arizona	6.7	North Dakota	7.8
California	5.4	Kentucky	6.7	West Virginia	7.9
Minnesota	5.5	Rhode Island	6.7	Oklahoma	8.0
Oregon	5.5	Alaska	6.8	Michigan	8.1
Texas	5.5	Montana	6.9	Arkansas	8.3
Washington	5.5	Wisconsin	6.9	North Carolina	8.4
Iowa	5.8	Kansas	7.0	Georgia	8.7
Colorado	6.0	Nebraska	7.0	South Carolina	9.0
Nevada	6.0	Florida	7.2	Tennessee	9.0
New Jersey	6.1	Hawaii	7.2	Alabama	9.3
New York	6.1	Virginia	7.2	Delaware	9.6
Vermont	6.2	Pennsylvania	7.3	Louisiana	9.8
Connecticut	6.4	Indiana	7.7	District of Columbia	11.4
New Mexico	6.4	Maryland	7.7		

Source: https://downloads.lww.com/wolterskluwer_vitalstream_com/sample-content/9780781777766_Pillitteri/samples/Chapter01.pdf.

Table 1.3 shows the ranking of the United States compared with other developed countries. One would expect that a country such as the United States, which has one of the highest gross national products in the world and is known for its technological capabilities, would have the lowest infant mortality rate. However, in 2000, the U.S. infant mortality rate was higher than that of 27 other countries.

Table 1.3. *Differences in Infant Mortality by the Month of Prenatal Care Began in the Southeastern US from 2005 to 2009*

Month Prenatal Care Began	Average Infant Mortality (per 100,000) (2005–2009)					
	Alabama	Florida	Georgia	Louisiana	Mississippi	US
No prenatal care	3891.23 ± 1258.15	3607.83 ± 109.01	3314.24 ± 827.48	4262.16 ± 1492.23	5281.83 ± 231.53*	3074.82 ± 505.11
1st month	893.38 ± 117.67	811.68 ± 60.22	666.79 ± 40.66	929.34 ± 69.34	935.60 ± 1.35	762.40 ± 83.20
2nd month	824.49 ± 46.12	553.09 ± 31.50	583.27 ± 119.41	890.63 ± 143.02	1028.82 ± 125.00	540.92 ± 40.07
3rd month	913.96 ± 31.36	561.68 ± 5.03	739.16 ± 106.19	889.18 ± 102.66	997.71 ± 64.32	533.57 ± 37.40
4th month	935.49 ± 62.49	571.24 ± 36.49	776.03 ± 107.61	1098.92 ± 214.20	1313.59 ± 138.71	611.74 ± 42.24
5th month	811.39 ± 222.35	718.12 ± 67.83	840.30 ± 149.83	1319.22 ± 51.66	1179.05 ± 193.38	709.32 ± 39.65
6th month	914.63	599.15 ± 73.28	720.61 ± 99.71	1146.26 ± 7.88	1516.92	635.48 ± 48.66

7th month	NA	531.54 ± 52.06	610.04 ± 121.25	NA	NA	571.98 ± 61.32
8th month	NA	422.98 ± 32.23	NA	NA	NA	546.13 ± 35.28

* $p < 0.05$, compared to the US.

Source: *He, X., Akil, L., Aker, W. G., Hwang, H. M., & Ahmad, H. A., (2015). Trends in infant mortality in United States: A brief study of the southeastern states from 2005–2009. International Journal of Environmental Research and Public Health, 12(5), 4908–4920. https://doi.org/10.3390/ijerph120504908.*

The quality of healthcare that is accessible is one element that could influence variations in infant mortality amongst countries. For instance, all citizens of Sweden are entitled to free maternity and child healthcare as part of a comprehensive healthcare program. Prenatal clinics offer financial incentives to women who visit them early in their pregnancies, which effectively ensures that all pregnant women will seek prenatal care. These people think that if there was a guaranteed healthcare system like this, the infant mortality rate in the US would go down. Thankfully, more pregnant women in the US are receiving prenatal care—roughly 80% of them start receiving it in the first trimester.

Early prenatal care is crucial because it helps identify possible risks and makes preventive measures possible, which can help lower pregnancy complications. The higher percentage of babies born to adolescent moms (30% of babies are born to mothers younger than 20 years of age) is another way that the United States varies from other nations. Adolescent pregnancy increases the risk of premature births, which could leave some newborns less equipped than others to deal with life outside the womb.

Issues that arise at birth or shortly after are the primary causes of early infant mortality in the United States. Major causes include respiratory distress syndrome, congenital anomalies, low birth weight, premature birth, and sudden infant death syndrome. The American Academy of Pediatrics recommended in 1992 that infants sleep on their backs or sides to reduce the risk of sudden infant death syndrome, though other factors may also play a role.

In the days before the development of antibiotics and formula sterilization techniques, infant mortality was primarily caused by gastrointestinal disorders. Healthcare professionals can mitigate the risk of gastrointestinal infections causing infant mortality by promoting breastfeeding and teaching mothers to strictly adhere to hygienic practices.

1.6.3.7. Childhood Morbidity Rate

These days, gastrointestinal issues, post-injury complications, and respiratory diseases (such as tuberculosis and asthma) are common health issues affecting a significant percentage of children. Common childhood communicable diseases are affecting fewer children in the United States as more vaccines become available. For example, due to widespread vaccination against poliomyelitis, the disease that used to kill a lot of children has become very rare—virtually nonexistent. Although the disease's incidence spiked in the early 1990s, measles was currently expected to be totally eradicated by 2010. This is crucial because measles encephalitis can be just as deadly and debilitating as poliomyelitis. It is also necessary to continue educating people about the advantages of being vaccinated against German measles, or rubella, as this type of measles can cause serious congenital defects in the unborn child. While it is encouraging that the overall incidence of childhood diseases that can be prevented is declining, in these communities and list barriers to high vaccination coverage up to 50% of children under four years old remain unvaccinated. If childhood infectious diseases are not kept at the top of the national priority list, there is a chance that they will spread once more.

The emergence of HIV has altered the way that care is provided in all fields, but it has particularly affected maternal and child health. Sexually active teenagers and childbearing women are particularly vulnerable to contracting HIV through blood and blood products, as well as through placental exchange, which allows an infected woman to pass the virus to a fetus during pregnancy. Adolescents and young adults need to be educated about safer sexual practices to help stop HIV from spreading. As in other areas of practice, standard precautions in maternal and child health must be strictly adhered to to protect other clients and healthcare providers.

The prevalence of syphilis, genital herpes, hepatitis A and B, and tuberculosis is also rising among infectious diseases. Lack of safer sex practices and an increase in non-monogamous relationships are likely to be blamed for the rise in genital herpes and syphilis cases. The use of contaminated injection equipment and drug abuse are the main causes of the rise in hepatitis B cases. Shared diaper changing areas in daycare centers are one factor contributing to the rise in hepatitis A cases. Once thought to be almost completely eradicated, tuberculosis has returned and is now striking young adults at a rate comparable to that of measles. One type affects HIV-positive individuals as an opportunistic illness that is especially resistant to standard treatment.

1.6.3.8. Childhood Mortality Rate

Like the infant mortality rate, the childhood mortality rate in the United States is also declining. In 1980, for example, the mortality rate was about 6.4% for children aged 1 to 4 years and 3.1% for children aged 4 to 14 years; today, it is 3.0% and 1.8%, respectively. The risk of death in the first year of life is higher than that in any other year before age 55. Children in the prepubescent period (age 5 to 14 years) have the lowest mortality rate of any child age group.

Motor vehicle accidents continue to be the leading cause of death for children Although many of these accidents are largely preventable through education about the value of car seats and seat belt use, the dangers of drinking or abusing drugs and driving, and the significance of pedestrian safety,. The high rate of suicide in the 15–24 age group (more girls than boys attempt suicide, but boys are more successful) is a particularly unsettling mortality statistic. Even though school-age kids and teenagers might not express their anger or sadness during a medical appointment, these underlying emotions might be the main cause for concern. Clinicians who are aware of signs of anger or depression can be useful in identifying these feelings and reducing the risk of suicide. Concerns are also growing over the high rate of homicide (which is 1% among school-age children and 20% among adolescents) and the rise in HIV infections among adolescents.

1.6.4. Trends in Healthcare Environment

The settings for maternal and child healthcare are changing to better meet the needs of increasingly well-informed and vocal clients

1.6.4.1. Cost Containment

Cost containment refers to healthcare delivery systems that closely monitor personnel costs, the use and brands of supplies, hospital stays, procedures performed, and the number of referrals requested in an effort to lower overall healthcare costs. Prior to the cost-containment movement gaining traction, health insurance covered each procedure or piece of equipment the patient received separately. No matter how many materials, techniques, or staff members are employed in the client's care, the agency is paid a set amount under managed care. Aiding in cost reduction is a crucial role in a managed care setting. Cost-effective ideas like using generic brands of supplies, avoiding opening supply kits to remove a single item, and encouraging the use of disposable supplies to reduce staff time spent cleaning and sterilizing are all appreciated.

Cost containment has drastically changed the way healthcare is provided, most notably by reducing the number of hospital days and redefining staff roles. Women used to spend three or four days in the hospital after giving birth before managed care; these days, they hardly ever stay more than 48 hours. Regardless of how minor or inexperienced the task, clinicians handled all patient care prior to managed care. In managed care, support staff (e.g., unlicensed assistive personnel) work under the nurse's supervision on a variety of duties. Because it holds registered clinicians (RNs) accountable for a wider range of patient services, this system is intended to elevate RNs to higher levels of function. The point-of-service care is highlighted. It also makes RNs more accountable and responsible for assigning work correctly. The new advanced practice position of case manager has been created as a result of managed care.

Understanding the legal ramifications of delegation as outlined in state practice acts is crucial because certain state laws pertain to particular duties and responsibilities that registered clinicians may or may not be able to assign. The nurse bears the responsibility for the task's completion and quality, so it is incumbent upon them to ascertain whether the patient's condition and the assistive person's skill level allow for safe delegation.

There are four rules to follow when delegating:

- Right task for the situation;
- Right person to complete the task;
- Right communication concerning what is to be done; and
- Right feedback or evaluation that the task was completed.

Because managed care restricts the amount of time and supplies available for care, it was initially thought to be a system that could result in low-quality treatment. However, because it encourages creativity, it has given clinicians more opportunities in environments where it functions well.

1.6.4.2. Alternative Settings and Styles for Healthcare

There have been many significant changes to maternity care settings over the past 100 years. The majority of births occurred in homes at the turn of the 19th century; only the extremely sick or impoverished gave birth in "lying-in" hospitals. Hospitals hosted roughly 40% of live births by 1940; today that number is closer to 98%. A less noticeable but still significant trend is emerging today: more and more families are choosing, once again, to give birth at home or in other non-hospital locations rather than in medical facilities. These non-hospital birth environments give families more control over the childbirth process and offer alternatives to hospital birth environments. This movement's encouragement of family participation in childbirth is one of its strong points. It also offers expanded roles for nurse practitioners, such as the nurse-midwife, and increases accountability for assessment and professional judgment. Currently, midwives are responsible for birthing of all births in the United States instead of doctors.

Hospitals have remodeled labor and delivery suites into birthing rooms, sometimes known as labor-delivery-recovery-postpartum (LDRP) or LDR rooms, in response to consumer demand for a more natural childbirth environment. The room is intended to feel like a home, so partners, family, and other supporters are welcome to stay and take part in the birthing process (Figure 1.5). Following delivery, couplet care—care provided by the primary nurse to both the mother and the infant—is advised. Many families who might have otherwise chosen against giving birth in a hospital find that LDRP rooms are appealing because they support a comprehensive, family-centered approach to maternity and child healthcare. Nevertheless, LDRPs are not perfect. There have been claims that they make it harder for clinicians to meet the needs of women during labor and after delivery, that they are less private for families in labor, and that they are generally less soothing for families that have recently given birth. Numerous medical facilities are still looking for the greatest options for childbirth, labor, and recovery. The idea is to maintain as much of a natural birthing process as possible while guaranteeing the safety that skilled nurse-midwives or doctors can offer, whether the delivery occurs at home, in a birthing center, or in a hospital.

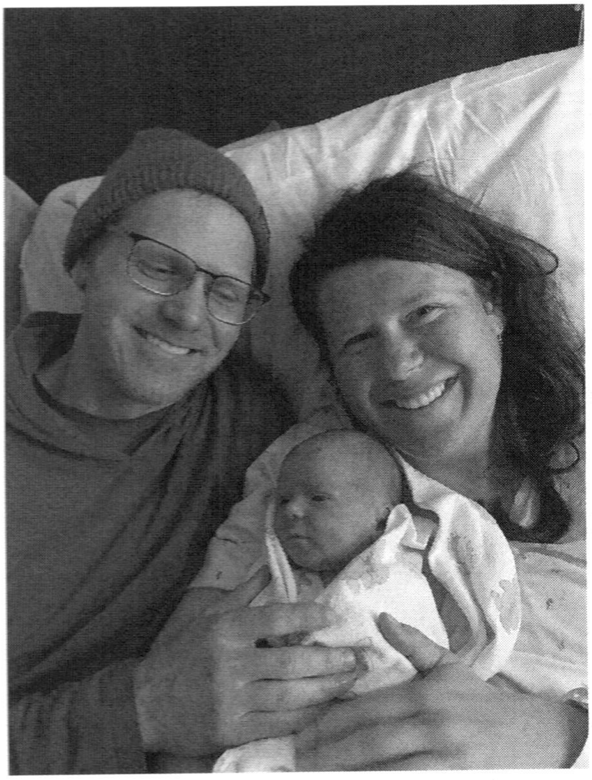

Figure 1.5. *Parenthood.*

Source: *By James.rybarsyk – Own work, CC BY-SA 4.0, https://commons.wikimedia.org/w/index.php?curid=106709873.*

Healthcare settings for children are evolving, with services now being offered in a variety of locations such as clients' homes, community centers, clinics, schools, and group homes. In these settings, clinicians can provide a range of services including immunizations, screenings, education on health and safety, counseling, crisis intervention for teens, parenting classes, and care for sick children and their families. Community-based care is a cost-effective way to promote health, prevent disease, and provide care to many children and families in a familiar environment.

1.6.4.3. Strengthening the Ambulatory Care System

The scope of the ambulatory care system is still expanding. An increasing number of patients who would have otherwise required hospital admissions are now receiving care at home or in ambulatory clinics. This choice has been shown to be crucial for the treatment of ill children as well as pregnant patients who wish to be released from the hospital soon after giving birth or who are experiencing pregnancy complications. It has been demonstrated that removing a child from their family while they are ill may be detrimental to their development, so any initiative to lessen the frequency of separation should be beneficial. It's also a better approach to care for pregnant women to avoid prolonged hospital stays, as this keeps family relationships intact.

1.6.4.4. Shortening Hospital Stays

An increasing number of hospitals can perform pediatric surgeries that don't require an overnight stay, such as tonsillectomy and repair of inguinal or umbilical hernias. When the parent and child arrive at the hospital early on the day of surgery, the child is given medication and undergoes a preoperative physical examination. Following surgery, the young patient is taken to a short-term observation unit and then a recovery room. Four hours after surgery, if the child is doing well and exhibits no complications, he or she can be released from the hospital. In a similar vein, women who start preterm labor are admitted to the hospital, where their labor is stopped, and then they are discharged home under strict supervision. After an easy birth, moms and babies typically spend two days in the hospital, if not less.

Intensive health education from the staff and follow-up from home care or community health clinicians are necessary for short-term hospital stays. Parents need to learn how to look out for warning indications in their children without getting alarmed. A pregnant woman experiencing a complication needs to be trained to recognize symptoms that call for quick care. Before the joy and exhaustion of giving birth have worn off, new parents need to be educated about the nutritional requirements of their infant, how to care for the umbilical cord, how to bathe their baby, and safety precautions. This kind of instruction is challenging because it entails not just teaching self-care facts but also offering encouragement and assurance that the client or their parents are capable of handling this degree of care.

1.6.4.5. Including the Family in Healthcare

When a child needs to be admitted for an extended period of time, the majority of hospitals have created policies that reduce the impact of being separated from their parents. Open visiting hours let parents spend as much time as possible with their kids and spend the night in a bed next to them. During a hospital stay, parents are also permitted and encouraged to provide all the care they want for their child, including feeding, bathing, and giving oral medication. Nonetheless, a parent spends the majority of their time just being nearby to offer a safe, comforting influence on their child. For similar reasons, room-in parents are encouraged to provide their healthy newborn with their whole attention while they are in a maternity unit. Family-centered care is essential because parents have a significant impact on their child's hospital stay and general well-being. As a result, the nurse's caseload will include more than just four kids—for instance, four kids and four sets of parents—or just one newborn and his or her two parents.

1.6.4.6. Increase in the Number of Intensive Care Units

Over the past 20 years, the care of infants and children has become extremely technical. It is generally assumed that newborns with a term birthweight (more than 2,500 g or 5.5 lb) will thrive at birth. However, many infants are born each year with birthweights lower than 2,500 g or who are ill at birth and do not thrive. Such infants are regularly transferred to a neonatal intensive care unit (NICU) or intensive care nursery (ICN). Children who are undergoing cardiac surgery or recovering from near-drownings or multi-injury accidents are cared for in a pediatric intensive care unit (PICU). Intensive care at this early point in life is one of the most costly types of hospitalization. Expenses of $1,000 a day, or $20,000 to $100,000 for a total hospital stay, are not rare for care during a high-risk pregnancy or care for a high-risk infant. As the number of these settings increases, the opportunities for advanced-practice clinicians also increase.

1.6.4.7. Regionalization of Intensive Care

It is standard procedure for communities to set up centralized maternity or pediatric health services to prevent duplication of care sites. This kind of planning results in a single location that is adequately manned and furnished for any eventualities. For instance, sick newborns might be taken to a central high-risk nursery for medical attention. Pregnant women at high risk and sick children can receive care in a community setting that has specialized resources for diagnosing and treating particular conditions. The family members left behind need a lot of support when a parent, older child, or newborn is admitted to a regional center. If medical staff doesn't keep them updated on their loved one's condition through phone calls and pictures, they might feel as though they have "lost" their baby, kid, or parent. They should also be urged to visit as soon as feasible.

Transporting the sick or premature newborn to the regional care facility was the preferred approach when regionalization concepts of newborn care were first accepted (Figure 1.6).

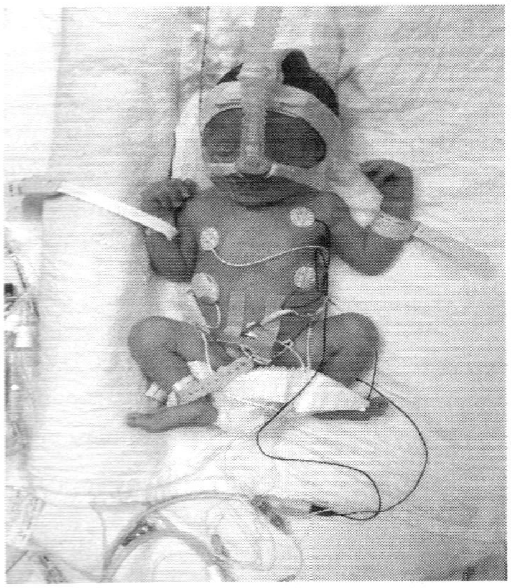

Figure 1.6. *A nurse prepares an infant transport incubator to move a premature infant to a regional hospital. Helping with safe movement of pregnant women and ill newborns to regional centers is an important responsibility.*

Source: By Lazarus000 - Own work, CC BY-SA 4.0, https://commons.wikimedia.org/w/index.php?curid=70407716.

Today, however, the uterus has advantages as a transport incubator that far outweigh those of any commercial incubator yet designed, so if it is known ahead of time that a child may be born with a life-threatening condition, it might be safer to transport the mother to the regional center during pregnancy.

The claim that children will experience homesickness in unfamiliar environments, become overwhelmed by the number of sick children they see, and become afraid because they are far from home is a significant argument against regionalizing pediatric care. Being away from her community and support system puts a lot of stress on the pregnant woman and her family and restricts the involvement of her own doctor in her care, which is a key argument against the regionalization of maternal care. These are crucial things to think about. More than any other medical profession, clinicians set the standard for hospitals, so they have to make sure that patients and their families are treated with the same warmth and hospitality in regional centers as they would have in a smaller facility. Enough staffing means that clinicians will have enough time to soothe scared kids, get them ready for new things, or help the expectant mother and her family. By recording the significance of these actions, the nurse's role is preserved and they can be included in important pathways.

1.6.4.8. Increased Reliance on Comprehensive Care Settings

The goal of comprehensive healthcare is to address all of a child's requirements in one location. Child care used to be more specialized in the past. For instance, a newborn suffering from a disease (e.g., cerebral palsy, myelomeningocele) may have been handled by a group of experts for every aspect of the issue. A neurologist, an orthopedic surgeon, a physical therapist, an occupational therapist, a psychologist for IQ testing, a speech therapist, and a special education teacher could be on this team. It may be necessary for the parents to locate a particular dentist who treats patients with a variety of disabilities. Instead of considering the child's development as a whole, each specialist would focus on a single aspect of the child's needs. Parents who don't have additional guidance may become disoriented in the confusing network of appointments with various medical professionals. They might not have been able to pay for all the required services at once if they had not been receiving financial assistance for the upbringing of their child. Determining which of the child's issues required urgent attention and which could wait without getting worse and becoming a permanent handicap may have been challenging. Specialists are still crucial to a child's care, but in the managed care setting of today, parents need a reliable primary care physician to assist in coordinating these specialized services. Often, an advanced-practice nurse, such as a family nurse practitioner, pediatric nurse practitioner, or women's health nurse practitioner, serves as this child's primary care provider, guiding them through all stages of care. In this way, clinicians can assist in ensuring that a primary healthcare provider can meet the needs of both parents and children.

1.6.4.9. Increased Use of Alternative Treatment Modalities

Families are increasingly turning to alternative therapy providers—such as acupuncturists or therapeutic touch practitioners—in addition to or instead of conventional medical professionals. The knowledge of complementary and alternative therapies, which may augment or diminish the efficacy of conventional therapy, is becoming more and more important for nurses.

Furthermore, medical professionals who are not aware of certain alternative therapy options may miss a significant chance to benefit from the advantages of that specific therapy. If a teenager is going to have a painful procedure, for example, it would be helpful to know that she has experience with meditation. Asking the teenager if she would like to meditate before the procedure could help her unwind. This may help the child feel less uncomfortable while also giving her a sense of control over an uncomfortable circumstance. As more people turn to herbal remedies, it's critical to inquire about them during a health evaluation to avoid medication interactions. For example, taking ginger frequently helps with morning sickness during pregnancy.

1.6.4.9.1. Increased Use of Technology

Every setting related to healthcare is using technology more and more. The field of reproductive assistance (e.g., in vitro fertilization), and the potential for stem cell study is opening up new avenues. Other examples include using a computer to chart, searching the Internet for information, and using Doppler ultrasound to track the heart rates of fetuses. Maternal and child health clinicians need to be knowledgeable about these technologies as well as able to communicate to clients how they work and why they are advantageous. If not, users might perceive new technologies as more frightening than beneficial.

A Closer Look

Maternal and Child Health

Although racial and ethnic disparities in education, housing, and socioeconomic status are evident in many spheres of society, maternal and child health is one area where these disparities are particularly noticeable. The risk of maternal mortality or a pregnancy-related death is three to four times higher for black women than for white women, despite the fact that the United States has the highest rate of maternal mortality among developed nations. Given that racism has a structural and systemic detrimental influence on the health of Black women, this illustrates how racism is a social justice and public health issue.

Analysis of variance shows the significant difference in infant mortality by the maternal race of mother in the Southeastern US from 2005 (**A**) to 2009 (**E**).

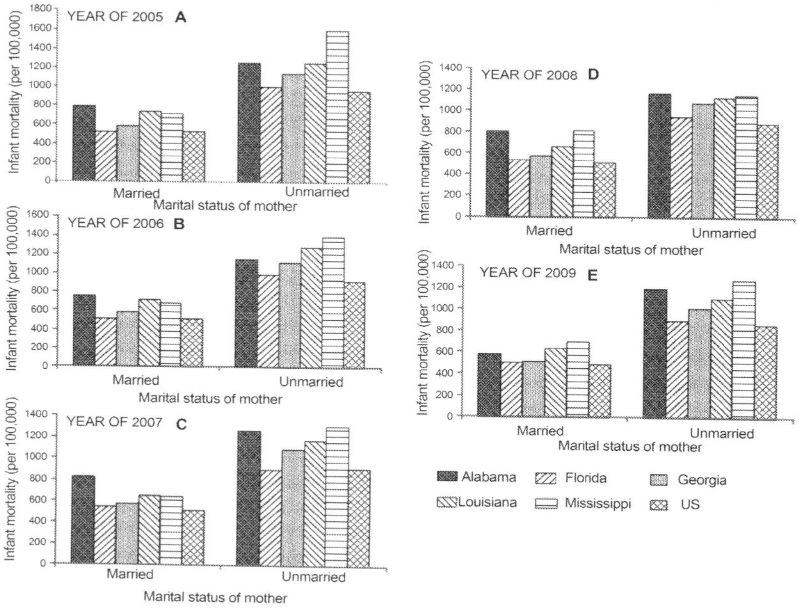

Source: *He, X., Akil, L., Aker, W. G., Hwang, H. M., & Ahmad, H. A., (2015). Trends in infant mortality in United States: A brief study of the southeastern states from 2005–2009. International Journal of Environmental Research and Public Health, 12(5), 4908–4920. https://doi.org/10.3390/ijerph120504908*

It is crucial to include pregnancy-associated mortality and severe maternal morbidity (SMM) in our discussion of the obstacles to attaining equitable maternal health, in addition to maternal mortality. Within a year of becoming pregnant, maternal deaths are included in pregnancy-associated mortality (SMM), which also considers the long-term health effects that pregnancy complications may have on a woman. These differences in SMM and pregnancy-related mortality also exist in our Massachusetts communities. Compared to white non-Hispanic women, black non-Hispanic women in the state have a twice as high risk of pregnancy-related mortality. When gathering or analyzing data, we must take into account both severe maternal morbidity and pregnancy-associated mortality. By broadening this focus, we can gain a more comprehensive understanding of the community and, consequently, recognize and comprehend the obstacles to equitable maternal health.

It is imperative that we acknowledge the multifaceted factors that contribute to the injustices experienced by African American women nationwide, and in Massachusetts particularly. These comprise (but are not restricted to) unequal distribution of resources from governmental structures, implicit biases in the medical field, disparities in access to quality prenatal care, and structural and institutional racism. To improve maternal health across the state, community coalitions and organizers must push for more equitable practices, policies, and research.

A bill aimed at mitigating racial disparities in maternal health, for instance, was presented to the state legislature slightly more than one year ago and is anticipated to be passed later this year. To address these disparities, community-driven strategies will be the primary focus of its investigation into many of these intricate factors. Community coalitions can help see through and support the equitable implementation of the programs and resource allocations outlined in these bills, even though supporting legislation like this is crucial to achieving equity.

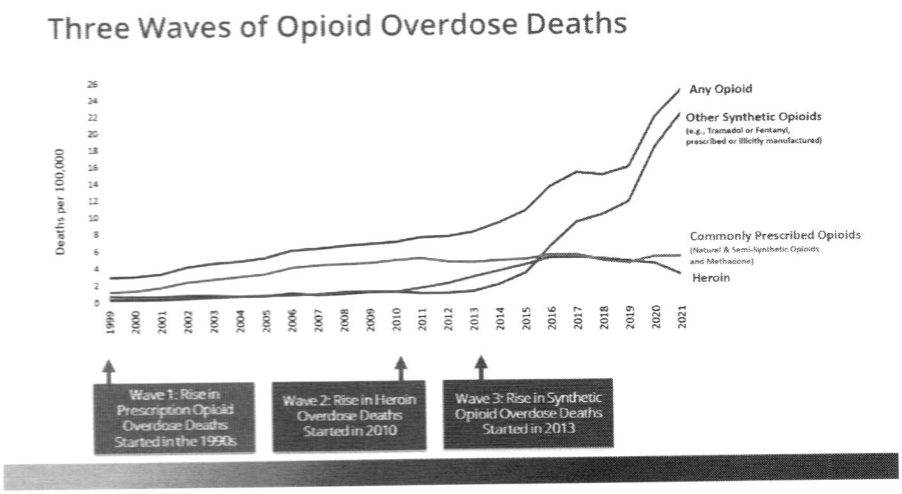

Source: *By en:Centers for Disease Control and Prevention. Understanding the Opioid Overdose Epidemic. See large image., Public Domain, https://commons.wikimedia.org/w/index.php?curid=134325455.*

It is crucial to take into account women who are addicted to substances when pursuing equitable maternity and child health. Despite having historically had a lower pregnancy-related death rate than the country as a whole, Massachusetts saw an alarming 33% increase in pregnancy-related deaths between 2012 and 2014. As a result, a committee known as the Massachusetts Maternal Mortality and Morbidity Review (MMMMR) was established to look into possible causes. They discovered that roughly 1 in 5 of the 199 pregnancy-related deaths in Massachusetts that took place between 2005 and 2014 had a substance abuse component. This is consistent with the rise in opioid overdose deaths that have occurred in Massachusetts over the same time period, as the state has seen a five-fold increase in opioid-related deaths in the last 20 years. The opioid crisis did not spare pregnant women; between 2011 and 2015, over one-third of deaths among women giving birth alive were related to fatal overdoses of opioids. One of the root causes of these disparities in maternal health is the widespread, particularly women. Community coalitions can address these issues by using advocacy, education, and awareness campaigns to fight stigma in their local communities. Racism and the stigma associated with substance-using women both contribute to severe health disparities, but they do so in different ways and shouldn't be viewed as interchangeable. But when it comes to maternal health, these problems can and do intersect, so coalitions must take intersectional approaches into account to address the health disparities they create.

Community coalitions can take steps to improve care for pregnant women with substance use disorders (SUD), even though the amount of data may seem overwhelming. The Massachusetts Perinatal Quality Collaborative's Maternal Opioid Use During Pregnancy Toolkit is one comprehensive attempt to address the disparity in maternal healthcare for women with SUD. This toolkit was created through a cooperative effort involving teams with a variety of disciplinary specialties. A wide range of resources are included in the toolkit itself to support and identify the unique treatment needs of SUD women during pregnancy and after giving birth. To address the special needs of pregnancy that are concurrent with SUD, it also highlights the significance of comprehensive care integration and cross-disciplinary partnerships in this work. Community coalitions should think about adopting a similar strategy and pushing for a more integrated model of care that deals with maternal health and SUD issues at the same time. Even though the differences in maternal health that black women and women with SUD face can seem overwhelming, it's important to keep in mind that changing policies and practices to be more equitable is a process and that even little steps taken in the community to address these disparities can have a big impact on one person's or one family's health.

Summary

- Maternal health refers to women's health during pregnancy, childbirth, and the postpartum period; each stage should be a positive experience, ensuring that mothers and their newborns realize their full health and well-being potential.
- Maternal and child health (MCH) is a global priority that has been continually discussed for many decades; it is one of the essential public health services.
- The revolution in health care involves the conflict between cost containment and quality of care. When health care became a profitable business industry, cost containment and managed care were born.
- Ensuring the well-being of mothers and children is paramount for the overall health and prosperity of any society. Numerous factors influence maternal and child health, ranging from access to healthcare services to socio-economic conditions and cultural practices.
- The philosophy of maternal and neonatal health revolves around the fundamental principle that every woman and newborn has the right to safe and dignified care during pregnancy, childbirth, and the postnatal period.
- The primary goal of maternal and child health care can be stated simply as the promotion and maintenance of optimal family health to ensure cycles of optimal childbearing and childrearing.
- Family is a fundamental social institution that plays a central role in shaping individuals' identities, values, and relationships. It serves as the primary unit for emotional support, socialization, and caregiving, providing a sense of belonging and security.
- Family-centered care refers to the collaborative partnership among the individual, family, and caregivers that exists to determine goals, share information, offer support, and formulate plans for health care.
- The importance a society places on human life can best be measured by the concern it places on its most vulnerable members—its elderly, disadvantaged, and youngest citizens.
- Evidence-based practice involves the use of research or controlled investigation of a problem in conjunction with clinical expertise as a foundation for action.
- Women's Health Issues (WHI) it is dedicated to improving the health and health care of all women throughout the lifespan and in diverse communities.
- Measuring maternal and child health is not as simple as defining a client as ill or well. Individual clients and health care practitioners may have different perspectives on illness and wellness.

References

1. Ahluwalia, I. B., et al. (2003). Who is breast-feeding? Recent trends from the Pregnancy Risk Assessment and Monitoring System. *Journal of Pediatrics, 142*(5), 486–491.
2. Callister, L. C. (2003). Toward evidence-based practice: U.S. trends in obstetric procedures, 1990–2000. *MCN: American Journal of Maternal/Child, 28*(1), 52.

3. Foster, J. (2004). Fatherhood and the meaning of children: An ethnographic study among Puerto Rican partners of adolescent mothers. *Journal of Midwifery and Women's Health, 49*(2), 118–125.

4. Hutchins VL. Maternal and Child Health Bureau: Roots. Pediatrics. 1994;94(5):695–699.

5. Kitchener, M., et al. (2005). Medicaid and community-based services: National program trends. *Health Affairs, 24*(1), 206–212.

6. Nelms, B. C. (2004). The joy of pediatrics: Working with children. *Journal of Pediatric Health Care, 18*(2), 55–56.

7. Oxtoby, K. (2003). Men in. *Times, 99*(32), 20–23.

8. Poole, J. H., & Long, J. (2004). Maternal mortality: A review of current trends. *Critical Care Clinics of North America, 16*(2), 227–230.

9. Porreco, R. P., et al. (2005). Expectation of pregnancy outcome among mature women. *American Journal of Obstetrics and Gynecology, 192*(1), 38–41.

10. Simpson, K. R., & Atterbury, J. (2003). Trends and issues in labor induction in the United States: Implications for clinical practice. *JOGNN: Journal of Obstetric, Gynecologic, and Neonatal, 32*(6), 767–779.

11. Turner, P. K. (2004). Mainstreaming alternative medicine: Doing midwifery at the intersection. *Qualitative Health Research, 14*(5), 644–662.

12. Weier, K. M., & Beal, M. W. (2004). Complementary therapies as adjuncts in the treatment of postpartum depression. *Journal of Midwifery and Women's Health, 49*(2), 96–104.

Chapter 2

ANATOMY AND PHYSIOLOGY OF PREGNANCY

Contents

Unit Introduction 48
2.1. Gravidity and Parity 50
2.2. Pregnancy Tests 51
2.3. Adaptations to Pregnancy 52
Summary 77
References 77

Unit Introduction

Significant physiologic and anatomical changes occur during pregnancy. All of the maternal physiological systems, in addition to the reproductive organs, adjust as necessary to support the growing fetus and preserve maternal homeostasis. All medical professionals who treat pregnant patients, including midwives, must have a solid understanding of these changes. An overview of the changes that occur in the reproductive organs, the impact of the main pregnancy hormones, fetal development, and maternal adaptations during pregnancy are given in this chapter.

A woman's body goes through a lot of changes during pregnancy to support the growth and development of the fetus. Pregnancy is a complicated physiological process. Pregnancy anatomy and physiology must be understood to guarantee the best possible outcomes for the health of the mother and the unborn child. Pregnancy starts with fertilization, which is the process by which a sperm enters an egg and forms a zygote. After going through several divisions, the zygote becomes a blastocyst, which implants itself into the uterine lining 6 to 12 days after fertilization. Human chorionic gonadotropin (hCG), which supports the corpus luteum in the ovary and aids in maintaining the pregnancy, is released in response to this implantation.

The mother's body undergoes a number of anatomical and physiological changes as the pregnancy goes on to make room for the developing fetus. For example, the uterus enlarges significantly to make room for the growing fetus. The proliferation of uterine muscle cells and the stretching of the uterine wall contribute to this enlargement. The cervix also changes, getting softer and more elastic in preparation for giving birth.

Pregnancy is a critical time for hormonal changes. During pregnancy, the placenta, a temporary organ, develops and secretes hormones including relaxin, progesterone, and estrogen. These hormones control a number of physiological functions, such as the fetus's growth and development, the maintenance of the uterine lining, and the relaxation of pelvic ligaments in before childbirth. The cardiovascular system also modifies itself to accommodate the heightened demands of gestation. To provide the growing fetus with oxygen and nutrients, there is a significant increase in blood volume and cardiac output. Hormonal shifts, especially an increase in progesterone and estrogen, lower blood pressure and cause vasodilation, which improves blood flow to the placenta and uterus.

Pregnancy also affects the respiratory system. Some pregnant women experience dyspnea due to the diaphragm being elevated by the expanding uterus. This is particularly common in the later stages of pregnancy when lung capacity is reduced. Hyperventilation and respiratory alkalosis are caused by hormonal changes, such as elevated progesterone levels, which activate the brain's respiratory center. To support the developing fetus and get ready for delivery, the musculoskeletal system also changes. The placenta secretes the hormone relaxin, which relaxes pelvic ligaments and joints to facilitate the baby's easier passage during childbirth. On the other hand, musculoskeletal pain and an elevated risk of injury can also result from this increased joint laxity. The mother's body undergoes numerous anatomical and physiological changes during pregnancy to support the fetus's growth and development. To ensure the health and well-being of mother and child, as well as to provide the best prenatal care possible, it is imperative to comprehend these changes.

Orientation and Directional Terms

Term	Definition	Illustration
Reproductive system	The reproductive system of an organism, also known as the genital system, is the biological system made up of all the anatomical organs involved in sexual reproduction.	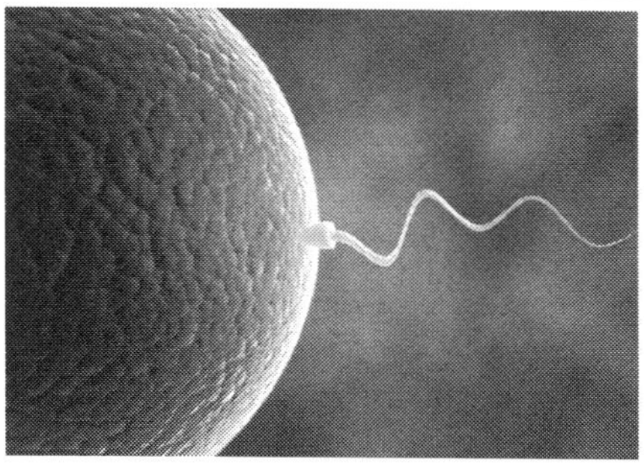
Pregnancy	Pregnancy is the period when a fertilized egg develops in a woman's uterus, from conception to birth.	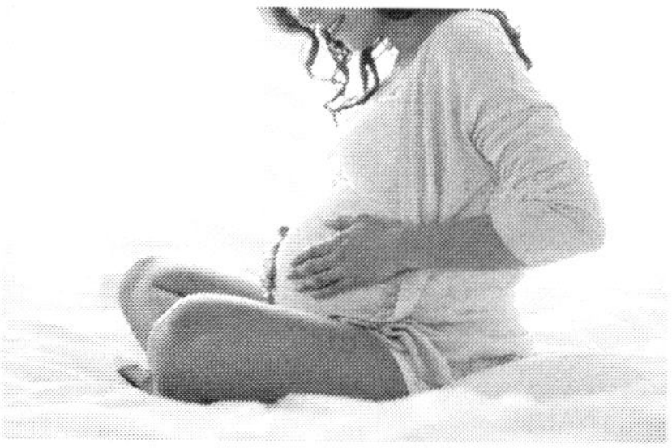
Human chorionic gonadotropin	Human chorionic gonadotropin (hCG) is a hormone that plays a key role in pregnancy and can also be used to diagnose some cancers.	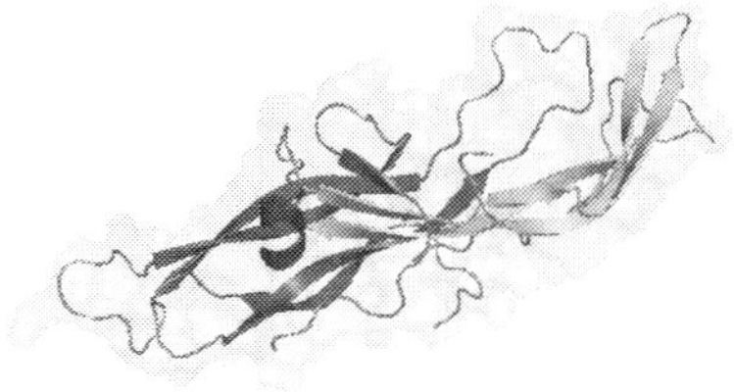
Cardiovascular system	The **cardiovascular system**, is a system of organs that delivers oxygen, nutrients, hormones, and other substances to the body's cells and organs.	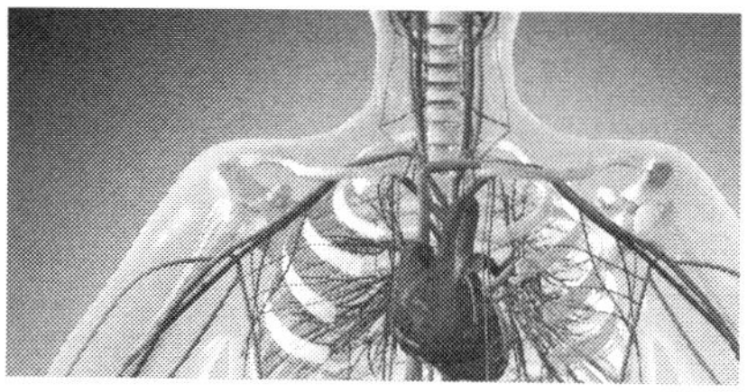
Dyspnea	Dyspnea is the medical term for shortness of breath, which is an uncomfortable feeling of difficulty breathing.	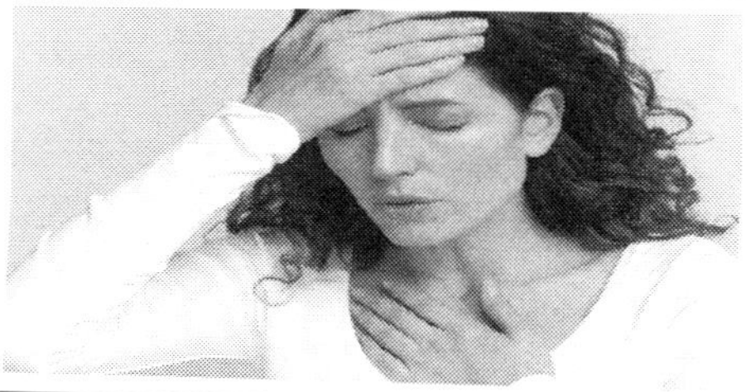

2.1. Gravidity and Parity

An understanding of the following terms used to describe pregnancy and the pregnant woman is essential to the study of maternity care:

- **Gravida:** A woman who is pregnant.
- **Gravidity:** Pregnancy.
- **Multigravida:** A woman who has had two or more pregnancies.
- **Multipara:** A woman who has completed two or more pregnancies to the stage of fetal viability.
- **Nulligravida:** A woman who has never been pregnant.
- **Nullipara:** A woman who has not completed a pregnancy with a fetus or fetuses who have reached the stage of fetal viability.
- **Parity:** The number of pregnancies in which the fetus or fetuses have reached viability when they are born, not the number of fetuses (e.g., twins) born. Whether the fetus is born alive or is stillborn (a fetus who shows no signs of life at birth) after viability is reached does not affect parity.
- **Postdate or Postterm:** A pregnancy that goes beyond 42 weeks of gestation.
- **Preterm:** A pregnancy that has reached 20 weeks of gestation but before completion of 37 weeks of gestation.
- **Primigravida:** A woman who is pregnant for the first time.
- **Primipara:** A woman who has completed one pregnancy with a fetus or fetuses who have reached the stage of fetal viability.
- **Term:** A pregnancy from the beginning of week 38 of gestation to the end of week 42 of gestation.
- **Viability:** Capacity to live outside the uterus; about 22 to 24 weeks since last menstrual period, or fetal weight greater than 500 g.

Information about gravidity and parity is gathered during history-taking interviews and can be entered into patient records in several ways. Using two numbers to represent gravidity and parity is one method. For instance, 1/0 indicates that a woman is conceiving her first child and has not yet brought her pregnancy to term. Another method that's frequently employed in maternity centers has five numbers that are divided by hyphens.

Additional precise parity information is provided by this system. The total number of pregnancies, including the current one (gravidity), is represented by the first digit; the total number of term births is represented by the second; the number of preterm births is indicated by the third; the number of abortions (miscarriages or elective terminations of pregnancy before viability) is represented by the fourth; and the number of children who are currently alive is represented by the fifth. For easier memory retention, the acronym GTPAL (gravidity, term, preterm, abortions, living children) can be used. For example, if a woman pregnant only once gives birth at week 34 and the infant survives, the abbreviation that represents this information is "1-0-1-0-1." During her next pregnancy, the abbreviation is "2-0-1-0-1." Additional examples are given in Table 2.1.

Table 2.1. *Effect of Pregnancy on Endocrine Function Tests [5]*

Hormone	Test	Result
FSH, LH	GnRH stimulation	Unresponsive from third gestation until several weeks postpartum.
Growth hormone	Insulin tolerance test	Response increases during first half of pregnancy and then normalizes until several weeks postpartum.
TSH	TRH stimulation	Response unchanged.
Pancreatic insulin	Glucose tolerance test	Peak glucose increases, and glucose concentration remains elevated for longer.
Adrenal cortisol	ACTH infusion	Exaggerated cortisol and aldosterone responses.
–	Metyrapone	Diminished response.
Mineralocorticoids	ACTH infusion	No deoxycorticosterone response.
–	Dexamethasone	No deoxycorticosterone response.

Source: https://en.wikipedia.org/wiki/Maternal_physiological_changes_in_pregnancy.

2.2. Pregnancy Tests

Early pregnancy detection enables early treatment to begin. The first biochemical indicator of pregnancy is human chorionic gonadotropin (hCG), and tests for pregnancy rely on detecting either the hCG or its beta (β) subunit. Beginning on the day of implantation, β-hCG production can be detected as early as 7 to 10 days after conception. The amount of hCG rises until it reaches a peak at roughly 60 to 70 days of gestation, after which it starts to fall until roughly 80 days into the pregnancy. It stays constant for around 30 weeks after which it progressively rises until term. Elevated hCG levels above normal can be a sign of ectopic pregnancy, aberrant gestation e.g., an unusually slow rise or fall in hCG levels may portend an imminent miscarriage, such as in the case of a fetus with Down syndrome or multiple gestations.

Pregnancy tests using serum and urine are conducted in clinics, offices, women's health centers, and lab settings. Urine tests can also be conducted at home. Tests on serum and urine can yield precise findings. For serum testing, a 7–10 ml venous blood sample is taken. Because first-voided morning urine has hCG levels that are similar to those in serum, it is typically required for urine tests. Urine samples drawn at random typically have lower levels. Compared to serum tests, urine tests are more affordable and yield results faster.

There are numerous pregnancy test options available. When using a test, the nurse should follow the instructions provided by the manufacturer. Pregnancy tests that measure the beta subunit of hCG in serum or urine samples using radioactive methods are called radioimmunoassay (RIA) tests. When using a test, the nurse should follow the instructions provided by the manufacturer. Pregnancy tests for the beta subunit of hCG in serum or urine samples are called radioimmunoassay (RIA) tests.

A serum test called the radioreceptor assay (RRA) gauges a blood sample's capacity to prevent radiolabeled hCG from binding to receptors. In the first six to eight days following conception, the test has an accuracy of 90% to 95%. The most widely used pregnancy test is the enzyme-linked immunosorbent assay (ELISA). It binds with hCG in urine by using a particular monoclonal antibody (anti-hCG) combined with enzymes. As early as seven days after conception, levels of hCG as low as 25 milli-international units/ml can be found, depending on the particular test. It takes less than five minutes to complete and can be done at home or in an office. A simple color change reaction indicates a positive test result. The majority of over-the-counter home pregnancy tests are based on ELISA technology. The woman typically applies urine to a strip for these one-step tests, and then reads the results. Instructions for gathering the specimen, conducting the test, and interpreting the findings are included with the test kits. Users can contact the toll-free number provided by the majority of kit manufacturers with any questions or concerns they may have regarding test procedures or results. When taking home pregnancy tests, the most frequent mistake is taking the test too early in the pregnancy.

Pregnancy test results must be interpreted with some discretion. The woman's medical history must be taken into account along with the type of pregnancy test and its level of sensitivity (ability to detect low levels of a substance) and specificity (ability to discern the absence of a substance). This contains the time of her most recent normal menstrual period (LNMP), the length of her typical cycle, and the outcomes of any prior pregnancy tests. It is critical to ascertain the woman's drug history and whether she abuses substances because certain drugs, like promethazine and diuretics, can produce false-negative results while anticonvulsants and tranquilizers can produce false-positive results. False results can also be caused by hormone-producing tumors, improper specimen collection, and laboratory mistakes. In cases where there is uncertainty, additional assessment or retesting may be necessary.

2.3. Adaptations to Pregnancy

The hormones associated with pregnancy and the mechanical pressures resulting from the growing uterus and other tissues are thought to be responsible for maternal physiologic adaptations. These adjustments safeguard the woman's regular physiological processes, fulfill the metabolic needs of pregnancy, and create a supportive environment for the growth and development of the fetus. Pregnancy is a normal phenomenon, but issues can arise.

2.3.1. Signs of Pregnancy

Some of the physiologic adaptations are recognized as signs and symptoms of pregnancy. Three commonly used categories of signs and symptoms of pregnancy are presumptive (those changes felt by the woman—e.g., amenorrhea, fatigue, nausea and vomiting, breast changes); probable (those changes observed by an examiner—e.g., Hegar sign, ballottement, pregnancy tests); and positive (those signs that are attributable only to the presence of the fetus—e.g., hearing fetal heart tones, visualization of the fetus, and palpating fetal movements). Table 2.2 summarizes these signs of pregnancy in relation to when they might occur and other causes for their occurrence.

Table 2.2. *Signs of Pregnancy*

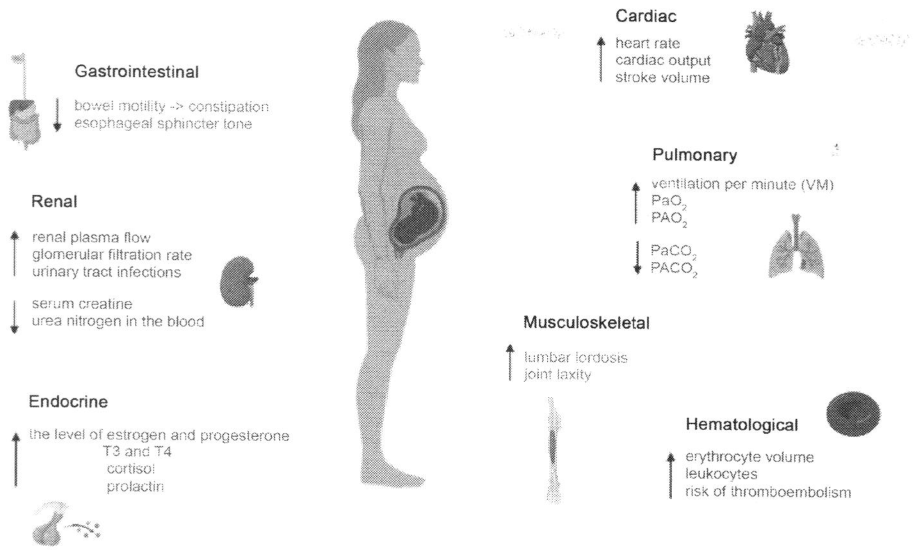

TIME OF OCCURRENCE (GESTATIONAL AGE)	SIGN	OTHER POSSIBLE CAUSE
PRESUMPTIVE SIGNS		
3-4 wk	Breast changes	Premenstrual changes, oral contraceptives
4 wk	Amenorrhea	Stress, vigorous exercise, early menopause, endocrine problems, malnutrition
4-14 wk	Nausea, vomiting	Gastrointestinal virus, food poisoning
6-12 wk	Urinary frequency	Infection, pelvic tumors
12 wk	Fatigue	Stress, illness
16-20 wk	Quickening	Gas, peristalsis
PROBABLE SIGNS		
5 wk	Goodell sign	Pelvic congestion
6-8 wk	Chadwick sign	Pelvic congestion
6-12 wk	Hegar sign	Pelvic congestion
4-12 wk	Positive result of pregnancy test (serum)	Hydatidiform mole, choriocarcinoma
6-12 wk	Positive result of pregnancy test (urine)	False-positive results may be caused by pelvic infection, tumors
16 wk	Braxton Hicks contractions	Myomas, other tumors
16-28 wk	Ballottement	Tumors, cervical polyps
POSITIVE SIGNS		
5-6 wk	Visualization of fetus by real-time ultrasound examination	No other causes
6 wk	Fetal heart tones detected by ultrasound examination	No other causes
16 wk	Visualization of fetus by radiographic study	No other causes
8-17 wk	Fetal heart tones detected by Doppler ultrasound stethoscope	No other causes
17-19 wk	Fetal heart tones detected by fetal stethoscope	No other causes
19-22 wk	Fetal movements palpated	No other causes
Late pregnancy	Fetal movements visible	No other causes

Source: *Fiat, F., Merghes, P. E., Scurtu, A. D., Almajan, G. B., Dehelean, C. A., Varan, N., & Bernad, E., (2022). The main changes in pregnancy—therapeutic approach to musculoskeletal pain. Medicina, 58(8), 1115. https://doi.org/10.3390/medicina58081115.*

2.3.2. Reproductive System and Breasts

2.3.2.1. Uterus

2.3.2.1.1. Changes in Size, Shape, and Position

Elevated levels of progesterone and estrogen during the first trimester stimulate the amazing growth of the uterus. Increased vascularity and blood vessel dilatation, hyperplasia (the creation of new muscle fibers and fibroelastic tissue), hypertrophy (the enlargement of preexisting muscle fibers and fibroelastic tissue), and decidua development all contribute to early uterine enlargement. The uterus reaches its largest size of a large hen's egg at 7 weeks of gestation, doubles in size to that of an orange at 10 weeks, and reaches its largest size of a grapefruit at 12 weeks. Uterine enlargement beyond the third month is mostly caused by the growing fetus's mechanical pressure.

The uterus changes position and shape as it grows larger. The uterus resembles an upside-down pear at conception. The uterus becomes spherical or globular during the second trimester as the muscular walls thicken and become more elastic. Subsequently, the uterus grows larger and more ovoid as the fetus lengthens, emerging from the pelvis into the abdominal cavity.

After the 14th week, the pregnancy may "show," though this largely relies on the height and weight of the woman. When there is good abdominal muscle tone in the nullipara, abdominal enlargement might be less noticeable (Figure 2.1). The kind and extent of abdominal enlargement are also influenced by posture. The uterus grows during a normal pregnancy at a steady pace. Between the twelfth and 14th weeks of pregnancy, the uterus can be palpated above the symphysis pubis as it grows (Figure 2.2). At 22 to 24 weeks of gestation, the uterus rises gradually to the level of the umbilicus, and at term, it almost reaches the xiphoid process. Fundal height decreases between weeks 38 and 40 when the fetus starts to descend and engage in the pelvis (lightening) (*see* Figure 2.2, dashed line). Typically, lightening happens in the multipara at the beginning of labor and in the nullipara approximately two weeks prior to the onset of labor.

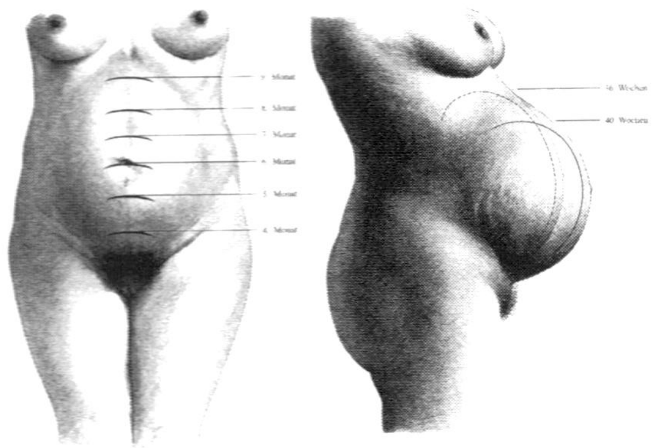

Figure 2.1. *Changes in pregnancy.*

Source: By Ernst Bumm and Albrecht Mayer – Grundriss zum Studium der Geburtshülfe 1902, Public Domain, https://commons.wikimedia.org/w/index.php?curid=30131762.

Fundal height, a measurement frequently used to estimate the length of pregnancy, is used to determine uterine enlargement. However, the accuracy of this estimation of the length of pregnancy can be affected by variations in the position of the fundus or the fetus, variations in the amount of amniotic fluid present, the presence of multiple fetuses, maternal obesity, and variations in examiner techniques.

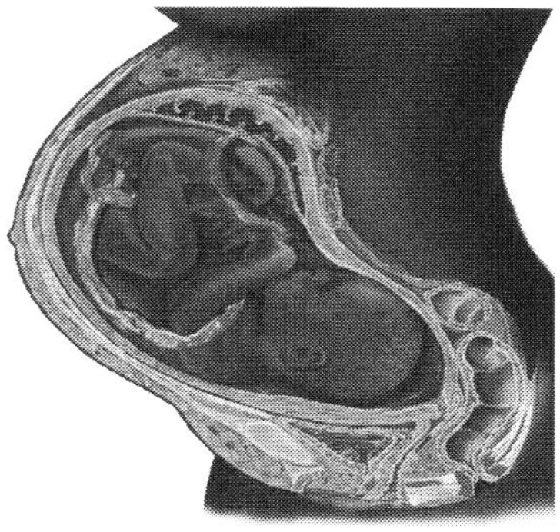

Figure 2.2. *Gestation.*

Source: By Chidiebere Ibe – https://twitter.com/ebereillustrate/status/1463552384702070799, CC BY-SA 4.0, https://commons.wikimedia.org/w/index.php?curid=113041281.

Because of the rectosigmoid colon on the left side, the uterus normally rotates to the right as it elevates, but the uterus remains in the midline due to the extensive hypertrophy (enlargement) of the round ligaments. The intestines eventually shift to either side of the abdomen as the expanding uterus touches the anterior abdominal wall (Figure 2.3). A pregnant woman's center of gravity is shifted because, when she stands, the majority of her uterus presses up against the anterior abdominal wall.

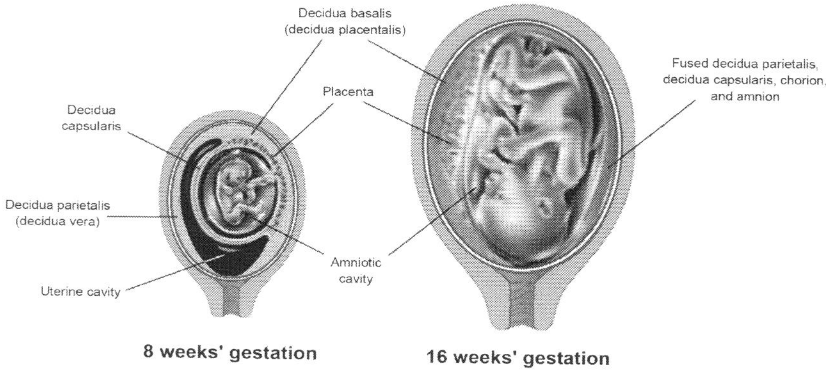

Figure 2.3. *Displacement of internal abdominal structures and diaphragm by the enlarging uterus at 4, 6, and 9 months of gestation.*

Source: *Ng, S. W., Norwitz, G. A., Pavlicev, M., Tilburgs, T., Simón, C., & Norwitz, E. R., (2020). Endometrial decidualization: The primary driver of pregnancy health. International Journal of Molecular Sciences, 21(11), 4092. https://doi.org/10.3390/ijms21114092.*

The lower uterine segment, or uterine isthmus, begins to soften and compress at around 6 weeks of gestation (Hegar sign) (Figure 2.4). Uterine anteflexion becomes excessive during the first trimester of pregnancy as a result of this. The woman experiences frequent urination as a result of the uterine fundus pressing on the bladder.

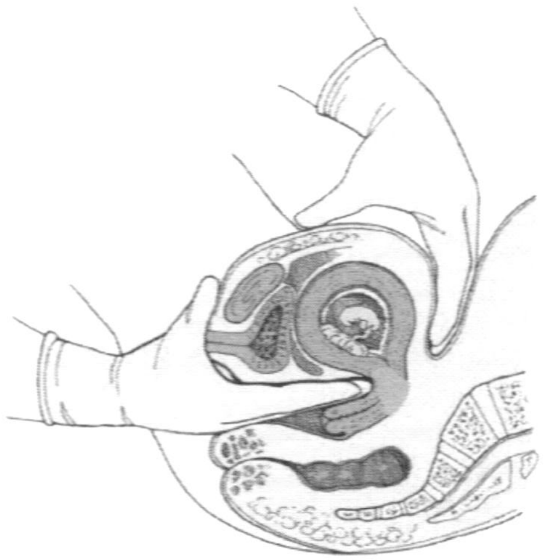

Figure 2.4. *Hegar sign. Bimanual examination for assessing compressibility and softening of the isthmus (lower uterine segment) while the cervix is still firm.*

Source: https://d3i71xaburhd42.cloudfront.net/349bfb309526ddbd7a73395e456b020f8283c469/8-Figure8-4-1.png.

2.3.2.1.2. Changes in Contractility

The abdominal wall begins to feel the force of uterine contractions shortly after the fourth month of pregnancy. The Braxton Hicks sign is the name given to these contractions. Throughout pregnancy, irregular, painless Braxton Hicks contractions happen sporadically. These contractions increase the amount of oxygen that reaches the fetus by facilitating the flow of uterine blood through the placenta's intervillous spaces. Some women find Braxton Hicks contractions annoying, despite the fact that they are not painful. These contractions become much more definite after the 28th week, but they usually stop when you walk or exercise. Although Braxton Hicks contractions don't increase in frequency or intensity or cause cervical dilation, they can be mistaken for actual labor.

2.3.2.1.3. Uteroplacental Blood Flow

The flow of blood from the mother to the uterus is necessary for placental perfusion. As the uterus gets bigger, blood flow increases quickly. The fetoplacental unit grows faster than the uterine blood flow, which increases 20-fold when this occurs. Consequently, in the later stages of pregnancy, more oxygen is drawn from the uterine blood. One-sixth of the mother's total blood volume is contained in the uterine vascular system during a typical term pregnancy. The average blood flow rate through the uterus is 500 ml/min, and the gravid uterus uses more oxygen to meet the needs of the growing fetus.

Three things that are known to reduce blood flow in women are low maternal arterial pressure, uterine contractions, and the supine position. Uterine blood flow may rise in response to estrogen stimulation. Uterine blood flow velocity can be measured with Doppler ultrasound examination, particularly in pregnancies at risk due to conditions like diabetes mellitus, intrauterine growth restriction, hypertension, and multiple gestations that are linked to decreased placental perfusion. The uterine souffle, which is the sound produced by blood in the uterine arteries that is synchronous with the mother's pulse, or the funic souffle, which is the sound produced by blood rushing through the umbilical vessels and synchronous with the fetal heart rate, can be heard by the healthcare provider using an ultrasound device or a fetal stethoscope.

2.3.2.1.4. Cervical Changes

About the start of the sixth week in a normal, unscarred cervix, a softening of the cervical tip known as the Goodell sign may be seen. The muscle and its collagen-rich connective tissue, which becomes loose, edematous, highly elastic, and increased in volume, are the causes of this sign, which is accompanied by increased vascularity, mild hypertrophy, and hyperplasia (increase in number of cells). Pregnancy gives the cervix its velvety appearance because the glands near the external ostium multiply beneath the stratified squamous epithelium. Increased friability can result in mild bleeding following deep penetration coitus or vaginal examination. The squamocolumnar junction, which is where cells are taken for cervical cancer screening, may also be farther from the cervix as a result of pregnancy. Evaluation of abnormal Papanicolaou (Pap) tests during pregnancy can be challenging due to all these changes. It is crucial to conduct a thorough examination of every expectant mother, though, as approximately 3% of cervical cancer cases are discovered during pregnancy.

The nullipara's cervix is rounded. Cervical lacerations practically invariably happen during childbirth. However, following childbirth, the cervix becomes more oval in the horizontal plane, with or without lacerations, and the external ostium appears as a transverse slit.

2.3.2.1.5. Changes Related to the Presence of the Fetus

Ballottement, or the passive movement of an unengaged fetus, is typically visible between weeks 16 and 18. Ballottement is a method of gently bouncing a floating structure and feeling its rebound to palpate it. When the examiner uses the palpation technique, the fetus rises to the surface of the vagina when the finger is gently tapped upward. A light tap on the finger is then felt as the fetus descends (Figure 2.5).

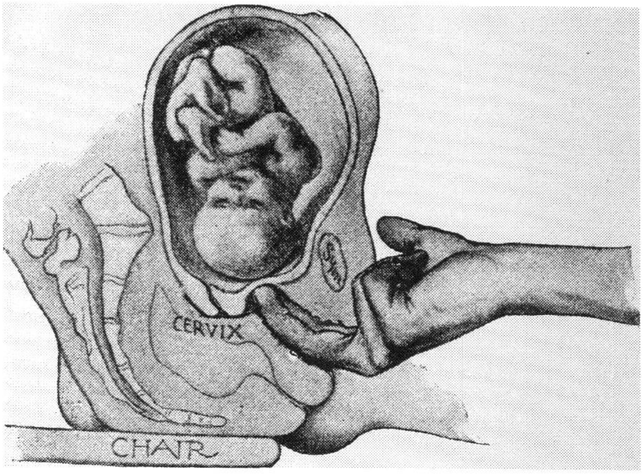

Figure 2.5. *Internal ballottement (18 weeks).*

Source: https://commons.wikimedia.org/wiki/File:The_diagnosis_of_diseases_of_women_%281905%29_%2814576778787%29.jpg.

A multiparous woman may notice her first fetal movements, or "feeling life," as early as the 14th or 16th week. These feelings might not become apparent to the nulliparous woman until the 18th week or later. Quickening is often characterized as a flutter and can be challenging to differentiate from peristalsis. Fetal movements progressively become more frequent and intense. The week that quickening takes place offers a rough indication for estimating the length of gestation.

2.3.2.2. Vagina and Vulva

Pregnancy hormones cause the vaginal mucosa to thicken, the connective tissue to loosen, the smooth muscle to hypertrophy, and the vaginal vault to lengthen, preparing the vagina for stretching during labor and delivery. The cervix and vaginal mucosa have a violet-bluish tint due to increased vascularity. Known as the Chadwick sign, the deepened color can be seen as early as the sixth week of pregnancy, but it is most noticeable by the eighth week.

A white or slightly gray mucoid discharge with a slight musty odor is known as leukorrhea. This abundant mucous fluid is a result of progesterone and estrogen stimulating the cervical cavity. Due to the hyperplasia of a typical pregnancy, there are a lot of exfoliated vaginal epithelial cells present, which is why the fluid is whitish. There is never any itching or bloodstaining from this vaginal discharge. Ferning typically does not occur in a dried cervical mucus smear due to the progesterone effect, unlike in an amniotic fluid smear. Rather, the dried mucus forms a pattern resembling beads or cells crystallizing. As a result of the mucus filling the endocervical canal, the mucous plug (operculum) forms (Figure 2.6). During pregnancy, the operculum functions as a barrier against bacterial invasion.

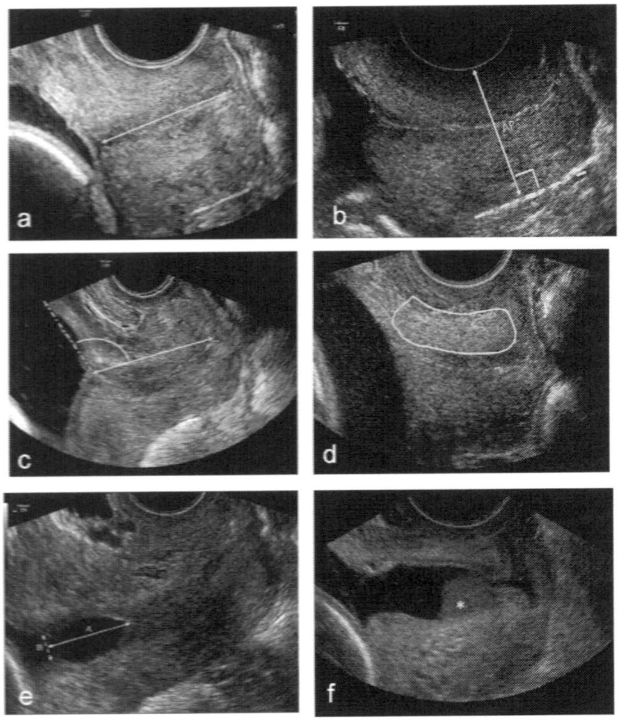

Figure 2.6. *Cervix during pregnancy.*

Source: *van der Merwe, J., Couck, I., Russo, F., Burgos-Artizzu, X. P., Deprest, J., Palacio, M., & Lewi, L., (2020). The predictive value of the cervical consistency index to predict spontaneous preterm birth in asymptomatic twin pregnancies at the second-trimester ultrasound scan: A prospective cohort study. Journal of Clinical Medicine, 9(6), 1784. https://doi.org/10.3390/jcm9061784.*

The pH of vaginal secretions increases (from approximately 3 to 6 [normal 4 to 7]) during pregnancy due to increased lactic acid production from *Lactobacillus acidophilus* action on glycogen in the vaginal epithelium, which is likely caused by elevated estrogen levels. Although the pregnant woman is better protected from some organisms by this acidic environment, she is more susceptible to other infections, particularly yeast infections because *Candida albicans* thrives in an environment rich in glycogen.

Sensitivity rises significantly as a result of the increased vascularity of the vagina and other pelvic viscera. A high level of sexual interest and arousal may result from the increased sensitivity, particularly in the second trimester of pregnancy. Edema and vulva varicosities may arise from the increased congestion, the relaxed blood vessel walls, and the heavy uterus. Usually, the varicosities and edema go away in the postpartum phase.

External structures of the perineum are enlarged during pregnancy because of an increase in vasculature, hypertrophy of the perineal body, and deposition of fat (Figure 2.7).

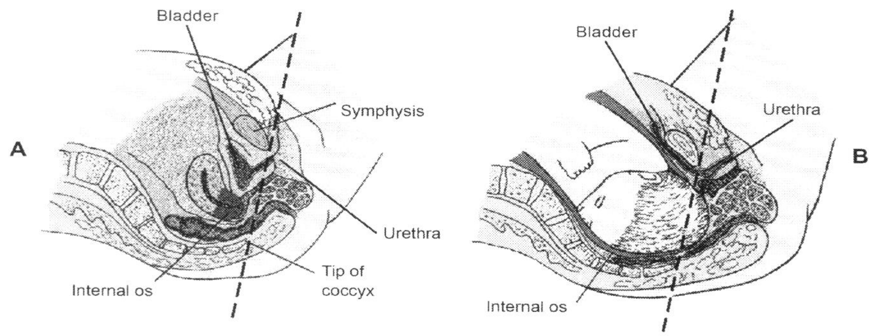

Figure 2.7. *(A) Pelvic floor in nonpregnant woman. (B) Pelvic floor at end of pregnancy. Note marked hypertrophy and hyperplasia below dotted line joining tip of coccyx and inferior margin of symphysis. Note elongation of bladder and urethra as a result of compression. Fat deposits are increased.*

Source: https://d3i71xaburhd42.cloudfront.net/349bfb309526ddbd7a73395e456b020f8283c469/9-Figure8-7-1.png.

The nullipara's labia majora approximate and conceal the vaginal introitus, whereas the parous woman's labia separate and gape following childbirth and vaginal or perineal trauma. (Figure 2.1) contrasts the nullipara and multipara's perineum with respect to the cervix, vulva, and pregnant abdomen.

2.3.2.3. Breasts

Early in the pregnancy, elevated levels of progesterone and estrogen cause the breasts to become fuller, more sensitive, tingly, and heavy. Breast sensitivity can range from a slight tingling sensation to intense pain. The pigmentation of the nipples and areolae increases, the nipples become more erectile, and secondary pinkish areolae form and extend beyond the primary areolae. Around the nipples, there may be hypertrophy of the sebaceous (oil) glands embedded in the primary areolae, which are known as Montgomery tubercles. These sebaceous glands may provide protection by maintaining the lubrication of the nipples during nursing.

The blood vessels beneath the skin enlarge due to the richer blood supply. The blood vessels, which were previously hardly perceptible, become apparent and frequently form an intricate blue network beneath the skin's surface. In primigravidas, venous congestion in the breasts is more noticeable. Striae gravidarum can show up on the breasts' external surfaces. Breast enlargement occurs gradually during the second and third trimesters, which is caused by the growth of the mammary glands. Pregnancy-related high levels of luteal and placental hormones stimulate the growth of the lobule-alveolar tissue and lactiferous ducts, resulting in a widespread, coarse nodule when the breasts are palpated. The tissue gets softer and looser as a result of glandular tissue dislodging connective tissue.

Lactation is not permitted until after the birth, even though the mammary glands have fully developed by midpregnancy. This is due to a drop in estrogen levels. By the third month of pregnancy, a thin, transparent, viscous secretory material called precolostrum is visible in the acini cells. As early as 16 weeks of gestation, the nipples may release the creamy, white to yellowish to orange premilk fluid known as colostrum.

2.3.3. General Body Systems

2.3.3.1. Cardiovascular System

Pregnancy causes significant anatomical and physiological changes in the cardiovascular system in mothers. Cardiovascular adaptations safeguard the woman's regular physiological processes, fulfill the metabolic demands placed on her body during pregnancy, and attend to the growth and development of the fetus. Due to the increased cardiac output and blood volume, there is likely some secondary cardiac hypertrophy. After delivery, the heart reverts to its original size. The expanding uterus causes the diaphragm to be displaced upward, elevating the heart and rotating it forward to the left (Figure 2.8). The apical impulse, a point of maximal intensity (PMI), is shifted upward and laterally about 1 to 1.5 cm. The degree of shift depends on the duration of pregnancy and the size and position of the uterus.

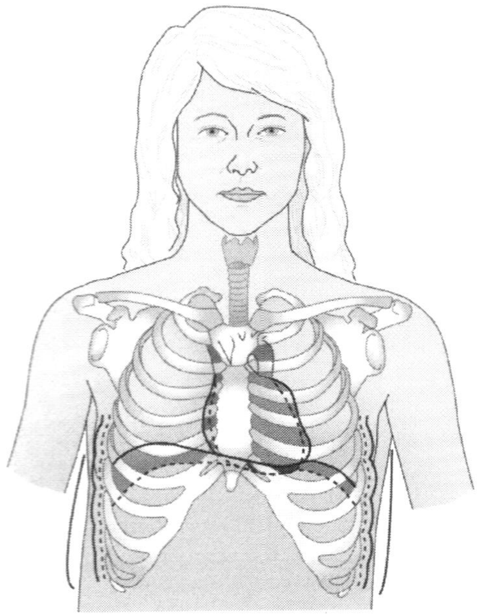

Figure 2.8. *Changes in position of heart, lungs, and thoracic cage in pregnancy. Broken line, nonpregnant; solid line, change that occurs in pregnancy.*

Source: https://d3i71xaburhd42.cloudfront.net/349bfb309526ddbd7a73395e456b020f8283c469/10-Figure8-8-1.png.

Auscultatory changes that are common during pregnancy are caused by changes in the size and position of the heart as well as increases in blood volume and cardiac output. After 20 weeks of gestation, S3 can be clearly heard, and S1 and S2 are more audibly split. Moreover, murmurs in the systolic and diastolic phases can be perceived over the pulmonic region.

These are temporary, going away soon after the woman gives birth. The pulse increases by 10 to 15 beats per minute between weeks 14 and 20 of pregnancy, and it continues to do so until term. Palpitations could happen. The mother's heart rate rises dramatically during the third trimester of a twin pregnancy. There could be an irregular heartbeat.

Premature ventricular systole, premature atrial contractions, and sinus arrhythmia are possible symptoms for the expectant mother. Therapy is not necessary for a healthy woman who has no underlying heart disease, but pregnant women who already have a heart condition will require close obstetric and medical supervision.

2.3.3.1.1. Blood Pressure

The following factors influence arterial blood pressure (brachial artery): age, activity level, health issues, and circadian rhythm. Pregnancy requires the consideration of additional factors. These variables include the size and kind of the blood pressure device, the mother's posture, and her level of anxiety. Anxiety in mothers can improve readings. The woman is given time to rest and the reading is repeated if an elevated reading is discovered.

The position of the mother influences readings. With the exception of some women who experience supine hypotensive syndrome, a woman's brachial blood pressure is highest when she is sitting, lowest when she is lying in the lateral recumbent position, and intermediate when she is supine. For this reason, the woman should be in the same position and use the same arm to get the reading at every prenatal visit. Recording the reading and the arm used should go hand in hand.

A correctly sized cuff is a must for accurate readings. The cuff should be 20% wider than the arm's diameter when wrapped around an average-sized person, or roughly 12 to 14 cm, and 18 to 20 cm for an obese person. When a cuff is too small, it produces a false high reading and when it is too large, a false low reading occurs. Additionally, there may be differences between auscultatory and oscillatory blood pressure readings, so caution should be used when comparing them. While it may slightly drop as pregnancy progresses, systolic blood pressure typically stays constant with prepregnancy levels. In the first trimester, diastolic blood pressure starts to fall; it keeps going down until 24 to 32 weeks; after that, it gradually rises and reaches prepregnancy levels by term.

Calculating the mean arterial pressure (MAP) (mean of the blood pressure in the arterial circulation) can increase the diagnostic value of the findings. Normal MAP readings in the nonpregnant woman are 86.4 mm Hg ± 7.5 mm Hg. MAP readings for a pregnant woman are slightly higher. One way to calculate a MAP is illustrated in Box 1.

Box 2.1. Calculation of mean arterial pressure

Blood pressure: 106/70 mm Hg

Formula: $$\frac{(\text{systolic}) + 2(\text{diastolic})}{3}$$

$$\frac{(106) + 2(70)}{3}$$

$$\frac{106 + 140}{3}$$

$$246/3 = 82 \text{ mm Hg}$$

The version of the MAP equation multiplying 0.412 by pulse pressure and adding diastolic blood. All women who lie flat on their backs during the second half of pregnancy experience some degree of vena cava compression. Some women see a drop in systolic blood pressure of over 30 millimeters of mercury. The woman experiences a half reduction in cardiac output, reflex bradycardia, and fainting after 4 to 5 minutes. We call this syndrome supine hypotensive syndrome. Increased venous pressure and decreased blood flow in the legs result from the uterus compressing the iliac veins and inferior vena cava (unless the woman is in the lateral position). These changes play a role in the development of hemorrhoids, varicose veins in the vulva and legs, and dependent edema in the later stages of term pregnancy (Figure 2.9).

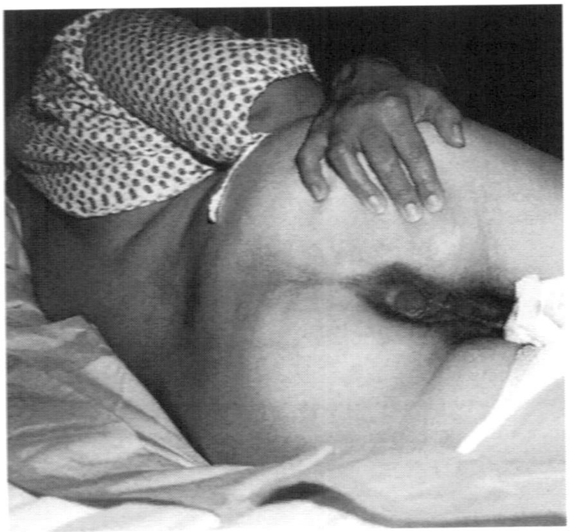

Figure 2.9. *Hemorrhoids.*

Source: https://d3i71xaburhd42.cloudfront.net/349bfb309526ddbd7a73395e456b020f8283c469/11-Figure8-9-1.png.

2.3.3.1.2. Blood Volume and Composition

There are wide variations in the amount of blood volume expansion. About 1500 ml, or 40–45%, more blood is produced than there would be without pregnancy. This increase is made up of 450 ml of red blood cells (RBCs) and 1000 ml of plasma. Around the tenth or twelfth week, the blood volume begins to rise, peaks between the 32nd and 34th week, and then somewhat declines at the 40-first week. When there are multiple gestations, the volume increases more than when there is only one fetus. Volume increase serves as a defense mechanism. It is necessary to supply the blood volume required by the enlarged uterus's hypertrophied vascular system, to sufficiently hydrate the tissues of the fetus and the mother when she is in an erect or supine position, and to provide a fluid reserve to make up for blood lost during childbirth and the puerperium. Despite the increased blood volume during pregnancy, peripheral vasodilation keeps blood pressure within normal limits.

During pregnancy there is an accelerated production of RBCs (normal, 4.2 to 5.4 million/mm^3). The percentage of increase depends on the amount of iron available. The RBC mass increases by about 20% to 30%.

Normal hemoglobin levels (12 to 16 g/dl blood) and hematocrit levels (37 to 47%) are declining because the increase in plasma outpaces the increase in RBC production. Physiologic anemia is the term used to describe this hemodilution state. Since the rapid expansion of blood volume occurs during the second trimester, when RBC production is slower, the decrease is more apparent during this time. The woman is deemed anemic if her hemoglobin level falls to 10 g/dl or less, or if her hematocrit falls to 35% or less. During the second trimester, the total white cell count rises and peaks in the third trimester. The granulocyte count is the main source of this increase, while the lymphocyte count remains relatively constant during pregnancy. See Table 2.3 for laboratory values during pregnancy.

Table 2.3. *Laboratory Values for Pregnant and Nonpregnant Women*

VALUES	NONPREGNANT	PREGNANT
HEMATOLOGIC		
Complete Blood Count (CBC)		
Hemoglobin, g/dl	12-16*	>11*
Hematocrit, PCV, %	37-47	>33*
Red blood cell (RBC) volume, per ml	1600	1500-1900
Plasma volume, per ml	2400	3700
RBC count, million per mm^3	4.2-5.4	5.0-6.25
White blood cells, total per mm^3	5000-10,000	5000-15,000
Neutrophils, %	55-70	60-85
Lymphocytes, %	20-40	15-40
Erythrocyte sedimentation rate, mm/hr	20	Elevated in second and third trimesters
Mean corpuscular hemoglobin concentration (MCHC), g/dl packed RBCs	32-36	No change in hemoglobin concentration
Mean corpuscular hemoglobin (MCH), pg	27-31	No change per pg (less than 1 ng)
Mean corpuscular volume (MCV), μm^3	80-95	No change per μm^3
Blood Coagulation and Fibrinolytic Activity†		
Factor VII	65-140	Increase in pregnancy, return to normal in early puerperium
Factor VIII	55-145	Increases during pregnancy and immediately after birth
Factor IX	60-140	Increase in pregnancy returns to normal in early puerperium
Factor X	45-155	
Factor XI	65-135	Decrease in pregnancy
Factor XII	50-150	Increase in pregnancy, returns to normal in early puerperium
Prothrombin time (PT), sec	11-12.5	Slight decrease in pregnancy
Partial thromboplastin time (PTT), sec	60-70	Slight decrease in pregnancy and decrease during second and third stage of labor (indicates clotting at placental site)
Bleeding time, min	1-9 (Ivy)	No appreciable change
Coagulation time, min	6-10 (Lee/White)	No appreciable change
Platelets, per mm^3	150,000-400,000	No significant change until 3-5 days after birth and then a rapid increase (may predispose woman to thrombosis) and gradual return to normal
Fibrinolytic activity	Normal	Decreases in pregnancy and then abruptly returns to normal (protection against thromboembolism)
Fibrinogen, mg/dl	200-400	Increased levels late in pregnancy
Mineral and Vitamin Concentrations		
Vitamin B_{12}, folic acid, ascorbic acid	Normal	Moderate decrease
Serum Proteins		
Total, g/dl	6.4-8.3	5.5-7.5
Albumin, g/dl	3.5-5	Slight increase
Globulin, total, g/dl	2.3-3.4	3.0-4.0
Blood glucose		
Fasting, mg/dl	70-105	Decreases
2-hr postprandial, mg/dl	<140	<140 after a 100-g carbohydrate meal is considered normal

VALUES	NONPREGNANT	PREGNANT
HEMATOLOGIC—cont'd		
Acid-base Values in Arterial Blood		
Po_2, mm Hg	80-100	104-108 (increased)
Pco_2, mm Hg	35-45	27-32 (decreased)
Sodium bicarbonate (HCO_3), mEq/L	21-28	18-31 (decreased)
Blood pH	7.35-7.45	7.40-7.45 (slightly increased, more alkaline)
HEPATIC		
Bilirubin, total, mg/dl	≤1	Unchanged
Serum cholesterol, mg/dl	120-200	Increases from 16 to 32 weeks of pregnancy; remains at this level until after birth
Serum alkaline phosphatase, units/L	30-120	Increases from week 12 of pregnancy to 6 weeks after birth
Serum albumin, g/dl	3.5-5.0	Slight increase
RENAL		
Bladder capacity, ml	1300	1500
Renal plasma flow (RPF), ml/min	490-700	Increase by 25%-30%
Glomerular filtration rate (GFR), ml/min	88-128	Increase by 30%-50%
Nonprotein nitrogen (NPN), mg/dl	25-40	Decreases
Blood urea nitrogen (BUN), mg/dl	10-20	Decreases
Serum creatinine, mg/dl	0.5-1.1	Decreases
Serum uric acid, mg/dl	2.7-7.3	Decreases
Urine glucose	Negative	Present in 20% of pregnant women
Intravenous pyelogram (IVP)	Normal	Slight-to-moderate hydroureter and hydronephrosis; right kidney larger than left kidney

Source: https://d3i71xaburhd42.cloudfront.net/349bfb309526ddbd7a73395e456b020f8283c469/13-Table8-4-1.png.

2.3.3.1.3. Cardiac Output

By the 32nd week of pregnancy, cardiac output has increased from 30% to 50% over the nonpregnant rate; by the 40th week of gestation, it has decreased to about a 20% increase. This increased cardiac output is a reaction to increased oxygen demands in the tissue and is mostly caused by an increase in heart rate and stroke volume. In late pregnancy, the lateral recumbent position significantly increases cardiac output compared to the supine position. The big, heavy uterus frequently obstructs the venous return to the heart while a woman is supine, which lowers blood pressure. Any exertion, including childbirth and labor, increases cardiac output. Table 2.4 summarizes cardiovascular changes in pregnancy.

Table 2.4. *Cardiovascular Changes in Pregnancy*

Heart rate	Increases 10-15 beats/min
Blood pressure	Remains at prepregnancy levels in first trimester Slight decrease in second trimester Returns to prepregnancy levels in third trimester
Blood volume	Increases by 1500 ml or 40%-50% above prepregnancy level
Red blood cell mass	Increases 17%
Hemoglobin	Decreases
Hematocrit	Decreases
White blood cell count	Increases in second and third trimesters
Cardiac output	Increases 30%-50%

Source: https://poliklinika-harni.hr/images/uploads/271/anatomija-i-fiziologija-trudnoce.pdf

2.3.3.1.4. Circulation and Coagulation Times

By week 32, there is a slight decrease in the circulation time. In the near future, it returns to almost normal. Pregnancy increases the tendency for blood to coagulate, or clot, due to elevated levels of several clotting factors, including fibrinogen, factors VII, VIII, IX, and X. This works to reduce the risk of bleeding but also increases the woman's risk of thrombosis, particularly after cesarean delivery, because fibrinolytic activity, or the breaking up or dissolving of a clot, is decreased during pregnancy and the postpartum period.

2.3.3.2. Respiratory System

Pregnancy causes structural and respiratory changes that are necessary to meet the needs of the fetus and the mother. The need to add to the tissue mass in the uterus and breasts, along with the acceleration of metabolic rate, causes a rise in maternal oxygen requirements. The fetus also needs a means of exhaling carbon dioxide and oxygen.

Increased chest expansion is possible due to the relaxation of rib cage ligaments brought on by elevated estrogen levels (*see* Figure 2.8). The thoracic cage experiences a 2 cm increase in transverse diameter and a 6 cm increase in circumference. The lower rib cage appears to flare out as the costal angle rises. After giving birth, the chest might not revert to its prepregnant state. When a woman is pregnant, her diaphragm can move up to 4 cm. As pregnancy progresses, abdominal breathing gives way to thoracic (costal) breathing, which makes it harder for the diaphragm to descend during inspiration. Rather than the costal muscles, the diaphragm is the main muscle involved in thoracic respiration.

Elevated estrogen levels cause the upper respiratory tract to become more vascular. Edema and hyperemia appear in the nose, throat, larynx, trachea, and bronchi as the capillaries swell. Many conditions that are common during pregnancy are caused by this congestion within the tissues of the respiratory tract. These conditions include stuffiness in the nose and sinuses, epistaxis (nosebleed), changes in voice, and a marked inflammatory response that can progress into a mild upper respiratory infection. Increased vascularity in the upper respiratory tract can also result in swelling of the tympanic membranes and eustachian tubes, which can cause hearing loss, ear pain, or an earful feeling.

2.3.3.2.1. Pulmonary Function

Pregnancy-related modifications to the chest wall and diaphragm elevation are linked to respiratory changes. A decreased carbon dioxide threshold is the result of modifications to the respiratory center. It is thought that progesterone and estrogen function to enhance the respiratory center's sensitivity to carbon dioxide. Furthermore, women who are expecting experience an increased awareness of the need to breathe; some may even experience dyspnea during rest, particularly during the third trimester (*see* Table 2.5 for respiratory changes in pregnancy). While pregnancy does not affect pulmonary function, respiratory tract illnesses can worsen during this time. The higher need for oxygen could be one of the major causes of this.

Table 2.5. *Respiratory Changes in Pregnancy*

Respiratory rate	Unchanged or slightly increased
Tidal volume	Increased 30%-40%
Vital capacity	Unchanged
Inspiratory capacity	Increased
Expiratory volume	Decreased
Total lung capacity	Unchanged to slightly decreased
Oxygen consumption	Increased 15%-20%

Source: https://d3i71xaburhd42.cloudfront.net/349bfb309526ddbd7a73395e456b020f8283c469/14-Table8-5-1.png.

2.3.3.2.2. Basal Metabolic Rate

During pregnancy, the basal metabolic rate (BMR) rises. This increase varies significantly based on the woman's nutritional status prior to pregnancy and the size of the fetus. After giving birth, the BMR reaches nonpregnant levels five to six days later. Pregnancy-related increases in BMR are caused by the uterine-placental-fetal unit's higher oxygen demands as well as the mother's increased cardiac work. The extra heat produced by the elevated BMR during pregnancy is dissipated by peripheral vasodilation and an increase in sweat gland activity. Some women find heat intolerance in pregnant women to be annoying. Many pregnant women in their early stages of pregnancy experience lassitude and fatigability after only mild exertion. These sensations might last longer and result in a stronger desire to sleep; these could be partly attributed to the elevated metabolic activity.

2.3.3.2.3. Acid-Base Balance

The partial pressure of carbon dioxide (PCO_2) decreases by approximately 5 mm Hg by the tenth week of pregnancy. Progesterone may be in charge of making the respiratory center receptors more sensitive, which leads to an increase in tidal volume, a decrease in PCO_2, a decrease in the base excess (HCO_3 or bicarbonate), and a slight increase in pH. These changes in the acid-base equilibrium suggest that pregnancy is a compensatory respiratory alkalosis state. These modifications also make it easier for the fetus to transfer CO_2 and for the mother to release O_2.

2.3.3.3. Renal System

The kidneys are in charge of controlling the volume of extracellular fluid, eliminating waste, preserving vital nutrients, and preserving the equilibrium of electrolytes and acid-base.

2.3.3.3.1. Anatomic Changes

Increased blood volume, pressure from an expanding uterus, and hormonal activity (progesterone and estrogen) all contribute to changes in renal structure during pregnancy. The ureters and renal pelves begin to dilate as early as the tenth week of pregnancy. Because the ureters are compressed between the uterus and the pelvic brim, their dilation is more noticeable above the pelvic brim. The ureters in women below the pelvic brim are typically of normal size. The smooth muscle walls of the ureters experience hyperplasia, hypertrophy, and relaxation of muscle tone. The ureters lengthen, curve into single or double curves, and become tortuous. The sigmoid colon shifts the heavy uterus to the right during the later stages of pregnancy, causing the renal pelvis and ureter to dilate more on the right side than the left.

Because of these changes, a larger volume of urine is held in the pelves and ureters, and the urine flow rate is slowed. The resulting urinary stasis or stagnation has the following consequences:

- A lag occurs between the time urine is formed and when it reaches the bladder. Therefore clearance test results may reflect substances contained in glomerular filtrate several hours before.
- Stagnated urine is an excellent medium for the growth of microorganisms. In addition, the urine of pregnant women contains more nutrients, including glucose, thereby increasing the pH (making the urine more alkaline). This makes pregnant women more susceptible to urinary tract infections.

During the early stages of pregnancy, bladder irritation, nocturia, and frequent and urgent urination (without dysuria) are frequently observed. In the near future, bladder symptoms could come back, particularly after lightning. Urinary frequency is caused by bladder compression (*see* Figure 2.7) and increased bladder sensitivity at first. The bladder rises into the abdomen during the second trimester from the true pelvis. When the bladder is moved upward, the urethra lengthens to 7 and a half centimeters. The bladder and urethra's hyperemia is a reflection of the pelvic congestion that arises during pregnancy. Because of its increased vascularity, the bladder mucosa is more prone to trauma and bleeding. The bladder can hold up to 1500 ml when bladder tone decreases. Concurrently, the expanding uterus compresses the bladder, causing the urge to urinate even in cases where the bladder is only partially full of urine.

2.3.3.3.2. Functional Changes

Normal pregnancy causes significant changes to renal function. Early in pregnancy, there is an increase in both renal plasma flow (RPF) and glomerular filtration rate (GFR). Pregnancy hormones, an increase in blood volume, the woman's posture, her level of physical activity, and her diet all contribute to these changes. The increased metabolic and circulatory demands of the mother's body, along with the excretion of fetal waste products, must be handled by the kidneys of the woman. When a woman lies in the lateral recumbent position, her renal function is at its peak, and when she assumes a supine position, it is at its lowest. Lying on one's side improves renal perfusion, which in turn boosts urine production and reduces edema. The vena cava and aorta are compressed by the weight of the pregnant woman's uterus when she lies supine, which lowers cardiac output. Consequently, the kidneys and uterus suffer as a result of the blood flow to the brain and heart being maintained at the expense of other organs.

2.3.3.3.3. Balance of Fluid and Electrolytes

No matter how much is consumed or lost through perspiration, diarrhea, or vomiting, the balance of sodium and water in the body is maintained by selective renal tubular reabsorption. To meet the needs of the fetus, 500–900 mEq of sodium is typically retained during pregnancy. The mother kidneys experience a major adaptation in which they increase tubular reabsorption to prevent excessive sodium depletion. More sodium is required to maintain an isotonic state and expand fluid volume due to the increased maternal intravascular and extracellular fluid volume. Even though the kidneys are highly efficient, they can become overworked if sodium intake is excessive, restricted, or taken with diuretics. The use of diuretics during pregnancy can result in two things: severe hypovolemia and decreased placental perfusion.

Early in pregnancy, the ability of the kidneys to excrete water is more effective than it is later in the pregnancy. Due to the increased rate of water loss in the early stages of pregnancy, some women experience thirst. Renal blood flow and GFR are reduced by the accumulation of fluid in the legs towards the end of pregnancy. There is no cure for this blood clotting in the lower legs, which is also known as dependent or physiologic edema. When the woman lies down, especially on her side, the fluid that has accumulated returns to the general circulation, causing the normal diuretic response to the water load. Nearly all of the glucose and other nutrients found in the plasma filtrate are typically reabsorption by the kidney.

However, tubular reabsorption of glucose is compromised in pregnant women, resulting in variable times and intensities of glucosuria. Within the normal range of 0 to 20 mg/dl, urine can be positive or negative at any given time of day. Before glucose is "spilled" into the urine by non-pregnant women, it needs to be at 160 to 180 mg/dl (not reabsorbed). Glycosuria, or glucosuria during pregnancy, is the result of a mother's blood glucose levels falling below 160 mg/dl. It is unclear why pregnant women lose out on glucose and other nutrients like amino acids, and the precise mechanism is still unknown. While two levels of glucosuria may be observed with elevated anxiety states in normal pregnancies, it is important to consider the possibility of both gestational diabetes and diabetes mellitus.

Except for during labor or after delivery, proteinuria rarely happens during a typical pregnancy. Little amounts of protein may then be lost in the urine due to the inability of renal tubules to absorb the higher amount of amino acids that need to be filtered. During pregnancy, values of less than 300 mg per 24 hours or trace to 1 protein (dipstick assessment) are acceptable. Neither the amount of protein excreted nor an increase in protein excretion in a pregnant woman with a known renal disease necessarily indicates a progression in the disease. Both are indicators of the severity of renal disease. However, since she may be more likely to experience a negative pregnancy outcome, a pregnant woman with hypertension and proteinuria needs to be closely monitored (*see* Table 2.3).

2.3.3.4. Integumentary System

Several alterations in the integumentary system during pregnancy are caused by changes in hormonal balance and mechanical stretching. The anterior pituitary hormone melanotropin, which is elevated during pregnancy, stimulates hyperpigmentation. Around the 16th week of pregnancy, the nipples, areolae, axillae, and vulva begin to darken. Facial melasma, also known as chloasma or the "mask of pregnancy," is a blotchy, brownish hyperpigmentation of the skin that affects the forehead, nose, and cheeks. It is more common in pregnant women with dark complexion. Between 50% and 70% of expectant mothers develop chloasma, which starts after the 16th week and steadily increases until term. For women who are susceptible, the sun intensifies this pigmentation. Normal pregnancy-related chloasma typically goes away after delivery.

The black line (Figure 2.10) is a pigmented line that, before hormone-induced pigmentation, is known as the linea alba. It extends from the symphysis pubis to the top of the fundus in the midline. In multigravidas, the entire line frequently appears before the third month; in primigravidas, the linea nigra extends starting in the third month, keeping pace with the fundus's rising height. Not every pregnant woman experiences linea nigra, and some experience hair growth along the line concurrently with or in addition to the pigmentation shift.

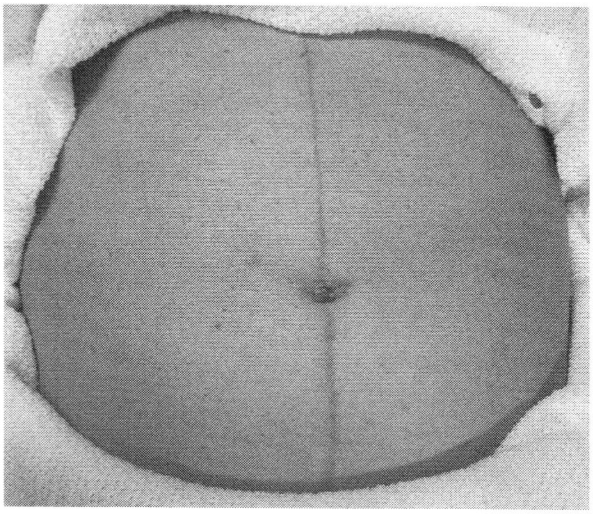

Figure 2.10. *Linea nigra.*

Source: By James Heilman, MD – Own work, CC BY-SA 3.0, https://commons.wikimedia.org/w/index.php?curid=24076795.

Stretch marks, or Striae gravidarum, which can show up in between 50% and 90% of expectant mothers in the second half of their pregnancy, could be brought on by adrenocorticosteroids. Striae are divisions found in the skin's underlying connective (collagen) tissue. These somewhat downward-sloping streaks typically appear over regions of maximum stretch, (i.e., breasts, thighs, and abdomen). There are instances when the stretching results in a feeling similar to itching. The occurrence of striae could run in the family. They usually start to fade after birth, but they never totally vanish. The color of the striae changes according to the skin tone of the expectant mother. In women with light skin, the striae appear pink, and in women with dark skin, they are paler than the surrounding skin. In the multipara, shimmering silvery lines (in women with lighter skin) or purplish lines (in women with darker skin) are frequently observed in addition to the striae of the current pregnancy. These stand in for the striae scars from earlier pregnancies. Vascular spiders is a common term used to describe angiomas. Usually located on the neck, thorax, face, and arms, these endoarteriolar lesions are small, pulsating, slightly elevated, and star-shaped or branched. They happen because there is more estrogen in the blood. The spiders don't blanch under pressure and have a bluish hue. Between the second and fifth month of pregnancy, vascular spiders are seen in approximately 65% of Caucasian women and 10% of African-American women. After birth, the spiders usually vanish.

About 60% of Caucasian women and 35% of African-American women experience pinkish-red, diffuse mottling or well-defined blotches over the palmar surfaces of their hands during pregnancy. The primary cause of these color changes, known as palmar erythema, is elevated estrogen levels. Certain dermatological conditions have been found to be specific to pregnancy or to occur more frequently during this time. During pregnancy, pruritus is a common dermatological symptom; the most common cause of pruritic rash is pregnancy-related cholestasis. Some forms are not common or rarely seen. The management's objective is to stop the itching. Although systemic steroids may be required, topical steroids are typically used as a form of treatment. Usually, the issue is resolved during the postpartum phase. Skin conditions that already exist may make pregnancy more difficult or better.

Gum hypertrophy could happen. An easily bleedable red, raised nodule on the gums is called an epulis (gingival granuloma gravidarum). This lesion typically keeps getting bigger as the pregnancy goes on, starting to appear about the third month. Usually, it can be controlled by preventing gum trauma (e.g., employing a gentle toothbrush). After birth, an epulis typically regresses on its own. Nail growth might quicken. Some women may observe that their nails are becoming softer and thinner. During pregnancy, greasy skin and acne vulgaris are possible. Some women have clearer, more radiant skin.

It is common to hear reports of hirsutism, which is defined as excessive or unusual hair growth. Fine hair growth may increase during pregnancy, but it usually stops growing after. On the other hand, coarse or bristly hair growth usually continues. During pregnancy, the rate of scalp hair loss slows down; postpartum hair loss may even increase. Perspiration increases as a result of an increased blood supply to the skin. Pregnancy makes women feel hotter, a condition that may be linked to an increase in body temperature brought on by progesterone and an increase in basal metabolic rate.

2.3.3.5. Musculoskeletal System

The pregnant woman's posture noticeably changes as a result of her body gradually changing and her weight increasing (Figure 2.11) as well as her gait. Late in pregnancy, the spinal curvature needs to realign due to the great abdominal distention that causes the pelvis to tilt forward, decreased abdominal muscle tone, and increased weight bearing. The woman moves forward in her center of gravity. To help her maintain her balance, a compensatory curvature in the cervicodorsal region (exaggerated anterior flexion of the head) develops, along with an increase in the normal lumbosacral curve, or lordosis. Upper extremity weakness, numbness, and aching could ensue. The lumbar and dorsal curves will be further emphasized by large breasts and a stoop-shouldered posture. Walking becomes more challenging, and Shakespeare is credited with coining the term "the proud walk of pregnancy" to describe the waddling gait of a pregnant woman. There may be significant strain on the middle and lower back's ligamentous and muscular structures. Musculoskeletal pain is frequently brought on by these and related changes, particularly in older women, those with back disorders, and those with impaired balance.

Pregnancy is a normal time for the pelvic joints to become slightly more mobile and relaxed. They are secondary to increased levels of circulating steroid sex hormones, particularly estrogen, which cause the connective and collagen tissue to soften and elongate excessively. An ovarian hormone called relaxin helps with this softening and relaxing. These modifications allow the pelvis to expand, which helps with labor and delivery. Although there is variation in the degree of relaxation, significant symphysis pubis separation and sacroiliac joint instability may result in pain and make walking difficult. Pelvic instability is often more prevalent in obese and multifetal pregnancies. As pregnancy goes on, peripheral joint laxity also rises, though the exact reason is unknown.

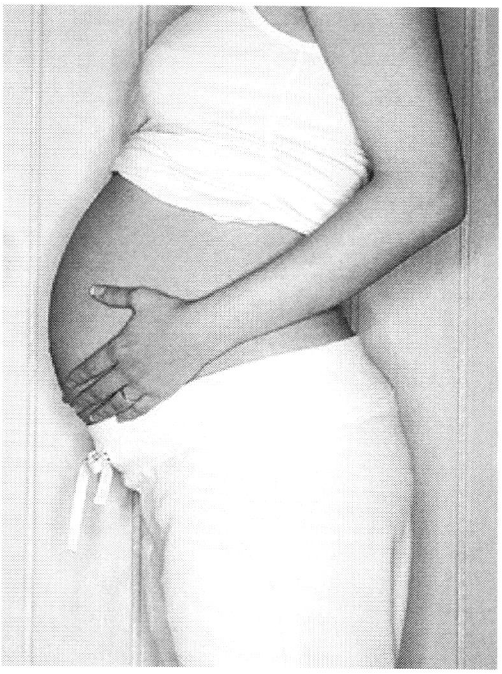

Figure 2.11. *Postural changes during pregnancy.*

Source: By Swangerschaft – Swangerschaft on Flickr.com, CC BY-SA 2.0, https://commons.wikimedia.org/w/index.php?curid=9443257.

The abdominal wall muscles stretch and eventually become less toned. The rectus abdominis muscles may split in the third trimester (Figure 2.12), causing the contents of the abdomen to bulge at the midline. The umbilicus expands or flattens. The muscles gradually regain tone after birth, but diastasis recti abdominis, or the separation of the muscles, may continue.

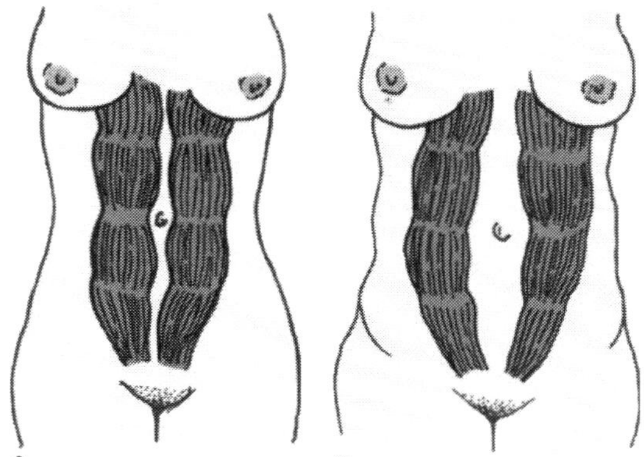

Figure 2.12. *Possible change in rectus abdominis muscles during pregnancy. (A) Normal position in nonpregnant woman. (B) Diastasis recti abdominis in pregnant woman.*

Source: https://d3i71xaburhd42.cloudfront.net/349bfb309526ddbd7a73395e456b020f8283c469/18-Figure8-12-1.png.

2.3.3.6. Neurologic System

Little is known regarding specific alterations in the functions of the neurologic system during pregnancy, aside from hypothalamic-pituitary neurohormonal changes. Specific physiologic alterations resulting from pregnancy may cause the following neurologic or neuromuscular symptoms:

- Compression of pelvic nerves or vascular stasis caused by enlargement of the uterus may result in sensory changes in the legs.
- Dorsolumbar lordosis may cause pain because of traction on nerves or compression of nerve roots.
- Edema involving the peripheral nerves may result in carpal tunnel syndrome during the last trimester. The syndrome is characterized by paresthesia (abnormal sensation such as burning or tingling) and pain in the hand, radiating to the elbow. The sensations are caused by edema that

compresses the median nerve beneath the carpal ligament of the wrist. Smoking and alcohol consumption can impair the microcirculation and may worsen the symptoms. The dominant hand is usually affected most, although as many as 80% of women experience symptoms in both hands. Symptoms usually regress after pregnancy. In some cases, surgical treatment may be necessary.

- Acroesthesia (numbness and tingling of the hands) is caused by the stoop-shouldered stance (*see* Figure 2.11(B)) assumed by some women during pregnancy. The condition is associated with traction on segments of the brachial plexus.
- Tension headaches are common when anxiety or uncertainty complicates pregnancy. However, vision problems, sinusitis, or migraine also may be responsible for headaches.
- "Light-headedness," faintness, and even syncope (fainting) are common during early pregnancy. Vasomotor instability, postural hypotension, or hypoglycemia may be responsible.
- Hypocalcemia may cause neuromuscular problems such as muscle cramps or tetany.

2.3.3.7. Gastrointestinal System

2.3.3.7.1. Appetite

A woman's appetite and food intake change during pregnancy. Some women experience morning sickness (vomiting and/or nausea) early in pregnancy; this condition may be caused by elevated hCG levels and changes in the metabolism of carbohydrates. Usually starting around week four or six of gestation, morning sickness, also known as nausea and vomiting of pregnancy (NVP), goes away by the end of the third month, or first trimester. The range of severity is from mild food aversion to more severe vomiting. The sight or smell of certain foods can set off the condition. The appetite rises by the end of the second trimester as a result of rising metabolic demands. NVP rarely has negative effects on the embryo, the fetus, or the mother; among the positive effects could be a decreased risk of miscarriage, early labor, or intrauterine growth restriction during these pregnancies. Further assessment is required and medical intervention is probably required if the vomiting is severe, lasts longer than the first trimester, or is accompanied by fever, pain, or weight loss.

Women may also experience changes in their taste perception, which can result in cravings and adjustments to their food intake. Some women experience pica, or cravings for things other than food, like ice, clay, and laundry starch. When a woman has proper nutrition and weight gain during her pregnancy, most of the subjects of these cravings are safe to consume in moderation.

2.3.3.7.2. Mouth

During pregnancy, the gums swell, become hyperemic, and become spongy. Their propensity for bleeding stems from the selective increase in vascularity and proliferation of connective tissue brought on by the rising estrogen levels. The gum line may become epulis (nonspecific gingivitis). Pregnant women may experience ptyalism, or excessive salivation, which can be brought on by eating starch, which stimulates the salivary glands, or by the woman's reduced unconscious swallowing when feeling queasy.

2.3.3.7.3. *Esophagus, Stomach, and Intestines*

Around 15% to 20% of pregnant women experience hiatal hernias, or herniations of the upper portion of the stomach, after the seventh or eighth month of pregnancy. This condition is brought on by the stomach moving upward, widening the diaphragmatic hiatus. It happens more frequently in older or obese women and multiparas. Reduced hydrochloric acid secretion due to increased estrogen production means that peptic ulcer development or flare-ups are rare during pregnancy and may even go better. Reduced smooth muscle tone and motility brought on by increased progesterone production results in esophageal regurgitation, delayed stomach emptying time, and reverse peristalsis. This can lead to "acid indigestion" or heartburn (pyrosis) in the woman, which can start in the first trimester and get worse by the third.

Pregnancy increases the need for iron, which causes the small intestine to absorb it more easily. Iron will continue to be absorbed in sufficient amounts for the fetus to have a normal hemoglobin level even in cases where the woman is deficient in it. Constipation may result from increased colonic water absorption brought on by increased progesterone, which also causes loss of muscle tone and decreased peristalsis. Hypoperistalsis (sluggishness of the bowel), dietary choices, dehydration, iron deficiency, reduced activity, distention of the abdomen by the pregnant uterus, and displacement and compression of the intestines are additional causes of constipation. When a pregnant woman strains at her stool and has hemorrhoids, the hemorrhoids may become everted or bleed.

2.3.3.7.4. *Gallbladder and Liver*

Due to the gallbladder's lowered muscle tone during pregnancy, it frequently becomes enlarged. Typical changes include longer emptying times and thicker bile due to prolonged retention. These characteristics, along with a small hypercholesterolemia brought on by elevated progesterone levels, could explain why gallstones form during pregnancy. Although it can be challenging to assess hepatic function during pregnancy, only slight alterations in liver function occur. Sometimes, in response to placental steroids, late pregnancy can cause intrahepatic cholestasis (retention and accumulation of bile in the liver, caused by factors within the liver). This condition can cause severe itching, known as pruritus gravidarum, with or without jaundice. These upsetting symptoms go away quickly after delivery.

2.3.3.7.5. *Abdominal Discomfort*

Changes in the intraabdominal space that can be uncomfortable include round ligament tension, flatulence, distention and cramping in the bowels, pelvic heaviness or pressure, and uterine contractions. The expanding uterus puts pressure on the intestines, which also raises the venous pressure in the pelvic organs. While the majority of stomach pain is a result of typical changes in a mother's body, the medical professional needs to be on the lookout for conditions like intestinal blockage or inflammation. Appendicitis may be difficult to diagnose in pregnancy because the appendix is displaced upward and laterally, high and to the right, away from McBurney's point (Figure 2.13).

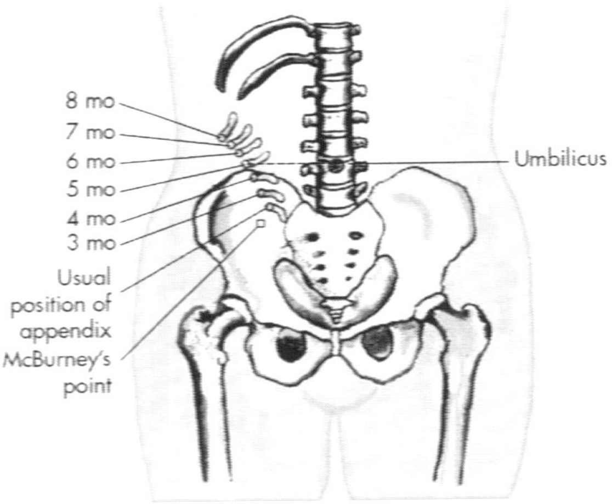

Figure 2.13. *Change in position of appendix in pregnancy. Note McBurney's point.*

Source: https://d3i71xaburhd42.cloudfront.net/349bfb309526ddbd7a73395e456b020f8283c469/20-Figure8-13-1.png.

2.3.3.8. Endocrine System

Profound endocrine changes are essential for pregnancy maintenance, normal fetal growth, and postpartum recovery.

2.3.3.8.1. Pituitary and Placental Hormones

During pregnancy, the anterior pituitary is unable to secrete luteinizing hormone (LH) and follicle-stimulating hormone (FSH) due to the elevated levels of progesterone and estrogen, which are produced by the placenta and the corpus luteum in the ovary until approximately 14 weeks of gestation. Ovulation and follicle maturation don't happen. While amenorrhea, or the lack of menses, affects most women, at least 20% experience mild, painless spotting in the early stages of pregnancy. Cervical friability-related bleeding following sexual activity and bleeding during implantation are both possible.

Following implantation, the fertilized ovum and the chorionic villi release hCG, which keeps the corpus luteum producing progesterone and estrogen until the placenta takes over. By reducing uterine contraction and preventing miscarriage, progesterone relaxes smooth muscles, which is crucial for preserving pregnancy. Maternal back, upper thighs, and abdomen all experience subcutaneous tissue fat deposits as a result of progesterone and estrogen. This fat is used as a store of energy during lactation and pregnancy. Additionally, estrogen increases vascularity, which results in vasodilation and encourages the enlargement of the breasts, uterus, and genitalia. The hormone estrogen relaxes the joints and ligaments in the pelvis. It also modifies the way that nutrients are metabolized by upregulating the metabolism of folic acid, raising the amount of total body proteins, and encouraging kidney tubules to retain water and salt. Digestive disturbances like nausea may be caused by hydrochloric acid and pepsin secretion being reduced by estrogen.

Early in the first trimester, the production of serum prolactin from the anterior pituitary starts to rise, and it continues to rise until term. It causes the first stages of lactation, but high estrogen and progesterone levels prevent lactation by delaying the binding of prolactin to breast tissue until after delivery. As the fetus grows older, the posterior pituitary produces more oxytocin. While high levels of progesterone delay contractions until close to term, this hormone can induce them during pregnancy.

After delivery, oxytocin also triggers the let-down or milk-ejection reflex in reaction to the newborn sucking on the mother's breast. It has been proposed that the placenta secretes human chorionic somatomammotropin (hCS), formerly known as human placental lactogen, which functions as a growth hormone and aids in the development of the breast. Its function is unclear, but it may also increase the amount of fatty acids needed for metabolic requirements and decrease the mother's metabolism of glucose.

2.3.3.8.2. Thyroid Gland

Hormone production and gland activity both rise during pregnancy. The thyroid gland has undergone a moderate enlargement due to hyperplasia of the glandular tissue and increased vascularity, which is indicative of increased activity. Elevated estrogen levels cause an increase in thyroxine-binding globulin (TBG). About 20 weeks into the pregnancy is when this increase starts. Between weeks six and nine of pregnancy, the level of total (free and bound) thyroxine (T_4) rises and reaches a plateau at week 18. After the first trimester, free triiodothyronine (T_3) and free thyroxine (T_4) return to nonpregnant levels. Pregnant women typically do not develop hyperthyroidism despite these changes in hormone production.

2.3.3.8.3. Parathyroid Gland

The metabolism of magnesium and calcium is regulated by parathyroid hormone. Due to the increased fetal need for calcium and vitamin D, pregnancy causes mild hyperparathyroidism. The peak level of parathyroid hormone is reached between weeks 15 and 35 of gestation, which coincides with the highest fetal skeleton growth requirements. After birth, levels return to normal.

2.3.3.8.4. Pancreas

Significant glucose intake is necessary for the fetus's growth and development. The fetus uses the mother's stored glucose as fuel, but it also reduces the mother's capacity to synthesize glucose by removing amino acids from the body. Blood glucose levels drop in mothers. The fetus does not receive maternal insulin through the placenta. For this reason, the pancreas produces less insulin in the early stages of pregnancy.

During pregnancy, the placenta expands and secretes increasing levels of hormones such as hCS, estrogen, and progesterone. The adrenal glands also boost cortisol production. These hormones collectively reduce the mother's insulin sensitivity. Cortisol prompts higher insulin production while also causing resistance to insulin in the body's tissues. This decrease in insulin sensitivity is a protective mechanism to ensure a sufficient glucose supply for the fetus. As a result, the mother's need for insulin rises steadily throughout pregnancy. Fortunately, the pancreas can effectively produce the necessary insulin to meet this demand.

2.3.3.8.5. Adrenal Glands

The adrenal glands change little during pregnancy. Secretion of aldosterone is increased, resulting in reabsorption of excess sodium from the renal tubules. Cortisol levels also are increased.

A Closer Look

Zygote

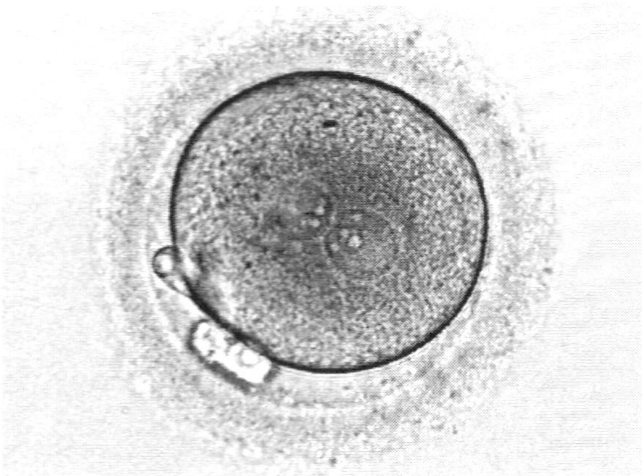

Source: By Nina Sesina – File:Zygote.tif, CC BY-SA 4.0, https://commons.wikimedia.org/w/index.php?curid=67459911.

The fertilized egg cell known as a zygote is the product of the union of a male gamete (sperm) and a female gamete (egg, or ovum). The zygote stage, which is short in the embryonic development of humans and other animals, is followed by cleavage, in which the single cell divides into smaller cells.

An organism with its own genetic makeup begins its development with the zygote. The zygote is diploid (carries two sets of chromosomes) because it is endowed with genes from two parents. Every organism—aside from bacteria—reproduces diploid zygotes through the joining of haploid gametes. This process is known as sexual reproduction.

All the necessary components for development are present in the zygote, but they only exist as an encoded set of instructions that are located in the genes of chromosomes. The new zygote's genes are actually not activated to produce proteins until multiple cell divisions lead up to cleavage. Through the process of mitosis, the relatively large zygote directly divides into numerous smaller cells of conventional size during cleavage (ordinary cell proliferation by division). These smaller cells, known as blastomeres, are appropriate for serving as the organism's initial building blocks. Human identical twins are produced from a zygote that divides into two distinct cell masses relatively early in the organism's life. These two masses develop into embryos despite having the same genetic makeup. Contrarily, fraternal twins are created from two distinct zygotes, which are two distinct eggs fertilized by two distinct sperm.

Summary

- Pregnancy is a time of profound anatomic and physiologic change. In addition to the reproductive organs, all maternal physiologic systems make adaptions needed to support the developing fetus and, at the same time, maintain maternal homeostasis.
- Early detection of pregnancy allows early initiation of care. Human chorionic gonadotropin (hCG) is the earliest biochemical marker for pregnancy, and pregnancy tests are based on the recognition of hCG or a beta (β) subunit of hCG.
- Maternal physiologic adaptations are attributed to the hormones of pregnancy and to mechanical pressures arising from the enlarging uterus and other tissues.
- In normal pregnancy, renal function is altered considerably. Glomerular filtration rate (GFR) and renal plasma flow (RPF) increase early in pregnancy. These changes are caused by pregnancy hormones, an increase in blood volume, the woman's posture, physical activity, and nutritional intake.
- The maturation of a follicle and ovulation do not occur. Although the majority of women have amenorrhea (absence of menses), at least 20% have some slight, painless spotting during early gestation.
- During pregnancy, gland activity and hormone production increase. The increased activity is reflected in a moderate enlargement of the thyroid gland caused by hyperplasia of the glandular tissue and increased vascularity.

References

1. Aminoff, M. (2004). Neurologic disorders. In R. Creasy, R. Resnik, & J. Iams (Eds.), *Maternal-Fetal Medicine: Principles and Practice* (5th ed.). Philadelphia: Saunders.
2. Berman, M., DiSaia, P., & Tewari, K. (2004). Pelvic malignancies, gestational trophoblastic neoplasia, and nonpelvic malignancies. In R. Creasy, R. Resnik, & J. Iams (Eds.), *Maternal-fetal Medicine: Principles and Practice* (5th ed.). Philadelphia: Saunders.
3. Buster, J., & Carson, S. (2002). Endocrinology and diagnosis of pregnancy. In S. Gabbe, J. Niebyl, & J. Simpson (Eds.), *Obstetrics: Normal and Problem Pregnancies* (4th ed.). New York: Churchill Livingstone.
4. Cole, K., et al. (2004). Accuracy of home pregnancy tests at time of missed menses. *American Journal of Obstetrics and Gynecology, 190*(1), 100–105.
5. Cunningham, F., Leveno, K., Bloom, S., Hauth, J., Gilstrap, L., & Wenstrom, K. (2005). *Williams obstetrics* (22nd ed.). New York: McGraw-Hill.
6. Furneaux, E., Langley-Evans, A., & Langley-Evans, S. (2001). Nausea and vomiting of pregnancy: Endocrine basis and contribution to pregnancy outcome. *Obstetrical and Gynecological Survey, 56*(12), 775–782.
7. Gibbs, R., Sweet, R., & Duff, W. (2004). Maternal and fetal infectious disorders. In R. Creasy, R. Resnik, & J. Iams (Eds.), *Maternal-Fetal Medicine: Principles and Practice* (5th ed.). Philadelphia: Saunders.

8. Gordon, M. (2002). Maternal physiology in pregnancy. In S. Gabbe, J. Niebyl, & J. Simpson (Eds.), *Obstetrics: Normal and Problem Pregnancies* (4th ed.). New York: Churchill Livingstone.
9. Harman, C. (2004). Assessment of fetal health. In R. Creasy, R. Resnik, & J. Iams (Eds.), *Maternal-Fetal Medicine: Principles and Practice* (5th ed.). Philadelphia: Saunders.
10. Hermida, R., Ayala, D., Mojon, A., & Fernandez, J. (2001). Time-qualified reference values for ambulatory blood pressure monitoring in pregnancy. *Hypertension, 38*(3 Pt 2), 746–752.
11. Jewell, D., & Young, G. (2003). Interventions for nausea and vomiting in early pregnancy. (Cochrane Review). In *The Cochrane Library*, Issue 2, 2004. Chichester, UK: John Wiley & Sons.
12. Lawrence, R., & Lawrence, R. (2004). The breast and the physiology of lactation. In R. Creasy, R. Resnik, & J. Iams (Eds.), *Maternal-Fetal Medicine: Principles and Practice* (5th ed.). Philadelphia: Saunders.
13. Liu, J. (2004). Endocrinology of pregnancy. In R. Creasy, R. Resnik, & J. Iams (Eds.), *Maternal-Fetal Medicine: Principles and Practice* (5th ed.). Philadelphia: Saunders.
14. Malone, F., & D'Alton, M. (2004). Multiple gestation: Clinical characteristics and management. In R. Creasy, R. Resnik, & J. Iams (Eds.), *Maternal-Fetal Medicine: Principles and Practice* (5th ed.). Philadelphia: Saunders.
15. Monga, M. (2004). Maternal cardiovascular and renal adaptation to pregnancy. In R. Creasy, R. Resnik, & J. Iams (Eds.), *Maternal-Fetal Medicine: Principles and Practice* (5th ed.). Philadelphia: Saunders.
16. Padua, L., Aprile, I., Caliandro, P., Carboni, T., Meloni, A., Massi, S., et al. (2001). Symptoms and neurophysical picture of carpal tunnel syndrome in pregnancy. *Clinical Neurophysiology, 112*(10), 1946–1951.
17. Pagana, K., & Pagana, T. (2003). *Mosby's diagnostic and laboratory test reference* (6th ed.). St. Louis: Mosby.
18. Rapini, R. (2004). The skin and pregnancy. In R. Creasy, R. Resnik, & J. Iams (Eds.), *Maternal-Fetal Medicine: Principles and Practice* (5th ed.). Philadelphia: Saunders.
19. Seidel, H., Ball, J., Dains, J., & Benedict, G. (2003). *Mosby's guide to physical examination* (5th ed.). St. Louis: Mosby.
20. Stewart, F. (2004). Pregnancy testing and management of early pregnancy. In R. Hatcher et al (Eds.), *Contraceptive technology* (18th ed.). New York: Ardent Media.
21. Whitty, J., & Dombrowski, M. (2004). Respiratory diseases in pregnancy. In R. Creasy, R. Resnik, & J. Iams (Eds.), *Maternal-Fetal Medicine: Principles and Practice* (5th ed.). Philadelphia: Saunders.

Chapter

PRENATAL CARE

3

Contents

Unit Introduction 79
3.1. An Overview of Antenatal Care 81
3.2. Nutrition During Pregnancy 86
3.3. Common Health Problems During Pregnancy 88
3.4. Psychological Changes in Pregnancy 92
3.5. Planned Intervention for the Alleviation of Psychological Difficulties During the Perinatal Period 94
3.6. Psychosocial Effects of the Actual Provision of Prenatal Care 99
3.7. Routine Screening and Diagnostic Tests 100
3.8. Fetal Assessment 105
Summary 118
References 118

Unit Introduction

Antenatal care, another name for prenatal care, is a subset of preventive medicine. It is given in the form of medical examinations, which include advice on leading a healthy lifestyle and medical information on biological changes, physiological changes in pregnant mothers, and prenatal nutrition, including prenatal vitamins. This helps to avert potential health issues throughout the pregnancy and supports the health of both the mother and the unborn child. Prenatal screening and diagnosis, along with routine care, have contributed to a decrease in the incidence of low birth weight, infections in newborns, miscarriages, maternal deaths, and other avoidable health issues.

Traditional prenatal care in high-income countries generally consists of:

- Monthly visits during the first two trimesters (from the 1st week to the 28th week);
- Fortnightly visits from the 28th week to the 36th week of pregnancy;
- Weekly visits after 36th week to the delivery, from the 38th week to the 42nd week;
- Assessment of parental needs and family dynamics.

Orientation and Directional Terms

Term	Definition	Illustration
Antenatal care	Prenatal care is the health care a woman receives during pregnancy, including checkups and testing.	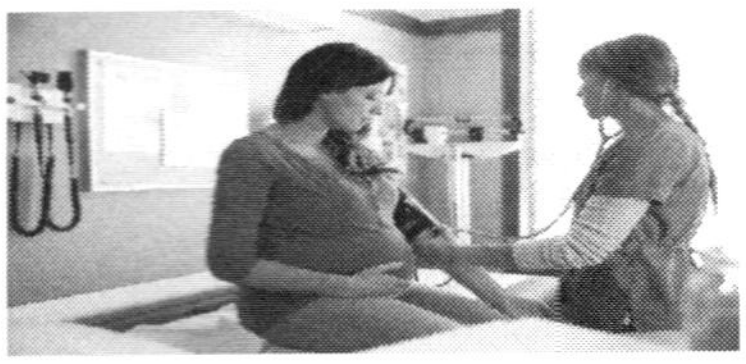
Foetal Heart Sound (FHS)	FHS stands for fetal heart sounds, and it's a valuable source of information about the health of the fetus and mother.	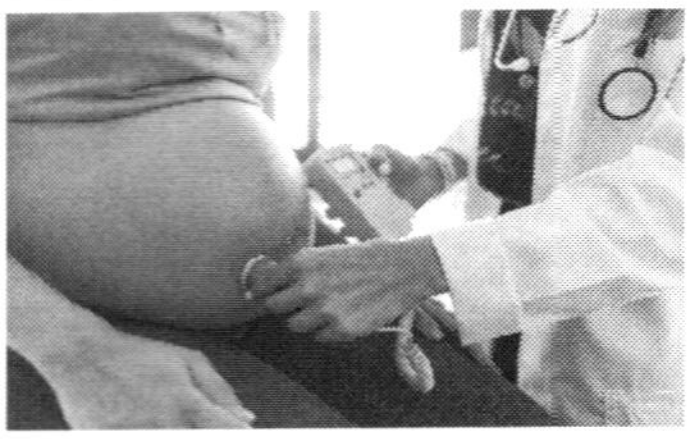
post-partum period	The postpartum period is the time after giving birth when a mother's body returns to its pre-pregnancy state.	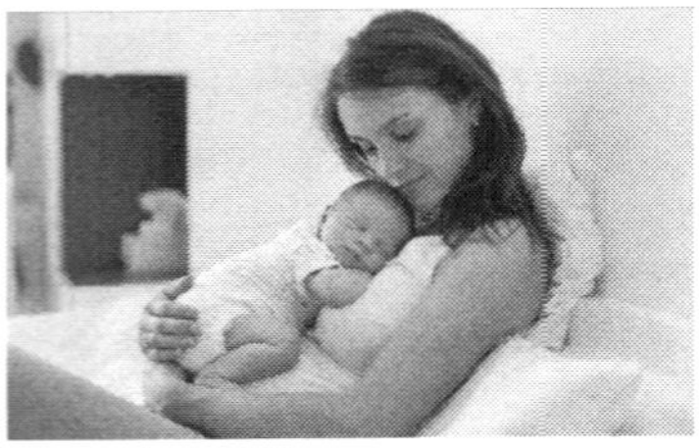
Child Protection	Child protection is the prevention of or response to the abuse, exploitation, violence, and neglect of children.	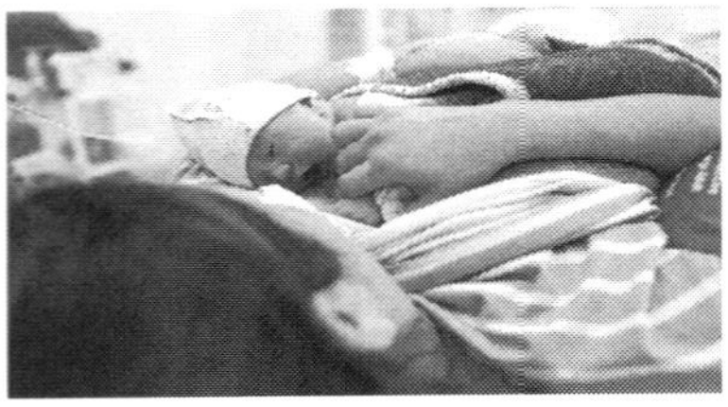
Pregnancy nutrition	Nutrition and pregnancy refers to the nutrient intake, and dietary planning that is undertaken before, during and after pregnancy.	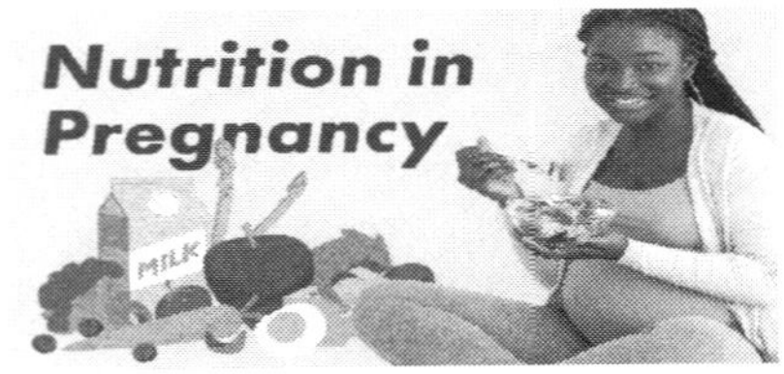

3.1. An Overview of Antenatal Care

Antenatal care, also known as prenatal care, is a part of preventive medicine. It involves medical check-ups, advice on maintaining a healthy lifestyle, and information on the physical and physiological changes in pregnant women, as well as prenatal nutrition and vitamins. This helps prevent potential health problems during pregnancy and promotes the well-being of both the mother and the unborn child. Prenatal screening, diagnosis, and regular care have played a role in reducing the occurrence of low birth weight, infections in newborns, miscarriages, maternal mortality, and other preventable health issues.

But it's important to understand that no matter how good the screening methods are, it is impossible to predict which woman will experience pregnancy-related problems during or right after giving birth.

You must therefore:

- Recognize that 'Every pregnancy is special and every pregnant woman must receive special care.'
- Complications being unpredictable may happen in any pregnancy/childbirth and we should be ready to deal with them if and whenever they happen.
- Ensure that ANC is used as an opportunity to detect and treat existing problems, e.g., essential hypertension.
- Prepare the woman and her family for the eventuality of an emergency.
- Make sure that services to manage obstetric emergencies are available on time.

Quality ANC has several components, which are described below.

1. A Few Primary Steps:
   - Ensure early registration and see to it that the first check-up is conducted within 12 weeks (first three months of pregnancy).
   - Track every pregnancy for conducting at least four antenatal check-ups (including the first visit for registration), keeping in mind all the essential components listed under section B.
   - Administer two doses of TT injection.
   - Provide at least 100 tablets of IFA.
2. Essential Components of Every Antenatal Check-Up:
   - Take the patient's history.
   - Conduct a physical examination–measure the weight, blood pressure and respiratory rate and check for pallor and edema.
   - Conduct abdominal palpation for fetal growth, fetal lie and auscultation of Foetal Heart Sound (FHS) according to the stage of pregnancy.
   - Carry out laboratory investigations, such as hemoglobin estimation and urine tests (for sugar and proteins).

3. Desirable Components:
   - Determine the blood group, including the Rh factor.
   - Conduct the Venereal Disease Research Laboratory (VDRL)/ Rapid Plasma Reagin (RPR) test to rule out syphilis.
   - Test the woman for Human Immunodeficiency Virus (HIV).
   - Check the blood sugar.
   - Carry out the Hepatitis B Surface Antigen (HBsAg) test.
4. Counselling:
   - Help the woman to plan and prepare for birth (birth preparedness/micro birth plan). This should include deciding on the place of delivery and the presence of an attendant at the time of the delivery.
   - Advantages of institutional deliveries and risks involved in home deliveries.
   - Advise the woman on where to go if an emergency arises, and how to arrange for transportation, money and blood donors in case of an emergency.
   - Educate the woman and her family members on signs of labor and danger signs of obstetric complications.
   - Emphasize the importance of seeking ANC and PNC.
   - Advise on diet (nutrition) and rest.
   - Inform the woman about breastfeeding, including exclusive breastfeeding.
   - Provide information on sex during pregnancy.
   - Warn against domestic violence (explain the consequences of violence on a pregnant woman and her foetus).
   - Promote family planning.
   - Inform the woman about the Janani Suraksha Yojana (JSY)/ any other incentives offered by the state.

3.1.1. Early Registration

3.1.1.1. Timing of the First Visit/ Registration

As soon as a pregnant woman is suspected of being pregnant, she should have her first appointment or register with ANC. It is important to encourage all women who are of reproductive age to see their doctor if they think they may be pregnant. The first appointment should ideally happen within a month. Nonetheless, a woman should be registered and receive care based on her gestational age even if she arrives for registration later in her pregnancy. It is advisable to counsel her husband and mother-in-law to provide support during her pregnancy, delivery, post-partum period, and following an abortion.

Early detection of pregnancy is important for the following reasons:

- It facilitates proper planning and allows for adequate care to be provided during pregnancy for both the mother and the fetus.
- Record the date of the Last Menstrual Period (LMP), and calculate the Expected Date of Delivery (EDD).
- The health status of the mother can be assessed and any medical illness that she might be suffering from can be

detected and also to obtain/recording baseline information (on blood pressure, weight, hemoglobin, etc.)

- Helps in the timely detection of complications at an early stage and manages them appropriately by referral as and where required.
- This also helps in providing the woman with the option of an early abortion. If so, then refer the woman at the earliest to a 24-hour PHC or First Referral Unit (FRU) (whichever is closer) that provides safe abortion services. It is important to find out as early as possible whether the woman wants to go in for an abortion so that the procedure can be done safely as per the legal provisions laid down under the Medical Termination of Pregnancy (MTP) Act, 1972.
- If a pregnancy is detected early and the woman is provided care from the initial stage, it facilitates a good interpersonal relationship between you and her. She will thus, be more likely to express her particular needs and wants while planning for the delivery.

3.1.2. Detection of Pregnancy

Using a pregnancy test kit to examine your urine is the easiest way to determine whether you are pregnant in the first trimester. Any woman in the reproductive age range who comes to you with symptoms of pregnancy or a history of amenorrhea should be offered the pregnancy test. The "Nischay" pregnancy test kit is now accessible throughout the nation thanks to the GoI. There are additional test kits on the market. These kits use the hormone human chorionic gonadotrophin (hCG) found in urine to identify pregnancy.

This test is easy to administer and can be done shortly after a missed period. It just takes two drops of the woman's urine and five minutes. Additionally, Accredited Social Health Activists (ASHAs) and link workers in your area have been given pregnancy test kits, which they may use on community visits. Make sure they have access to the kits and that they notify you of any successful outcomes. The woman needs to receive the proper counseling regarding the test results.

3.1.3. Number and Timing of Visits

- Ensure that every pregnant woman makes at least four visits for ANC, including the first visit/registration. It should be emphasized that this is only a minimum requirement and that more visits may be necessary, depending on the woman's condition and needs.
- Suggested schedule for antenatal visits
- **1st Visit:** Within 12 weeks—preferably as soon as pregnancy is suspected—for registration of pregnancy and first antenatal check-up
- **2nd Visit:** Between 14 and 26 weeks
- **3rd Visit:** Between 28 and 34 weeks
- **4th Visit:** Between 36 weeks and term

During the 28–34-week period, the pregnant woman should schedule a third visit with the MO at the PHC for an antenatal checkup. Besides this, she may also be advised and guided to avail investigation facilities, which are not available with you like Blood Grouping, etc. at the nearest PHC/CHC/FRU.

3.1.4. Seek Help for Early Registration and Antenatal Check-Up

The ANM is primarily in charge of registering every pregnancy within 12 weeks. It is important to make the most of opportunities like the Village Health and Nutrition Day (VHND) to guarantee early registration and prenatal check-ups.

Many individuals can assist you in updating your list as they are probably aware of the pregnant women in the village. These comprise Anganwadi Workers (AWWs), ASHAs, and other community-based workers, including members of panchayat and village health committees, Mahila Mandals, Self-Help Groups (SHGs), and NGOs. Educators and other influential members of the community may also possess inside information.

3.1.5. Estimate the Number of Pregnancies in Your Area

- To ensure complete registration, it is essential that you know the estimated number of pregnancies to be registered annually in your area.
- Calculating the expected number of annual pregnancies in your area will help you judge how good your pregnancy registration is. In case the number of pregnancies registered is less than that of the estimated pregnancies, you need to track down the pregnancies you have missed with the help of ASHAs and AWWs.
- Estimating the number of pregnancies will also help you judge whether you have an adequate stock of the supplies required to provide routine ANC (such as TT injections, IFA tablets and ANC record forms) and tackle any complications that arise during this period.

The following steps may be followed to calculate the expected number of pregnancies annually:

- You must know the birth rate and population size of the area under your jurisdiction.
- The birth rate of your area can be obtained from the MO at the PHC or you can consult the available district/state/national figures. It is advisable to use the available local figures for the birth rate for correct estimation.
- To know the exact population of the area under your jurisdiction, use the latest demographic data/census reports.
- If the number of women registered with you is less than expected, then you should approach community leaders and key people mentioned earlier, to ensure that more pregnant women are registered and come for ANC. The matter should also be communicated to the ASHA/link worker so that she can visit every house in the area and ensure that all pregnant women are registered.
- Some women may be receiving ANC from the private sector. Ensure that their names together with the names of the facilities where they are registered are mentioned in your antenatal register.

3.1.6. Keep a Track of All Pregnant Women by Name

- As the ANM, you must refer to your register to keep track of all pregnant women in your area. In case a woman who is registered with you does not return for her antenatal check-up, then she must be followed up at her home and counseled to go for regular antenatal check-ups.

- An antenatal check-up after a missed appointment should include all the components of the missed visit(s) as well as those that correspond to the present visit. For example, the woman should be given her TT injection and supply of IFA tablets, her weight and blood pressure should be checked and recorded and she should be counseled besides being screened for complications.
- It is very likely that women might not come for ANC early in their pregnancy. You should take the help of the AWWs, ASHAs, panchayat members and so on to track pregnant women who have not come for their antenatal check-ups.
- Once such women have been tracked down, arrangements should be made to give them ANC as soon as possible. These women should also be counseled on the importance of complete ANC for the better health of the baby and the mother.
- A policy decision has been taken for a name-based tracking system whereby pregnant women and children can be tracked for their ANCs and immunization along with a feedback system for the ANM, ASHA etc. This has been done to ensure that all pregnant women receive their ANCs and PNCs and children receive full immunization. This will also help in tracking and ensuring ANC/PNC for missed/left-out cases.

3.1.7. Record Keeping

For record keeping, the following must be done:

- A Mother and Child Protection Card should be duly completed for every woman registered by you. The case record should be handed over to the woman. She should be instructed to bring the record with her during all subsequent check-ups/visits and also to carry it along with her at the time of delivery. (Annexure l – Mother and Child Protection Card).
- This card has been developed jointly by the Ministry of Health and Family Welfare (MoHFW) and the Ministry of Women and Child Development (MoWCD) to ensure uniformity in record keeping. This will also help the service provider to know the details of previous ANCs/PNCs both for routine and emergency care.
- The information contained in the card should also be recorded in your antenatal register as per the Health Management Information System (HMIS) format.

3.1.8. Antenatal Check-Up

3.1.8.1. Preparing for and Conducting Antenatal Check-Ups

- Before beginning each antenatal check-up at your SC or during the VHND, ensure that all the required instruments and equipment are available and are in working condition. These include a stethoscope, blood pressure apparatus, weighing scale, inch tape, foetoscope, thermometer, Mother and Child Protection Card and register, watch, gloves, 0.5% chlorine solution, syringes and needles, hub cutter, spirit swabs, IFA tablets, TT injections, and equipment for testing hemoglobin and urine.
- You must greet every pregnant woman in a friendly manner at each visit.
- Listen to the woman's problems and concerns, and counsel her and her relatives.

- The antenatal examination should be carried out at an appropriate place where there is enough privacy for conducting abdominal palpation.
- All findings must be accurately recorded.

3.2. Nutrition During Pregnancy

The Academy of Nutrition and Dietetics recommends the following key components of a healthy lifestyle during pregnancy:

- Appropriate weight gain;
- A balanced diet;
- Regular exercise;
- Appropriate and timely vitamin and mineral supplementation.

3.2.1. Dietary and Caloric Recommendations

It takes about 300 extra calories per day to keep a pregnancy healthy. A balanced diet rich in protein, fruits, vegetables, and whole grains should provide these calories. Limiting sweets and fats is a good idea. A nutritious, well-balanced diet can also aid in the reduction of certain pregnancy side effects, like nausea and constipation.

3.2.2. Fluid Intake During Pregnancy

Fluid intake is also an important part of pregnancy nutrition. Follow these recommendations for fluid intake during pregnancy:

- You can take in enough fluids by drinking several glasses of water each day, in addition to the fluids in juices and soups. Talk to your healthcare provider or midwife about restricting your intake of caffeine and artificial sweeteners.
- Avoid all forms of alcohol.

3.2.3. Ideal Foods to Eat During Pregnancy

The following foods are beneficial to your health and fetal development during pregnancy (Figure 3.1):

- **Vegetables:** Carrots, sweet potatoes, pumpkin, spinach, cooked greens, tomatoes, and red sweet peppers (for vitamin A and potassium).
- **Fruits:** Cantaloupe, honeydew, mangoes, prunes, bananas, apricots, oranges, and red or pink grapefruit (for potassium).
- **Dairy:** Fat-free or low-fat yogurt, skim or 1% milk, soymilk (for calcium, potassium, vitamins A and D).
- **Grains:** Ready-to-eat cereals/cooked cereals (for iron and folic acid).
- **Proteins:** Beans and peas; nuts and seeds; lean beef, lamb and pork; salmon, trout, herring, sardines and pollock.

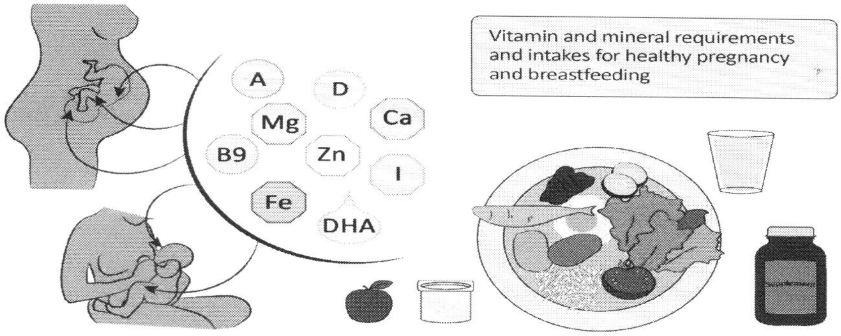

Figure 3.1. *Nutrition in pregnancy.*

Source: *Jouanne, M., Oddoux, S., Noël, A., & Voisin-Chiret, A. S., (2021). Nutrient requirements during pregnancy and lactation. Nutrients, 13(2), 692. https://doi.org/10.3390/nu13020692.*

3.2.4. Foods to Avoid During Pregnancy

Avoid eating the following foods during pregnancy:

- Unpasteurized milk and foods made with unpasteurized milk (soft cheeses, including feta, queso blanco and fresco, Camembert, brie or blue-veined cheeses—unless labeled "made with pasteurized milk").
- Hot dogs and luncheon meats (unless they are heated until steaming hot before serving).
- Raw and undercooked seafood, eggs and meat.
- Refrigerated pâté and meat spreads.
- Refrigerated smoked seafood.

3.2.5. Guidelines for Safe Food Handling

Follow these general food safety guidelines when handling and cooking food:

- **Wash:** Rinse all raw produce thoroughly under running tap water before eating, cutting or cooking.
- **Clean:** Wash your hands, knives, countertops and cutting boards after handling and preparing uncooked foods.
- **Cook:** Cook beef, pork or poultry to a safe internal temperature verified by a food thermometer.
- **Chill:** Promptly refrigerate all perishable food.

3.2.6. Prenatal Vitamin and Mineral Supplements

Before or soon after conception, the majority of medical professionals and midwives will recommend a prenatal supplement to ensure that all of your nutritional requirements are satisfied. Prenatal supplements, however, do not take the place of a balanced diet.

3.2.6.1. The Importance of Folic Acid

The U.S. Public Health Service recommends that all women of childbearing age consume 400 micrograms (0.4 mg) of folic acid each day. Folic acid is a nutrient found in:

- Some green leafy vegetables;
- Most berries, nuts, beans, citrus fruits and fortified breakfast cereals;
- Some vitamin supplements.

Birth defects of the brain and spinal cord known as neural tube defects can be prevented in part by taking folic acid. Different degrees of paralysis, incontinence, and occasionally intellectual disability can result from neural tube defects. Since most neural tube defects occur in the first 28 days after conception, folic acid is most beneficial during this time.

Unfortunately, it's possible that you won't become aware of your pregnancy until 28 days. As a result, you should start taking folic acid before getting pregnant and keep doing so all the way through your pregnancy. Your midwife or doctor will advise you on the right dosage of folic acid based on your unique requirements.

3.3. Common Health Problems During Pregnancy

Your feelings and thoughts could shoot through the roof when you find out you're expecting. You may be equally as nervous about something going wrong as you are about this new person you are bringing into the world.

Although most pregnancies progress smoothly, approximately 8% of pregnancies experience complications that can pose risks to the mother or baby if left untreated. These complications can arise from pre-existing health issues or unexpectedly. It is natural to feel scared when a complication is diagnosed, worrying about the health of the baby and yourself, and feeling guilt about possibly causing it. However, it is important to know that these complications are not your fault and are treatable. Seeking prenatal care from a trusted provider is crucial for early detection and proper management of complications, ultimately increasing the likelihood of a healthy outcome for both you and your baby.

Pregnancy can cause health issues for some women. These issues may pertain to the health of the fetus, the mother, or both. Problems can arise even in healthy women before they become pregnant. These issues could turn the pregnancy into a high-risk one. By allowing medical professionals to identify, treat, or manage conditions before they worsen, receiving early and consistent prenatal care can help lower the risk of issues. Identification of pregnancy-related mental health issues like anxiety and depression is another benefit of prenatal care. Some common complications of pregnancy include but are not limited to, the following.

3.3.1. High Blood Pressure

Reduced artery flow from the heart to the body's organs results in high blood pressure, also known as hypertension. The arteries' pressure rises as a result. This can make it more difficult for blood to get to the placenta during pregnancy, which gives the fetus oxygen and nutrition. Decreased blood flow can cause the fetus to grow more slowly and increase the mother's risk of preterm labor and preeclampsia (Figure 3.2).

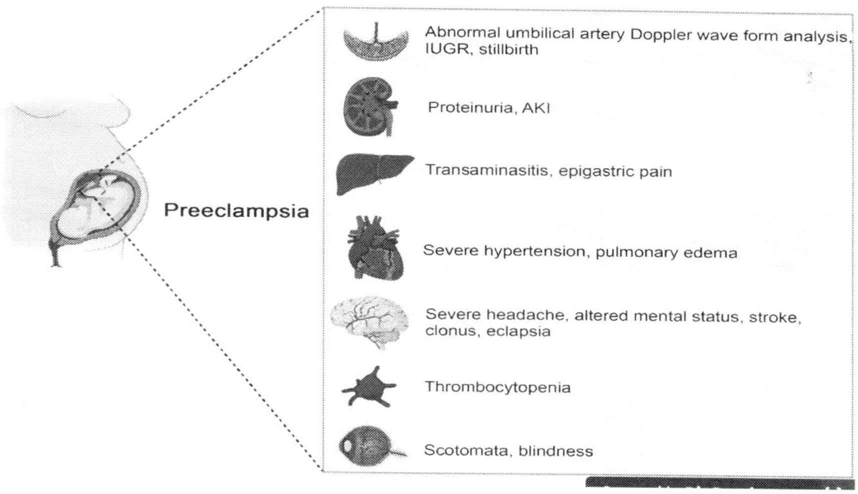

Figure 3.2. *Gestational hypertension.*

Source: *Longhitano, E., Siligato, R., Torreggiani, M., Attini, R., Masturzo, B., Casula, V., Matarazzo, I., Cabiddu, G., Santoro, D., Versino, E., et al., (2022). The hypertensive disorders of pregnancy: A focus on definitions for clinical nephrologists. Journal of Clinical Medicine, 11(12), 3420. https://doi.org/10.3390/jcm11123420.*

Pregnant women with high blood pressure will need to keep an eye on it and manage it during their pregnancy, possibly with medication. Gestational hypertension is a term used to describe high blood pressure that occurs during pregnancy. Gestational hypertension usually manifests in the second half of pregnancy and resolves postpartum.

3.3.2. Gestational Diabetes

When a woman who had never had diabetes before becomes pregnant and becomes pregnant with the disease, this is known as gestational diabetes. Normally, when food is broken down by the body, glucose—a type of sugar—is produced. Your body uses glucose as its primary energy source. The glucose enters your bloodstream after digestion and provides your body with energy. Your pancreas produces the hormone insulin, which helps your body absorb glucose from the blood and use it in its cells. Gestational diabetes is a condition in which the body either produces insufficient insulin or uses it improperly due to hormonal changes brought on by pregnancy. Instead, diabetes, also referred to as high blood sugar, is brought on by an accumulation of glucose in the blood.

Controlling gestational diabetes through adherence to a physician's prescribed treatment plan is the most effective means of mitigating or averting complications linked to elevated blood sugar levels during pregnancy. If left unchecked, it can result in preeclampsia, which raises blood pressure, and having a big baby, which raises the risk of cesarean delivery.

3.3.3. Infections

During pregnancy and/or delivery, infections, including certain STIs, can occur. These infections can cause complications for the pregnant woman, the pregnancy, and the baby after delivery. Certain infections can spread from mother to child through the birth canal during childbirth, while other infections can affect a developing fetus during pregnancy. With the right prenatal, perinatal, and postpartum care, many of these infections can be avoided or treated.

Some infections in pregnancy can cause or contribute to:

- Pregnancy loss/miscarriage (before 20 weeks of pregnancy);
- Ectopic pregnancy (when the embryo implants outside of the uterus, usually in a fallopian tube);
- Preterm labor and delivery (before 37 completed weeks of pregnancy);
- Low birth weight;
- Birth defects, including blindness, deafness, bone deformities, and intellectual disability;
- Stillbirth (at or after 20 weeks of pregnancy);
- Illness in the newborn period (first month of life);
- Newborn death;
- Maternal health complications.

Consult your healthcare provider about receiving vaccinations against chickenpox, also known as varicella, and rubella, also known as German measles, as well as booster shots before becoming pregnant if you intend to become pregnant. Additionally, you can receive certain vaccinations, like the flu shot, while you are expecting. To improve your chances of a successful pregnancy, discuss any infections you may have, such as STIs, with your doctor before becoming pregnant.

If an infection can be treated with medication, it can be detected early in pregnancy through testing for STIs and other infections. Alternatively, as soon as possible during your pregnancy, disclose any infections you are aware of to your healthcare provider. The risk to the fetus and baby is reduced with early intervention. You and your healthcare provider can take precautions to safeguard your health and the health of your infant even in the event that the infection cannot be cured.

3.3.4. Preeclampsia

Blood pressure that is dangerously high is a symptom of preeclampsia. If treatment is not received, it may be fatal. After 20 weeks of pregnancy, preeclampsia usually develops in women who have never had high blood pressure before. Preeclampsia symptoms can include pain beneath the ribs, a strong headache, and vision changes. Many women, though, do not experience symptoms immediately. Usually, the first warning sign is when a woman with high blood pressure shows up for a routine prenatal visit. In those circumstances, to distinguish between preeclampsia and high blood pressure, your doctor will perform tests to assess liver and kidney function.

Preeclampsia is a serious medical condition that can lead to preterm delivery and death. Its cause is unknown, but some women are at an increased risk. Risk factors include:

- First pregnancies;
- Preeclampsia in a previous pregnancy;

- Existing conditions such as high blood pressure, diabetes, kidney disease, and systemic lupus erythematosus;
- Being 35 years of age or older;
- Carrying two or more fetuses;
- Obesity.

Preeclampsia cannot be avoided, but maintaining good health may help during pregnancy. Experts advise seeing your obstetrician before getting pregnant or very early in the pregnancy if you have risk factors so you and your doctor can talk about ways to lower your risk. For instance, after the first trimester, many women who are at risk for preeclampsia are prescribed a baby aspirin. The best way to manage preeclampsia is through routine prenatal visits. Your blood pressure will be taken by your doctor during those scheduled visits. If it's high, additional testing can identify the ailment and begin the necessary treatment.

The best course of treatment for preeclampsia is delivery since the condition only goes away after the baby is born. On the other hand, premature birth increases the baby's risk of health issues. The decision regarding your course of treatment will be primarily based on the stage of pregnancy. Hospitalization might be necessary so that your team can keep a close eye on both you and your infant. Your physician will talk to you about the advantages and disadvantages of an early delivery vs. extending the pregnancy and attempting to treat the preeclampsia for as long as possible using alternative techniques. The condition will go away after delivery, but you will have a higher chance of developing heart disease in the future. Discuss with your physician the steps you can take to mitigate and control those risks.

3.3.5. Preterm Labor

Labor that starts earlier than 37 weeks of pregnancy is known as preterm labor. The final weeks before a full-term delivery (39 to 40 weeks) are when organs like the brain and lungs finish developing, so any baby born before 37 weeks is usually at risk for health issues. Preterm labor can result from several conditions, such as infections, shortened cervix development, or preterm births in the past. In certain cases, progesterone, a hormone that is naturally produced during pregnancy, may be used to help prevent preterm birth.

3.3.6. Depression and Anxiety

Studies reveal that up to 13% of U.S. Anxiety co-occurs in as many as 43% of depressed pregnant and postpartum women, and women reported frequent depressive symptoms following childbirth, making pregnancy-related anxiety and depression among the more common pregnancy complications. The mother's and her child's health may be significantly impacted by these medical conditions. The good news is that these illnesses are medically treatable.

3.3.7. Pregnancy Loss/Miscarriage

A pregnancy lost due to natural causes before 20 weeks of pregnancy is referred to as a miscarriage. Symptoms may include cramping, tissue or fluid leaking from the vagina, or vaginal spotting or bleeding. Vaginal bleeding, however, does not indicate that a miscarriage is occurring or will occur.

If a woman notices this symptom at any stage of her pregnancy, she should speak with her doctor.

3.3.8. Stillbirth

A stillbirth occurs when a pregnancy ends after the 20th week of gestation. Medical professionals are unable to determine the cause of the loss in about half of all cases that are reported. However, chromosomal abnormalities, placental issues, low fetal growth, long-term mother health problems, and infection are among the medical conditions that can lead to stillbirth.

3.3.9. Other Complications

Other complications of pregnancy may include the following:

- **Severe, Persistent Nausea, and Vomiting:** Although having some nausea and vomiting is normal during pregnancy, particularly in the first trimester, some women experience more severe symptoms that last into the third trimester.

The cause of the more severe form of this problem, known as hyperemesis gravidarum (pronounced *HEYE-pur-EM-uh-suhss grav-uh-DAR-uhm*), is not known. Women with hyperemesis gravidarum experience nausea that does not go away, weight loss, reduced appetite, dehydration, and feeling faint.

Affected women may need to be hospitalized so that they can receive fluids and nutrients. Some women feel better after their 20th week of pregnancy, while others experience the symptoms throughout their pregnancy.

- **Iron-Deficiency Anemia:** Because they are producing more blood than usual, pregnant women require more iron than usual. Low iron levels in the body during pregnancy can lead to iron-deficiency anemia, which is linked to low birth weight and preterm delivery. Flushing or feeling lightheaded, having trouble breathing, and turning pale are signs of an iron deficiency. To lessen the risk of iron-deficiency anemia, ACOG suggests taking 27 milligrams of iron daily, which is present in most prenatal vitamins. Certain women might require additional iron through supplementation. If you have iron-deficiency anemia, your doctor may screen you for it and suggest iron supplements if necessary.

3.4. Psychological Changes in Pregnancy

We will start by talking about the typical psychological changes that occur during pregnancy, which are thought to be particularly significant for medical and psychological practice. Our focus is on the potential role that psychological and psychosocial variables may play in the development of obstetric complications and, in turn, the morbidity that befalls newborns.

The first authors to acknowledge the intricacy of the psychological challenges associated with pregnancy and motherhood were psychoanalytic writers. Pregnancy brings with it aspects of narcissistic fulfillment, regressive tendencies, anxiety, psychological difficulties, and resurgence of conflicts from previous developmental stages. Bibring (1959) was one of the first to assert that, regardless of a mother's psychological condition, pregnancy is a psychobiological crisis that affects all expectant mothers. Like all "normal" crises that mark a turning point in life, it causes an acute disequilibrium but, given the right circumstances, can lead to a new degree of psychological development and integration. The resolution of this crisis has a significant impact on the woman's life as well as the early mother-child bond.

Subsequently, several empirical studies were conducted that provided information on the behavioral, cognitive, and emotional changes that occur during pregnancy. Although there has been little evidence of significant mental illness during pregnancy, tension, ambivalence, elevated anxiety, exhaustion, and elevated depression are frequently reported symptoms. Individual experiences with these emotional states, however, differ widely.

Due to the wide range of emotional changes that can occur during pregnancy, there has been a greater focus on the potential impact that psychological disorders may have on the course of pregnancy, labor, and delivery, as well as the child's development after birth. Pregnancy symptoms like backache, dizziness, fatigue, gastrointestinal discomforts, nausea, and pernicious vomiting were found to be indicative of ambivalence toward the pregnancy and of high anxiety levels; prolonged labor time was found to be positively correlated to maternal anxiety; prematurity and low birth weight were significantly associated with anxiety, and several correlational studies have shown that psychological and psychosocial factors during pregnancy are associated with an increased risk of physical complications. The study also found that pseudocyesis was a function of a simultaneous strong unconscious mother wish and fear of pregnancy; habitual spontaneous abortion was linked to anxiety, immaturity, and dependency, as well as uncertainty concerning the husband.

However, it should be highlighted that a large number of the existing research, particularly the older ones, have methodological flaws that lower the validity of their conclusions. Their retrospective design, willingness to draw conclusions about causality from merely correlations, univariate methodology, disdain for a third variable that might explain the apparent relationship between a predictor and an outcome variable, haphazard assessment of anxiety, and inability to categorize complications have all drawn criticism. Nonetheless, a number of studies have made an effort to address the methodological concerns expressed, using multivariate approaches, prospective designs, and hidden variable control.

Therefore, despite methodological flaws, the overall strength of the data does point to the possibility that psychosocial factors—of which anxiety and life stress are the most frequently mentioned—may either cause or influence obstetrical difficulties. Examining mediating factors that could modify the positive linear impact of life stress and anxiety on obstetrical complications has been a significant area of research. As a result, mediating factors have been proposed, such as the person's perception of stress, their degree of readiness to handle stress, or the existence of different degrees of psychosocial support. We will go into more detail about this latter variable.

It's challenging to define "social support," and it undoubtedly varies depending on the culture. Cobb (1976) has provided a rather satisfactory definition, though, equating support with information that makes the subject feel loved and cared for, respected, and a part of a network of mutual obligations. The degree of postpartum depression symptoms was predicted by many perceived social support dimensions that were measured during pregnancy, including emotional support, understanding, and instrumental assistance. Nuckolls, Cassel, and Kaplan as well as Norbeck and Tilden looked into the relationship between life stress, social support, and obstetrical complications. Nuckolls and associates. demonstrated that women with high psychosocial assets had a third of the obstetrical complication rate compared to women with low psychosocial assets, even in the face of increasing life stress before and during pregnancy. Similarly, Norbeck and Tilden's use of a prospective, multivariate design supported the hypothesis that complications related to pregnancy and infant conditions can be predicted by high levels of life stress, high levels of emotional disequilibrium, and low levels of tangible social support.

However, social support has also been investigated as a component of a planned intervention meant to strengthen mothers' own resources for a successful pregnancy and labor, in addition to its potential as a stress-reducing variable. Given the data linking perinatal complications to a higher lifetime risk of mental illness in people with a genetic predisposition, social support during pregnancy could play a significant role in mental health prevention, a topic that is becoming more and more important.

3.5. Planned Intervention for the Alleviation of Psychological Difficulties During the Perinatal Period

Chalmers has indicated that social support systems, including family education, healthcare, doctors, and nurses, need to be both present and of high quality. This is because research has shown that expectant mothers' perception of interpersonal support appears to buffer the potential effects of life stress. To prevent potential pregnancy complications, social support personnel must conduct a realistic examination of fears and psychological issues during pregnancy. Horsley even goes so far as to say that psychological management of pregnancy is likely to be insufficient if it doesn't start at the first prenatal visit.

3.5.1. Antenatal Classes

Participating in prenatal education classes offers a chance to address psychological issues that arise during pregnancy. The loss of women's customary informal networks of support and the thinning of communication lines between them have had a significant impact on prenatal education. Prenatal classes come in a variety of forms. Some begin early in pregnancy and concentrate mainly on self-care and hygiene; others, held in the final trimester of pregnancy, essentially prepare women for labor; still others, primarily teach mother craft skills.

But all of them have one thing in common: they all teach knowledge, skills, and problem-solving techniques. The Dick-Read method, which originated in England, and the Lamaze method are essentially the two methods that represent the use of psychological or physical, non-pharmaceutical modalities for the prevention of pain during childbirth. This field of study has a pioneering history in prenatal education.

According to Dick-Read, fear, passed down through the generations from mother to daughter, is what initiates the process of anxiety. Anxiety, in turn, causes tension in the uterine circular muscle fibers, which causes stiffness at the cervix opening and, ultimately, the experience of pain. His approach includes teaching pregnancy hygiene, the anatomy and physiology of labor and delivery, breathing and relaxation techniques, and fitness drills. This education is justified by the idea that delivery-related anxiety is eliminated and replaced with a more carefree attitude.

Although the French obstetrician Lamaze (1970) is credited with giving rise to the Lamaze method of childbirth preparation, the technique actually began in the Soviet Union towards the end of the 1950s and is based on Pavlov's theory of conditioning. The principles of Pavlov's theory were applied: verbal stimuli are just as effective as any other form of reinforcement; a stimulus acting on a specific area of the brain irradiates the specialized centers while the surrounding areas become nonresponsive to other incoming stimuli; and conditioned reflexes are formed within the nervous system and become associated by a temporary neurological bond that is subsequently reinforced by repetition. As a result, if an individual experiences fear or pain in response to the stimulation of uterine contractions, it is likely a learned or conditioned response that can be suppressed or substituted with a more positive emotion. In addition, the breathing exercises women use during labor produce such a potent activation that other parts of the cerebral cortex are prevented from reacting to stimuli coming from the uterus, which would be perceived as painful. Lastly, women can be trained to minimize pain, discomfort, and fear in response to verbal cues during labor. Small groups receive instruction in Lamaze training, which includes topics such as anatomy and physiology, breathing exercises, conditioned relaxation, cognitive restructuring, and social support from medical professionals and a "coach."

Katona (1981) the development of prenatal education and notes how the focus has shifted over time from the psychosocial aspects of reproduction to labor pain, medication use, and other aspects of labor. Historically, women's experiences have been undervalued and knowledge provision has been overestimated in preventive strategies. The more modern approaches to prenatal education place a greater emphasis on topics like the emotional changes of pregnancy, the underlying mechanisms of pregnancy symptoms, the relationship with the partner, sexuality patterns, the preparation of the other children in the family, enhanced self-esteem and satisfaction, accepting a new role, and a smooth postpartum adjustment, even though the physiological aspects of the reproductive process are undoubtedly useful. Prenatal classes may also be directed towards the partner of the mother. There is now a need for men to be prepared for child care and birthing due to the sharp increase in the number of men attending births. Men want to know how childbirth works, how it might make them and their wives feel, and what to anticipate during the postpartum phase.

Kitzinger (1988) developed a type of childbirth preparation class that is representative of the more modern approach. Having researched childbearing in a variety of cultural contexts, including the Caribbean, the US, and Africa, Kitzinger has created her own "psychosexual approach" to childbirth, accounting for women's emotional states as well as the network of relationships and the specific culture in which they are entangled. Women experience pain differently, according to Kitzinger, because it is always interpreted and situated within a personally and culturally predetermined framework. Prenatal education now addresses a much wider range of consumers and covers a far wider spectrum of ideologies, methods, content, and scope because it is no longer solely focused on pain reduction.

3.5.2. The Effectiveness of Antenatal Classes

It makes sense that there would be special interest in determining how effective prenatal classes are. Numerous factors play a role in determining this effectiveness, including the type and caliber of teachers, the teaching methodology used, the subject matter covered in the classes, and the attendance patterns.

It appears that no research has been done to link the characteristics of teachers or their methods of instruction to how well students apply their newly acquired knowledge in the workplace. Research indicates that the majority of attendees are women who are pregnant for the first time and those who have previously only had unsuccessful pregnancies. These are the characteristics of the attendees. Additionally, several socioeconomic factors and attendance have a strong correlation.

The demographics of women who do not attend classes include being younger, being poorer, having dropped out of school earlier, and having a lower likelihood of getting married. The middle classes have been the primary audience for prenatal education.

However, since prenatal classes are now regularly provided in more clinics, it is envisaged that lower-class women will also begin to gain from them. Only 12 of the 24 survey countries were able to provide estimates of the percentages of pregnant women attending classes; these estimates range from 10% to 90% of pregnant women, according to having a baby in Europe (1985) study. We are unable to provide estimates for attendance in the United States at this time, but in the late 1960s, very few expectant mothers were using childbirth preparation.

While there is little evidence that traditional classes improve the mechanical aspects of labor and delivery, Katona notes in her review of the literature on prenatal education that measuring the emotional effects has received less attention. Nonetheless, some research indicates that prenatal classes positively impact physiological and psychological outcome variables. It should be noted that there are significant methodological challenges in conducting a sufficient trial of prenatal childbirth preparation. The study conducted by Timm (1979) in Pittsburgh with 146 very low-income women is the only example of a three-group design that includes non-trained controls, placebo controls, and trained women; random assignment of women stratified for age, race, and parity to each group; and raters' ignorance of women's specific membership. The women who had taken prenatal classes, according to the results, utilized considerably fewer painkillers during labor and delivery.

Results from additional research also show that women who had received prenatal childbirth education were more likely to have spontaneous deliveries and that pain medication was used much less frequently and in smaller doses. Other obstetrical benefits of prenatal education have also been recognized: trained women had a significant reduction in cesarean sections, postpartum infections, premature births, cases of pregnancy-related toxemia, postpartum hemorrhage, and peritoneal tears compared to controls; additionally, their babies had higher Apgar scores at both the one- and five-minute mark.

Attendees showed more positive views toward pregnancy, labor, and delivery, themselves, their partners, and their children, according to the findings of studies looking at how prenatal training affected mothers' attitudes toward the self, the father, the baby, and the entire process. Women had significantly lower recollections of pain in all three studies, and they also typically took less medication, had fewer general anesthesias, and had less than half as many local anesthesias. Happiness during childbirth and less pain are not entirely independent, as the research by Norr, Block, Charles, Meyering, and Meyers and Charles, Norr, Block, Meyering, and Meyers make clear. A more positive experience of labor and delivery in women who had attended prenatal classes in comparison to non-attenders is also mentioned by Davenport-Slack and Boylan, Enkin et al., and Huttel et al.

A decrease in anxiety related to childbirth was noted in women who followed childbirth preparation classes, while Zax et al. and Klusman found that trained women had significantly lower anxiety levels both before and after the training.

There hasn't been much study done on how successful male preparation programs are. While Felton and Segelman tested men in the final class but before the birth, they discovered that they had shifted toward seeing themselves more in control to a greater extent than untrained men. Manion reports that men who had attended prenatal classes participated more in labor and delivery than those who did not. Contrarily, Wente and Crockenberg discovered that fathers who had gone to childbirth education classes did not report having an easier time adjusting compared to controls.

Studies have been conducted on the relationship between information provision, respiration, conditioned relaxation, cognitive restructuring, and social support as potential psychological mechanisms linked to the positive effects of prenatal training. The specific elements of prenatal education that are involved in lowering anxiety and discomfort are outlined in a review by Wideman and Singer: information sharing during labor preparation was found to have a strong positive association with attitudes toward the newborn and the number of painkillers used during labor. However, rather than merely describing the objective aspects of the impending event, this relationship seems to be more likely if the information is descriptive/sensory, involving a thorough explanation of the sensations likely to be experienced during the procedure. Controlled breathing can significantly lower autonomic reactivity to a stressful stimulus; however, no research has been done on this topic in relation to getting ready for childbirth. An additional theory regarding respiration is that it could cause the body to secrete endogenous analgesics, which include enkephalins and endorphins, which have been demonstrated to have morphomimetic properties. There hasn't been any research done on these amino acid chains and pregnancy in humans, though. A counterconditioning program of systematic desensitization, in which the progression of contractions is met with a relaxation response, and techniques that contrast tense muscles with a state of relaxation form the basis of the relaxation regimen taught during childbirth preparation training. Lastly, research has looked at social support's ability to mitigate the negative effects of stress. On those studies, we previously reported. Even though social support has been shown to have positive effects, there are still unanswered questions about the mechanisms underlying these findings.

Though many of the results are based on self-report measures and anecdotal reports, methodological issues have been raised again regarding the systematic documentation of the benefits of antenatal education; measurement techniques have not always been satisfactory; findings are not consistently confirmed; attitudinal changes are likely secondary to decreased medication use; observer biases are present; and, generally, it is very difficult to design well-controlled studies.

3.5.3. Controlled Trials of Explicit Social and Psychological Support in the Perinatal Period

Prenatal classes may include general social and psychological support for expectant and new mothers, but it's also possible that this kind of care could be provided as part of routine prenatal care. Provisions like intensive prenatal care, more frequent check-ups, home visits, phone calls, a 24-hour hotline, family-centered care, emotional support, education about health-related behavior and signs of preterm labor, information/feedback sharing, and free transportation could all be included in this general support package, etc.

Elbourne, Oakley, and Chalmers (1989) reviewed 14 controlled trials of the kind described above pertaining to increased social and psychological support during pregnancy. Giving social and psychological support was the main goal of six of those studies; in the other eight, this goal was stated explicitly but was not the primary focus of the trial. These later studies mostly concentrated on information sharing and feedback, care organization, or getting ready for pregnancy, childbirth, and parenthood.

Overall, the evidence from those trials of increased social and psychological support points to several positive psychological and behavioral effects: mothers who received support were more likely than controls to report feeling "in control" of their pregnancies, to attend antenatal classes, to feel happy, nervous, and worried during their pregnancies, and to be satisfied with the antenatal care they had received. They were also less likely to have negative feelings about the impending birth. Moreover, women who received support were also more likely to report that their labor was worry-free and to have a companion with them. Following delivery, the women who had received more support during their pregnancy were less likely than the controls to feel unhappy, to be nursing their baby when they were discharged from the hospital, and to have their partner help with baby care.

Finally, six weeks after giving birth, the experimental group's mothers were more likely than the controls to continue to breastfeed, to feel "in control," and to have started feeding the infant solid foods. At six weeks postpartum, women in the experimental group were less likely than controls to be feeling physically ill, and their babies were less likely to have concerning health issues. This was a physical manifestation of the positive psychological effects. Lastly, no adverse effects of increased social and psychological support during pregnancy were noted in any of these controlled trials.

Rae Grant cites another recent review of 30 publications detailing supportive prevention programs that span the prenatal and early infancy periods in North America, England, and Australia. It was determined that the programs with the biggest effects were those that included a variety of elements, lasted a long time—between two and five years—started early in pregnancy, and included home visits as a key element. Numerous beneficial effects, both immediate and long-term, were discovered. Better physical health, better nutrition from parents, fewer low birth weight babies, fewer feeding issues, fewer accidents and ER visits, and a lower incidence of child abuse were the short-term effects on children, while better social support networks, increased confidence, better parenting skills, improved parent-child relationships, fewer child abuse incidents, longer intervals between pregnancies, and more frequent, appropriate service use were the short-term effects on parents. Long-term effects of prenatal/pregnancy programming included decreased school aggression and distractibility, decreased delinquency, improved school attitudes, improved social functioning, and higher rates of prosocial attitudes in children. Mothers who had taken part in these programs had greater levels of education, and family employment rates were higher.

Currently underway is a new multicultural controlled supportive prenatal/infancy program, funded by the European Communities and started by the World Health Organization's Regional Office for Europe. Specific supportive intervention techniques are being tested in several Mediterranean countries (Cyprus, Greece, New Yugoslavia, Portugal, Slovenia, and Turkey) to promote the psychosocial development of children. These techniques are administered by primary healthcare workers to mothers at eight different time points, ranging from the last trimester of pregnancy to the child's 24 months of life. The ultimate objective is to encourage the application of the developed intervention strategies across the primary healthcare network in the participating nations.

Although the focus of this paper is pregnancy, it is important to note that continuous human support during labor and delivery can also have significant positive effects on the perinatal stage. In the past, standard birth practices have included women providing continuous social support to one another during labor in a large number of cultures. In studies designed by Sosa, Kennell, Klaus, Robertson, and Urrutia as well as Klaus, Kennell, Robertson, and Sosa, continuous support during labor was implemented. The perinatal complications, such as meconium staining, stillbirths, cesarean sections, forceps deliveries, and oxytocin augmentation, as well as the number of depressed newborns and neonates admitted to neonatal intensive care, were considerably lower in the women who had supportive female companions during labor than in the control group. The women who labored with a companion experienced a significantly shorter labor period than those who did not. Furthermore, compared to unsupported moms, supported mothers behaved differently with their newborns, showing them more affection through stroking, talking, and smiling. The authors concluded that the companion's presence might explain why the obstetrician performed fewer interventions, but they appear to prefer theories that focused more on the companion's potential effects on the mother. Social support may shorten the labor's duration by reducing anxiety in women who are in labor and preventing an increase in catecholamine concentrations, which would otherwise cause uterine muscle contractions to increase. Based on research on animals, where stress can lower uterine and placental blood flow and subsequently oxygenate the fetus, the authors hypothesize that social support could lower the number of newborns admitted to intensive care. Replication is necessary, though, to investigate the mechanisms by which support affects physiological processes in more detail.

3.6. Psychosocial Effects of the Actual Provision of Prenatal Care

Social circumstances have an impact on women's health, prenatal care utilization, and response to it. Women with less favorable sociodemographic traits typically receive less appropriate prenatal care. Low-risk women typically attend antenatal clinics earlier and more frequently, according to research conducted in various nations with widely disparate prenatal care systems, including the United States, the United Kingdom, and France. These are typically older, married, primiparae, and socioeconomically more affluent women.

The women who need it most, those from socially disadvantaged backgrounds, do not appear to have benefited most from the advancements in prenatal care. One common excuse for nonattendance is a lack of acceptance or access to antenatal clinics. Socially marginalized women frequently exhibit low confidence in the services they receive, feel ashamed of their precarious circumstances, find it difficult to communicate with caregivers, and frequently fail to heed advice. Furthermore, compared to middle-class women, women from lower socioeconomic classes indicate a desire for more information. Because all pregnancies have the potential to be pathological, the idea that all pregnant women should receive the same care has become increasingly prevalent in prenatal care across many nations. As a result, the opinions of women regarding the procedures and their execution have frequently been ignored in prenatal care research. Throughout the past 10 years, researchers—particularly those in the UK—have focused on women's satisfaction with the various aspects of care due to the realization that disgruntled customers make ineffective prenatal attendants. Pregnant women generally view prenatal care as important, but they do not appear to feel that they personally benefit much from it, and they are unable to articulate why they should attend. According to all the studies, women want more personal care—less waiting time, more visits with the same doctor, improved communication with medical staff, more opportunities to ask questions and get clear answers, and more consideration for their needs and concerns. The women give two explanations for their incapacity to ask questions: either they perceive the doctors as hurried or as intimidating. However, medical professionals often believe that women ask questions because they are anxious, and that the primary goal of responding to them is to allay their fears rather than to impart knowledge. Furthermore, there is evidence to suggest that a portion of the communication breakdown stems from the mismatch between what doctors consider important and what women consider to be threatening. Last but not least, some prenatal care literature may create unrealistic expectations in women, making them anticipate a level of individualized attention that they are unlikely to receive.

There is more data on how women view interventions used during labor and delivery than there are studies that explain how they feel about the various procedures they undergo during pregnancy. Oakley documents the professionals' unwillingness to adequately explain the reasoning behind the various procedures carried out during pregnancy, as well as the ensuing outcomes and the resulting increase in women's anxiety. When it comes to the ultrasound scan's impact, women who are still struggling to accept their pregnancy will benefit the most since it lends the event more realism. However, the closer proximity to the fetus may also make the mother feel more vulnerable to the pregnancy's outcome, which could lead to worry. Regarding amniocentesis, it has been observed that women experience anxiety before the test because they fear it could harm the fetus or result in miscarriage. However, once the results are known, this anxiety subsides for the remainder of the pregnancy.

The role that pregnant women have in their own care is a last but crucial point to consider. Most of the time, they merely follow directions and have little to no control over the officially approved care they get. The increasing involvement of women in identifying their health needs, organizing their services, and selecting how they will be used is an area that will require experimentation in the future.

3.7. Routine Screening and Diagnostic Tests

If you are pregnant, a variety of tests are available. These tests can both verify your pregnancy and track the growth of your unborn child inside you. Additionally, there are optional tests available that can reveal whether a pregnancy is impacted by a variety of conditions. Pregnancy care should include routine check-ups with your doctor or midwife, as well as guidance and information about the tests you and your unborn child may require.

The different kinds of tests available to pregnant women include tests (Figure 3.3):

- to confirm pregnancy;
- to monitor the health of the mother and the baby;
- maternal health screening;
- for specific medical problems (screening and diagnostic tests).

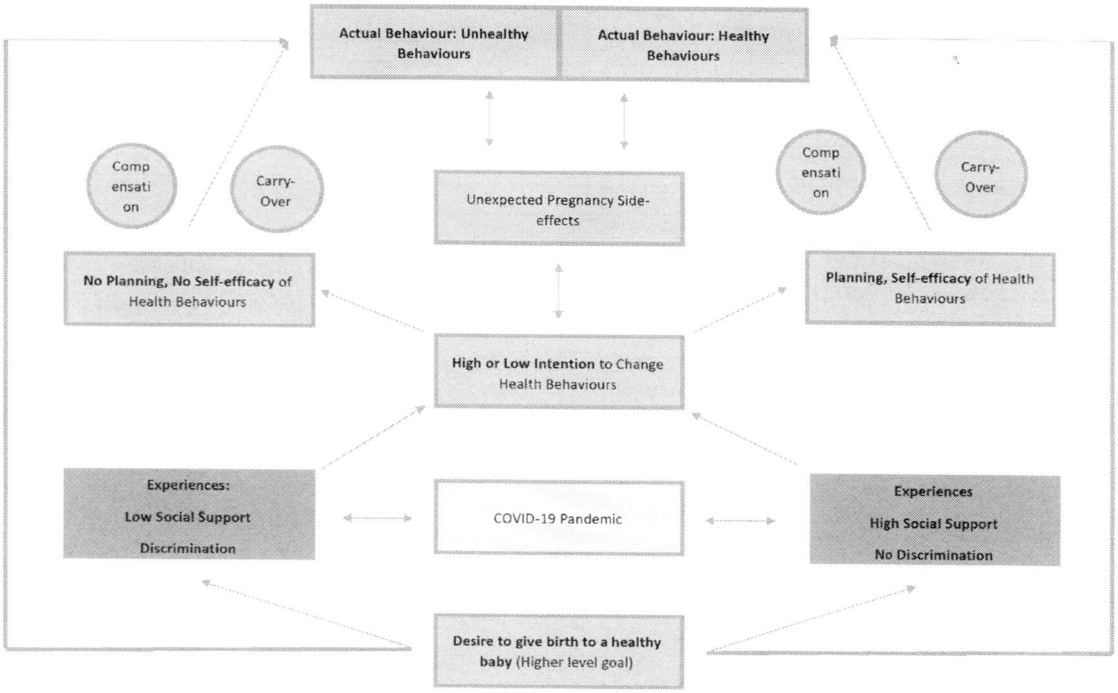

Figure 3.3. *Schematic illustration with the assumption of the compensatory carry-over action model (CCAM) for changes in pregnancy.*

Source: *Herzog-Petropaki, N., Derksen, C., & Lippke, S., (2022). Health behaviors and behavior change during pregnancy: Theory-based investigation of predictors and interrelations. Sexes, 3(3), 351–366. https://doi.org/10.3390/sexes3030027.*

3.7.1. Tests to Confirm Pregnancy

A missed menstrual period is usually the first sign of pregnancy. Tests to confirm pregnancy detect a pregnancy hormone called human chorionic gonadotropin (βhCG).

The various tests include:

- **Home Test Kit:** These are available from pharmacies. A typical kit includes special paper that is sensitive to the presence of βhCG in urine. It is important to use a home test kit according to the manufacturer's instructions, or false results can occur. Always confirm your results with your doctor. Pregnancy tests taken by your doctor are rarely inaccurate.
- **Urine Test at the Doctor's Office:** The doctor can test your urine for βhCG.
- **Blood Test:** A test of the βhCG levels in your blood can be accurate within one week or so of conception.

3.7.2. Prenatal Tests to Monitor the Health of the Mother and the Baby

To monitor your pregnancy and the growth of the unborn child, scheduling routine check-ups with your doctor or midwife is part of pregnancy care. This includes tests to monitor your health and the health of your unborn child, as well as tests to help rule out any possible pregnancy complications.

Routine prenatal tests may include:

- **Maternal Health Screening Blood Tests:** At different stages of the pregnancy, such as blood group, iron levels, checks for maternal diabetes, immunity to rubella and other infections.
- **Ultrasound (First Trimester):** A painless, non-invasive scan done within the first 3 months of pregnancy. This can be used to confirm the number of babies and helps to calculate the date you are due to give birth. This is known as your estimated due date.
- **Ultrasound (Second Trimester):** This is usually performed between 18 and 20 weeks. It is used to check the baby's development, and monitor the size and location of the placenta. The baby's sex can often be determined (if you wish to know), although this may not be 100% accurate.
- **Ultrasound (Third Trimester):** In the last 3 months of pregnancy, an ultrasound may be offered to check the baby's growth, fluid levels around the baby and the positioning of the placenta.

3.7.3. Tests for Specific Medical Conditions in Pregnancy

It is not required to get tested for certain medical conditions, such as Down syndrome, genetic disorders known to run in families, or neural tube abnormalities like spina bifida. Before deciding whether to move forward with these tests, a woman may want to talk through her options with her doctors or a genetic counselor.

3.7.4. Screening Tests and Diagnostic Tests in Pregnancy

Knowing the distinction between diagnostic and screening tests is crucial. Screening tests are unable to offer a definitive answer, but they can provide information about the likelihood that a baby may have a specific health issue. A diagnostic test provides a more definite result.

3.7.4.1. Routine Screening Tests

Screening tests are used to identify individuals who are more likely to have a health issue. This implies that individuals can receive treatment sooner, which may be more effective, or make well-informed decisions regarding their health. Screening exams aren't flawless. Some people will be informed that they or their unborn child are more likely to have a certain health condition, even though this is not the case. Furthermore, some individuals may receive information suggesting that they or their child have a lower likelihood of developing a health condition when, in reality, they do.

Screening tests can give an indication of the likelihood of a baby having certain conditions, but they are not diagnostic. If a screening test shows a higher chance of a particular condition, additional tests can be done to confirm the findings.

Examples of routine screening tests include:

- **Combined First-Trimester Screening:** This test combines information from a first-trimester ultrasound (e.g., a measurement taken from the back of the baby's neck known as the nuchal translucency) and a blood test from the mother (first-trimester maternal serum screening) to calculate the chance of a group of chromosome differences, including Down syndrome.

- **Second-Trimester Maternal Serum Screening:** This is a maternal blood test that helps to determine the chance of some conditions that may affect the unborn baby, such as chromosome differences (including Down syndrome) or neural tube defects (such as spina bifida).
- **Non-Invasive Prenatal Testing (NIPT, also known as Cell-Free DNA Screening):** It is a blood test that looks at the baby's genetic material (DNA), which can be found in the mother's bloodstream. It can provide information about the chance of conditions such as Down syndrome and some other chromosome differences and can be done any time from 10 weeks into the pregnancy. It is more accurate than combined first-trimester screening or second-trimester maternal serum screening, but it is more costly than the screening tests.

3.7.4.2. Diagnostic Tests

Certain pregnancies are known to carry a higher risk of a specific condition. For instance, the mother might be older (we know that the chance of having a baby with a chromosome difference such as Down syndrome increases with age) or there might be a family history of an inherited disorder. In other situations, a pregnancy screening test might have indicated a higher risk of a specific ailment. More precise information regarding the existence of a condition can be obtained through a diagnostic test. Certain diagnostic tests involve taking a sample of placenta or amniotic fluid with a needle, and there is a slight chance of complications, such as miscarriage (Figure 3.4).

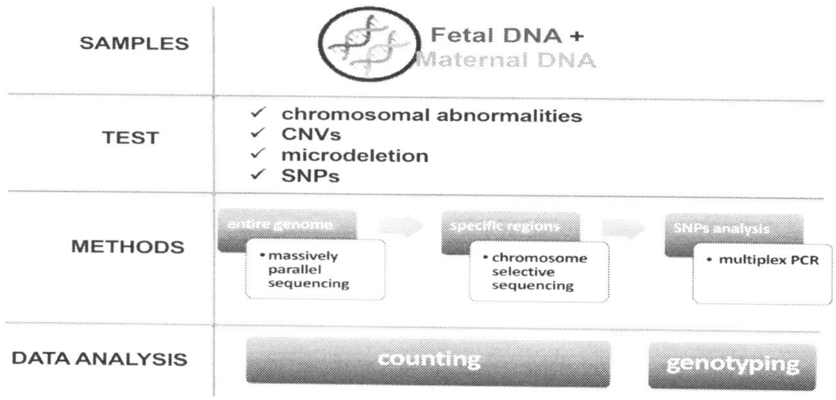

Figure 3.4. *Non-invasive prenatal test (NIPT) analysis. [CNVs: copy number variations, SNPs: single nucleotide polymorphisms].*

Source: *Carbone, L., Cariati, F., Sarno, L., Conforti, A., Bagnulo, F., Strina, I., Pastore, L., Maruotti, G. M., & Alviggi, C., (2021). Non-invasive prenatal testing: current perspectives and future challenges. Genes, 12(1), 15. https://doi.org/10.3390/genes12010015.*

Diagnostic tests include:

- **Ultrasound:** It may be used to check the health of the baby in the case of unusual pregnancy symptoms, such as vaginal bleeding or lack of fetal movement.

- **Chorionic Villus Sampling (CVS):** A test that checks for specific medical conditions by taking a sample of the placenta. The placenta was originally formed from the same cells as the baby, so testing a small sample of the placenta can provide information about the baby. To collect the sample, the doctor inserts a slender needle through the mother's abdomen. The needle is guided with the help of ultrasound. The tissue (known as a chorionic villus sample) is then examined in a laboratory.
- **Amniocentesis:** A doctor inserts a slender needle through the abdomen to withdraw a small amount of amniotic fluid, the fluid that surrounds the baby in the womb. This fluid sample contains some of the baby's cells which have been shed as the baby grows, and these are then examined in the laboratory.

3.7.5. Making Decisions About Diagnostic Testing in Pregnancy

One in 20 women are informed that their pregnancy may be complicated. Many women who have an increased chance result on a screening test will go on to have a normal pregnancy because these tests cannot provide conclusive information. The woman and her family, after consulting with her physician or midwife, decide whether to pursue additional testing to determine whether a condition is present.

Diagnostic tests may be considered for a range of reasons. For example, if a diagnostic test confirms the presence of a medical condition:

- Some abnormalities can be surgically corrected while the baby is still in the uterus.
- A woman and her baby may need specialist care before, during and after the birth.
- Knowing in advance that the baby has a particular condition may provide a family with time to prepare.
- Depending on the condition identified in diagnostic testing, some women or families may decide not to continue a pregnancy and arrange a termination of pregnancy (abortion).

3.7.6. Immunizations in Pregnancy

Immunizations can guard against a variety of infectious diseases for both you and your unborn child. Under the National Immunization Program, the seasonal influenza vaccine—often referred to as the "flu shot"—is advised and financially supported for all expectant mothers. The flu shot protects you and your unborn child for the first six months of life and is safe to receive at any point during pregnancy. Pregnant women can receive the whooping cough combination vaccine, commonly referred to as the "three-in-one dTpa vaccine," for free as early as week 20. The vaccination protects against tetanus, diphtheria, and whooping cough, commonly known as pertussis.

3.7.7. Best Practice for Health Professionals Talking to Families About Screening and Test Results

In a study about prenatal screening, Down Syndrome Australia discovered that 49% of families felt pressured to end their pregnancy by medical professionals, 42% thought they were misinformed about the condition, and 45% thought they were not receiving the right support during their pregnancy. Health professionals must give families timely access to accurate and well-balanced information before, during, and after prenatal screening and diagnostic testing so they can make an educated decision.

Medical practitioners must also:

- Deliver high chance or confirmed diagnosis results using neutral language (e.g., 'chance' rather than 'risk,' factual delivery of a diagnosis without emotive terms such as 'I'm sorry' or 'bad news').
- Provide up-to-date, evidenced-based information on Down syndrome and other conditions being screened for, both before screening and after results are given.
- Offer referrals to peer support services such as local Down syndrome associations.
- Offer non-directive counseling and support services both before and after a decision is made on whether to continue the pregnancy.
- Give respect for decisions made by families, and not revisit that decision once it has been communicated while making it clear that they have a right to change their mind.

3.8. Fetal Assessment

We can confirm an estimated due date and observe your baby's growth and development with this test. A sonographer with expertise in maternal-fetal medicine will conduct the ultrasound, and a physician with training in this field will review the findings.

3.8.1. Prenatal Diagnosis

Prenatal diagnosis refers to those testing modalities used during pregnancy to screen and diagnose fetal aneuploidies and anomalies.

3.8.1.1. Nuchal Translucency (NT)

The best time to perform an ultrasound measurement of the fetus's fluid behind its neck is between weeks 10 3/7 and 13 6/7. An increased risk for chromosomal abnormalities like trisomy 21 or 18 is correlated with an increase in the NT. Furthermore, even in cases where karyotype is normal, those gestations with increased NT have an increased risk of unfavorable pregnancy outcomes, such as intrauterine fetal death and fetal cardiac defects. Since trisomy 18 and 21 are difficult to detect with NT measurements alone, it is not advised to use them as the only method of aneuploidy screening.

3.8.1.2. Combined First-Trimester Screening

Nuchal translucency combined with a measurement of the maternal serum markers, free beta human chorionic gonadotropin (free β-hCG) and pregnancy-associated plasma protein A (PAPP-A), is used to calculate the risk for trisomies 18 and 21. It is performed between 10 3/7 and 13 6/7 weeks' gestation. It is an effective screening tool, with a detection rate of 82–87% for trisomy 21 at a 5% false-positive screen rate. Free β-hCG is elevated and PAPP-A is decreased in a pregnancy affected by Down syndrome.

3.8.1.3. Second-Trimester Screening

The quadruple screen (Quad screen) involves analyzing levels of maternal serum alpha-fetoprotein (MSAFP), total hCG, unconjugated estriol, and inhibin A between 15 and 21 weeks'= of gestation to calculate the risk for trisomies 18 and 21. In addition, it provides a risk assessment for open neural tube defects. For patients who present after 13 6/7 weeks or choose not to undergo first-trimester screening, the Quad screen is an option. In a pregnancy affected by Down syndrome, both MSAFP and unconjugated estriol are low and hCG and inhibin A are elevated. The Quad screen has a detection rate of 81% for Down syndrome at a 5% false-positive rate. Like first-trimester screening, the Quad screen requires an invasive test to confirm the diagnosis of a chromosomal abnormality (i.e., amniocentesis or chorionic villous sampling [CVS]). For those patients who chose to undergo first-trimester screening and/or CVS, neural tube defect screening in the form of a second-trimester MSAFP level should be offered. The MSAFP is elevated in the presence of an open neural tube defect. Evidence exists that focused ultrasound during the second trimester is an effective tool for detecting an open neural tube defect.

3.8.1.4. Integrated Screening and Sequential Screening (Independent, Step Wise, and Contingent)

These options involve a combination of first- and second-trimester screening.

1. **Integrated Screen:** The NT and maternal serum levels of PAPP-A are obtained in the first trimester, and the Quad screen is obtained in the second trimester. When the test does not include an NT measurement it is called serum integrated. With both full-integrated screening and serum screening the results are reported when all the tests are completed, yielding a detection rate for Down syndrome of 94% and 87%, respectively, at a 5% false-positive rate.
2. **Sequential Screening:** In the first trimester, NT, PAPP-A, and free β-hCG are measured; in the second trimester, a quad screen is performed. Under the independent approach, women who have an increased risk are offered invasive testing, and results are provided after the first trimester. With a high false-positive rate of 11% and a detection rate of 94%, a second-trimester screening is carried out and interpreted independently of first-trimester results if there is a low risk. Patients who are found to be at high risk following first-trimester screenings are offered invasive testing under the step-by-step approach. If not, the second trimester is finished, the results are presented, and the first trimester's results are added. There is a 5% false-positive rate with a 95% detection rate. When an elevated risk is detected, the contingent approach performs the first trimester of the sequential testing and then moves on to the quad screen. The second part is finished by those who are at intermediate risk. Those who are low risk, however, do not receive additional testing. The most economical screening method for trisomy 21 is contingent sequential screening, which offers a high detection rate and a low false-positive rate.

3.8.1.5. Ultrasound Testing

Uterine ultrasound examination is used in the following circumstances:

1. **Determination of Pregnancy Viability:** Fetal heart motion can be

detected at 6 weeks of gestation by an abdominal scan and a few days earlier by transvaginal ultrasound. Once the crown-rump length (CRL) is ≥5 mm, fetal heart motion should be seen. Ultrasound is also used in the case of a suspected fetal demise later in pregnancy.

2. **Calculation of Gestational Age:** Measurement of the CRL between 6 and 14 weeks' gestation allows for the most accurate assessment of gestational age, to within 5 days. After the first trimester, a combination of biparietal diameter, head circumference, abdominal circumference, and femur length is used to estimate gestational age and fetal weight. Measurements in the second trimester are accurate to within ⍰10–14 days and in the third trimester to within 14–21 days.
3. **Diagnosis of Multiple Pregnancy and Determination of Chorionicity and Amnionicity:** The determination of chorionicity and amnionicity is made by ultrasound examination of the fetal membranes and is best done as early as possible in the first trimester but after 6 weeks and prior to 14 weeks of gestation.
4. **Anatomic Survey:** A large number of congenital anomalies can be diagnosed reliably by ultrasonography, including anencephaly, hydrocephalus, congenital heart defects, gastroschisis, omphalocele, spina bifida, renal anomalies, diaphragmatic hernia, cleft lip and palate, and skeletal dysplasia. Identification of these anomalies before birth can help determine the safest method of delivery and the support personnel needed at delivery. Ultrasonography can also aid in determining fetal gender for patients in whom this determination impacts the likelihood of a known X-linked genetic disorder.
5. **Visual Guidance:** Ultrasound is used for guidance during procedures such as amniocentesis, CVS, percutaneous umbilical blood sampling (PUBS), and some fetal surgeries (e.g., placement of bladder or chest shunts).
6. **Assessment of Growth and Fetal Weight:** Ultrasonography is useful to detect and monitor both intrauterine growth restriction (IUGR; defined as an estimated fetal weight <10%) and fetal macrosomia (estimated fetal weight >4500 g). Evidence is accumulating that maternal physical size and race should be considered in customizing the fetal weight for the determination of IUGR. Estimation of fetal weight is also important in counseling patients regarding expectations after delivering a premature infant. Ultrasound assessment for fetal weight by an experienced sonographer is accurate within 10–20% of actual weight.
7. **Assessment of Amniotic Fluid Volume:** Amniotic fluid volume may be assessed objectively with ultrasound by measuring the maximum vertical pocket (MVP) or amniotic fluid index (AFI: total of cord-free deepest vertical pockets in four quadrants) in centimeters.
   - **Oligohydramnios:** Defined as an AFI of <5 cm, AFI <10% for gestational age, or MVP <2 cm. Oligohydramnios is associated with increased fetal morbidity and mortality with spontaneous rupture of membranes as the most common cause. Other causes include placental insufficiency, chronic hypertension, post-dates gestation, and fetal anomalies such as renal agenesis, bladder outlet obstruction, cardiac disease, and karyotypic abnormalities.
   - **Polyhydramnios:** Defined as an AFI >25 cm, AFI >95% for gestational age, or MVP >8 cm. Causes of polyhydramnios include diabetes, multiple gestation with twin-twin transfusion syndrome, nonimmune hydrops, and fetal anomalies such as open neural tube defects, cardiac diseases, and gastrointestinal obstruction.

Most cases of polyhydramnios are idiopathic; however, the risk for fetal anomalies increases with the severity of the polyhydramnios.

8. **Assessment of Placental Location and Presence of Retroplacental Hemorrhage:** This is useful in suspected cases of placenta previa or accreta. Most cases of abruptio placentae are not diagnosed by ultrasonography because abruption is a clinical diagnosis.
9. Assessment of Fetal Well-Being:
   - **Biophysical Profile:** Ultrasonography is used to assess fetal movements, fetal breathing, fetal tone, and amniotic fluid volume. See biophysical profile under antepartum tests of fetal well-being (Table 3.1).
   - **Doppler Studies:** Doppler ultrasonography of fetal vessels, particularly the umbilical artery, is a useful adjunct in the management of high-risk pregnancies, especially those complicated by IUGR. Changes in the vascular Doppler pattern (i.e., increased systolic/diastolic ratios and absent or reversed end-diastolic flow in the umbilical artery) signal elevations in placental vascular resistance. These abnormalities correlate with an increased risk for perinatal morbidity and mortality. In high-risk pregnancies, assessment of the middle cerebral artery is useful for evaluating the presence of fetal anemia, and Doppler assessment of the uterine artery may be useful in the prediction and evaluation of preeclampsia. The overall use of Doppler ultrasonography has been associated with a 29% decrease in perinatal mortality and fewer inductions of labor and cesarean deliveries in high-risk pregnancies; however, no benefit in using this technique has been demonstrated in screening a low-risk population.

Table 3.1. Biophysical Profile

Variable	Normal Response (2 points)
Fetal breathing	≥1 episode of continuous breathing movement of at least 30 seconds
Fetal gross body movements	≥3 body or limb movements
Fetal tone	≥1 extension of fetal extremity or spine with return to flexion, or opening of fetal hand
Amniotic fluid	≥1 pocket of amniotic fluid of >2 cm in two perpendicular planes
Nonstress test	Reactive

3.8.1.6. Amniocentesis

Amniotic fluid can be tested for chorioamnionitis, fetal blood type, hemoglobinopathies, karyotypic abnormalities, genetic disorders (for which testing is available), fetal lung maturity, and to monitor the degree of isoimmunization by measuring the amount of bilirubin in the fluid. Karyotypic abnormality testing is typically conducted between 16 and 20 weeks of gestation. A sample of amniotic fluid is extracted while being guided by ultrasonography. For genetic research, fetal cells in the fluid can be cultured in tissue culture. The pregnancy loss rate associated with amniocentesis is typically estimated using visual guidance from the ultrasound to be between 1 in 200 and 1 in 1600. Since early amniocentesis (before 14 weeks) is linked to a noticeably higher risk of fetal loss and limb abnormalities, it is usually not advised. Amniocentesis is indicated for women who have a history of aneuploidy or abnormal first- or second-trimester screening results; women who have previously given birth to a child with a chromosomal abnormality; women who may have an X-linked disorder; women who have autosomal recessive disorders, in which the trait in question is carried by both parents, and women who are being evaluated for inborn metabolic errors.

3.8.1.7. Chorionic Villus Sampling

Usually, CVS is carried out between weeks 10 and 12. Using a trans-cervical catheter or a needle inserted through the abdomen, chorionic villi are removed from the placenta. The resulting cells are then cultured and examined. The same indications apply as for amniocentesis. While highly operator-dependent, the rates of pregnancy loss following CVS are comparable to those following amniocentesis. CVS is usually not advised before 10 weeks of pregnancy because of the higher-than-expected incidence of limb abnormalities.

3.8.1.8. Percutaneous Umbilical Blood Sampling

A transabdominal needle is inserted into the fetal umbilical vein or artery under ultrasound guidance. Fetal blood samples can be obtained for hematocrit, platelet count, fetal blood type, karyotype, or viral studies. This offers a pathway for red blood cell or platelet transfusion during pregnancy as well. When a fetus has a severe hemolytic disease, either with or without hydrops, such as when it's caused by Rh or an atypical antibody isoimmunization, PUBS is typically used.

3.8.2. Antepartum Tests of Fetal Well-Being

Antepartum testing refers to those testing modalities used during pregnancy to assess fetal health and identify fetuses at risk for poor pregnancy outcomes.

3.8.2.1. Nonstress Test (NST)

The nonstress test is a straightforward, noninvasive procedure that measures the heart rate in response to fetal movements to assess the health of the developing fetus. If the fetal heart rate exhibits periodic accelerations and is normal at baseline, the condition of the fetus is confirmed.

The following guidelines can be used, although there may be variations between institutions:

1. **Reactive NST:** In a 20-minute monitoring period, there are ≥2 accelerations of the fetal heart rate 15 beats/min above the baseline, each lasting at least 15 seconds. In a fetus <32 weeks of gestation, the accelerations must reach 10 beats/min above the baseline and last at least 10 seconds. The perinatal mortality within 1 week after a reactive NST is □1.9 per 1000.
2. **Nonreactive NST:** Fetal heart rate does not meet the established criteria during a prolonged period of monitoring (usually at least 1 hour). There are many causes of a nonreactive NST besides fetal compromise, including fetal sleep cycle, chronic maternal smoking, and exposure to medications such as central nervous system depressants and propranolol. Because of this low specificity (the false-positive rate is □75–90%), a nonreactive NST should be followed by more definitive testing such as a biophysical profile or a contraction stress test.

3.8.2.2. Biophysical Profile (BPP)

The biophysical profile is an additional test that evaluates the health of the fetus. It entails doing an NST to measure the fetal heart rate and a 30-minute ultrasound to measure the fetal breathing movements, tone, and gross body movements (AFI). For every variable, two points are awarded if it is present during the observation period, and zero if it is not. A score of 8 to 10 is regarded as normal; a score of 6 is ambiguous and calls for a second BPP within 24 hours; a score of 0 to 4 is abnormal and typically indicates delivery. Fetal hypoxemia is the cause of alterations in the BPP parameters. Because it can also be impacted by other variables like gestational age, medications, and incorrect technique, caution is required. Institutions routinely track high-risk pregnancies using the BPP. Its use to track complex pregnancies is not supported by data from randomized clinical trials, though. Even though BPP's usefulness has only been investigated at later gestations, there is institutional variation in the gestational age at which it is performed, with some institutions starting as early as 24 weeks.

3.8.2.2.1. Modified Biophysical Profile

Test time has been reduced through modifications to the BPP scoring system. The most popular combination involves assessing just an NST and an AFI. Sometimes the modified BPP is used as a baseline test, and if the results are abnormal, further testing, such as a full BPP, is conducted. The stillbirth rate within 1 week of a normal BPP or a modified BPP is the same at 0.8 per 1000.

3.8.2.3. Contraction Stress Test (CST)

A fetus at risk for uteroplacental insufficiency is evaluated using the CST. Both the uterine contractions and the fetal heart rate are continuously observed. Three contractions lasting 40 to 60 seconds spread over 10 minutes is deemed an adequate test. If enough contractions don't happen on their own, oxytocin or nipple stimulation might be applied. The test is known as the oxytocin challenge test (OCT) if oxytocin is required to cause contractions for the CST. If contractions are followed by late decelerations, it could indicate the presence of uteroplacental insufficiency. Patients with placenta previa, those who have undergone a vertical incision cesarean section in the past, and those who have high-risk factors for preterm delivery (such as cervical insufficiency or premature rupture of membranes) may not be candidates for the CST.

Test results are interpreted as follows:

1. **Negative (Normal) Test:** No late decelerations occur. This result is associated with a very low perinatal mortality rate of 0.3 per 1000 in the week following the test.
2. **Positive (Abnormal) Test:** Late decelerations occur with at least 50% of the contractions. This result is associated with an increased risk of perinatal morbidity or mortality and indicates that delivery is usually warranted.
3. **Equivocal (Suspicious) Test:** Late decelerations occur but with <50% of the contractions. Prolonged fetal monitoring is usually recommended, and the CST should be repeated in 24 hours.

3.8.2.4. Doppler Studies

Doppler ultrasound is a relatively new technique to be applied to the study of feto-placental and/or uteroplacental circulatory dynamics.

Later observational research revealed that the typical waveform showed forward blood flow during the cardiac cycle and had a pattern consistent with the feto-placental circulation as a low resistance system. There was sometimes even a reversal of flow, from the placenta to the fetus, during diastole in certain pregnancies that were compromised (most notably those linked to fetal growth restriction). Observational data made it evident that many of the fetuses with highly abnormal waveforms did not have good outcomes. It was unclear, though, whether the extra data that Doppler ultrasonography would have brought to a clinical setting where there were already multiple indicators of a bad prognosis would have been beneficial. Furthermore, there was a strong chance that the Doppler ultrasound data could have been harmful; specifically, there was a wide range in the amount of time that a fetus with, say, absent end-diastolic velocities could exhibit further indications of severe compromise. As a result, in certain circumstances, the test might have encouraged an unnecessarily early delivery. It was urged that Doppler ultrasonography not be employed in clinical settings without first undergoing appropriate assessment. Since then, Doppler ultrasound use during pregnancy has been the subject of more randomized controlled trials than any other technique for fetal assessment.

3.8.2.5. Fetal Movement Counting

It has been suggested that maternal perception of fetal movement can be used as a gauge for fetal health. Various techniques have been assessed, such as "the count to 10," which entails keeping track of 10 fetal movements during a 2-hour period while the mother is at rest. Other methods include counting for a certain amount of time every day or on specific days of the week. However, there is disagreement over the usefulness of maternal kick counts as a predictor of stillbirth due to inconsistent findings from various studies published in the literature. Additional assessment is necessary in cases where mothers report abnormal fetal counting.

3.8.3. Intrapartum Tests of Fetal Well-Being

Intrapartum testing refers to those testing modalities used during labor to identify fetuses at risk for acidosis, adverse neonatal outcomes, or death.

3.8.3.1. Electronic Fetal Heart Rate Monitoring (EFM)

The advantages of EFM over intermittent fetal heart rate auscultation have been hotly debated, despite the technology's widespread adoption. The association between EFM and lower rates of early infant and neonatal mortality, Apgar scores <4 at 5 minutes, and neonatal seizures was not established until recently. The rates of both operative vaginal deliveries and cesarean sections are rising in relation to EFM. There are two types of fetal heart rate monitoring: external, where a monitor is affixed to the mother's belly, or internal, where an electrode is affixed to the fetal scalp.

The nomenclature and interpretation of EFM are based on the 2008 National Institute of Child Health and Human Development (NICHD) workshop report:

1. **Baseline Fetal Heart Rate (FHR):** It is the rate maintained for at least 2 minutes apart from periodic variations, rounded to the nearest 5 beats/min over a 10-minute period. The normal FHR is 110–160 beats/min. Fetal

tachycardia is present at >160 beats/min and fetal bradycardia at <110 beats/min. Causes of fetal tachycardia include maternal or fetal infection, fetal hypoxia, thyrotoxicosis, and maternal use of drugs such as parasympathetic blockers or β-mimetic agents. Causes of bradycardia include hypoxia, complete heart block, and maternal use of drugs such as β-blockers.

2. **Variability:** In the normal mature fetus, there are rapid fluctuations in the baseline FHR. This variability indicates a functioning sympathetic–parasympathetic nervous system interaction and is the most sensitive indicator of fetal well-being. An amplitude range from peak to trough of 6–25 beats/min indicates moderate variability and suggests the absence of fetal hypoxia. Marked variability occurs when >25 beats/min is noted. Minimal variability is quantified as <5 beats/min; absent variability refers to an undetectable amplitude range. Decreased variability may be caused by severe hypoxia, anencephaly and other fetal neurologic abnormalities, complete heart block, and maternal use of drugs such as narcotics or magnesium sulfate. In addition, variability is decreased during normal fetal sleep cycles.
3. **Accelerations:** These are often associated with fetal movement and are an indication of fetal well-being. The presence of accelerations suggests the absence of any acidosis.
4. **Decelerations:** There are three types of decelerations (Figure 3.5):
   - **Early Decelerations:** These result from physiologic head compression and occur secondary to an intact vagal reflex tone, which follows minor, transient fetal hypoxic episodes. These are benign and are not associated with fetal compromise. They appear as mirror images of the contraction pattern.
   - **Late Decelerations:** These are a result of uteroplacental insufficiency (UPI) and indicate the presence of fetal hypoxia. Potential causes include maternal hypotension, sometimes as a result of supine positioning or regional anesthesia, as well as uterine hypertonicity. More chronic causes of UPI, such as hypertension, postdate gestation, and preeclampsia may predispose a fetus to the development of late decelerations. Although by themselves they reflect only a decreased oxygen tension for the fetus, their persistence may lead to the development of fetal acidemia and eventual compromise. The nadir occurs after the contraction peaks, with the shape demonstrating a gradual decrease and slow return to baseline.
   - **Variable Decelerations:** These result from abrupt compression of the umbilical cord. They can also be seen as a consequence of cord stretch, as in phases of rapid fetal descent, and with a cord prolapse. Variable decelerations tend to increase in the setting of oligohydramnios. The majority of these decelerations are benign and not predictive of

an acidemic fetus. However, severe variable decelerations (those lasting >60 seconds), especially in the setting of decreased variability and/or tachycardia, may portend a compromised fetus. They have a V or W nonuniform shape with a rapid descent and return to baseline: time from baseline to the nadir of the deceleration is 30 seconds.

5. **Interpretation of Electronic Fetal Monitoring:** FHR patterns can be classified in one of three categories: I (Normal), II (Indeterminate), or III (Abnormal):
   - **Category I FHR Pattern:** This has 4 characteristics: normal baseline rate (110–160 beats/min), moderate variability (6–25 beats/min), absence of late or variable decelerations, and absence or presence of early decelerations or accelerations. In the setting of these findings, there is a high likelihood of a normally oxygenated fetus.
   - **Category III FHR Pattern:** Conversely, there are 4 FHR patterns predictive of abnormal fetal acid-base status grouped in category III.
   - **Sinusoidal Pattern:** These include a sinusoidal heart rate, defined as a pattern of regular variability resembling a sine wave, with a fixed periodicity of 3–5 cycles/min and amplitude of 5–40 beats/min. A sinusoidal pattern may indicate fetal anemia caused by fetomaternal hemorrhage or alloimmunization.
   - **Baseline FHR Variability is Absent:** The other three abnormal FHR patterns in category III are diagnosed when baseline FHR variability is absent and any one of the following is present:
   - Recurrent late decelerations;
   - Recurrent variable decelerations;
   - Bradycardia.
   - **Category II:** Comprises all FHR patterns not in category I or III. Category II tracings are not predictive of abnormal fetal acid-base status. When a category II tracing is identified, a fetal scalp stimulation test may help identify fetuses in which acid-base status is normal.

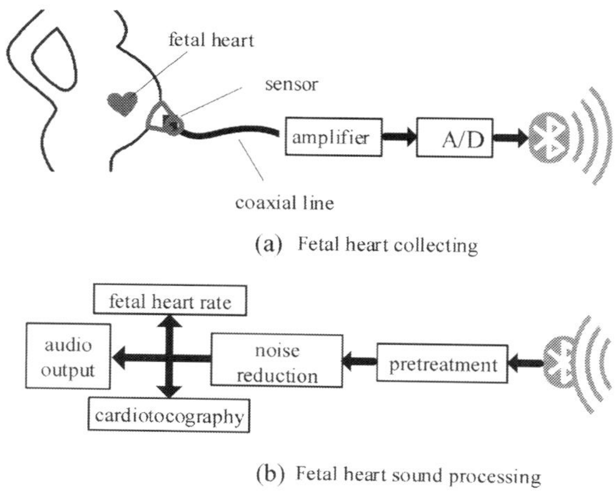

Figure 3.5. *Examples of fetal heart rate monitoring.*

Source: *Wei, J., Wang, Z., & Xing, X., (2021). A wireless high-sensitivity fetal heart sound monitoring system. Sensors, 21(1), 193. https://doi.org/10.3390/s21010193.*

3.8.3.2. Fetal Scalp Blood Sampling

When the fetal acid-base status was unclear or nonreassuring, the fetal heart rate (FHR) had been used to assess it during labor. The process of collecting the sample is unfamiliar to many practitioners, and noninvasive techniques like fetal scalp stimulation and vibroacoustic stimulation offer a similar level of comfort. It is not frequently utilized in clinical care as a result.

3.8.3.3. Scalp Stimulation/Vibroacoustic Stimulation

Fetal pH of >7.20 has been linked to an acceleration of heart rate (FHR) in response to vibroacoustic stimulation through the mother's abdomen or manual stimulation of the fetal presenting part. These tests are frequently used to assess the health of the fetus during labor; however, acidemia is not always indicated by a lack of fetal response to stimulation.

3.8.3.4. Fetal Pulse Oximetry

This technique was designed as an adjunct to FHR monitoring in labor and involves the placement of a fetal pulse oximeter transcervically next to the fetal cheek. Normal fetal oxygen saturation as measured by pulse oximetry (SpO_2) is 30–70%. Due to the lack of clinical significance, it is currently not recommended.

3.8.4. Tests of Fetal Lung Maturity

3.8.4.1. Testing Strategies

When considering delivery at < 39 weeks, fetal lung maturity testing is advised unless clinically indicated for reasons related to the mother or the fetus. Testing <32 weeks is not advised because the sample will probably be immature. Any fetal lung maturity test result that is mature suggests that the risk of neonatal respiratory distress syndrome (RDS) is extremely low. All of the tests have low positive predictive values (between 30% and 60%), suggesting that an immature result does not always correspond well with the presence of RDS. Testing options and availability for fetal lung maturity vary by institution.

3.8.4.2. Lecithin-Sphingomyelin (L-S) Ratio

Lecithin is a phospholipid that can be measured specifically in amniotic fluid. It is a principal active component of surfactant and is manufactured by type II alveolar cells. Sphingomyelin is a phospholipid found predominantly in body tissues other than the lungs. The L-S ratio compares levels of lecithin, which gradually increase after 28 weeks, to levels of sphingomyelin, which remain constant. An L-S ratio ≥2:0 is considered mature.

Some disorders are associated with delayed lung maturation including diabetes mellitus and Rh isoimmunization complicated by fetal hydrops. Acceleration of fetal lung maturity is seen in sickle cell disease, maternal narcotic addiction, prolonged rupture of membranes, chronic maternal hypertension, IUGR, and smoking. Differences may also occur in various racial groups. The L-S ratio measurement can be affected by the presence of blood or meconium. In addition, the L-S ratio is costly, difficult to perform, and time-consuming compared with other available tests.

3.8.4.3. Phosphatidylglycerol (PG)

About 35 weeks is when phosphatidylglycerol first appears in amniotic fluid, and levels peak between 37–40 weeks. Being the final surfactant to form in the fetal lung, this material serves as a helpful marker for lung maturation in the latter stages of pregnancy. It can be described as either present or absent, and its existence is a reliable indicator that RDS won't happen. PG levels can be measured on vaginal pool specimens from patients who have ruptured membranes and are unaffected by contamination with blood or meconium.

3.8.4.4. Surfactant/Albumin Ratio by TDx Fetal Lung Maturity (TDx FLM II)

This test (Abbott Laboratories, Abbott Park, IL) measures the relative concentrations of surfactant and albumin (milligrams of surfactant per gram of albumin) in amniotic fluid, which increases with increasing lung maturity. Like the L-S ratio, blood and meconium can interfere with the results. A value ≤39 mg/g is considered immature, 40–54 mg/g is indeterminate, and ≥55 mg/g is mature. TDx FLM II has several advantages over the L-S ratio: less technical expertise is required, it is performed more easily, and results are available quickly. Unfortunately, this test will no longer be available since it has been discontinued by the manufacturer.

3.8.4.5. Lamellar Body Count (LBC)

Following type II pneumocyte secretion, surfactant is encapsulated into lamellar bodies, which are granules used for storage. These lamellar bodies are counted in this test using a standard hematologic cell counter. More than 50,000 cells per microliter indicate lung maturity. This test yields faster results and is simpler to conduct than the L-S ratio at a sensitivity level that is comparable to or higher than the TDx FLM II. Blood and meconium have the potential to impact how this test is interpreted.

3.8.4.6. Cord Blood Banking

After the baby is born, stem cells from the umbilical cord are extracted and kept in private or public cord blood banks. On the day of delivery, the family is given a collection kit to bring. The blood is usually taken after the baby is delivered by the delivery provider. Following the clamping of the umbilical cord, a needle is used to extract the blood, which is then placed into a bag and sealed to complete the collection process. After that, the sample is brought to the cord blood bank. While there are advantages and disadvantages to cord blood banking, parents can choose to do so; it is not always advised. When there is a family member with a known illness that can be treated with a hematopoietic transplant, private cord blood banking should be taken into consideration. The likelihood of a person using their own cells to treat a particular disease is estimated to be 1:2700. Certain diseases, such as genetic disorders and inborn errors of metabolism, cannot be treated in the same person because the diseased cells contain the mutation.

A Closer Look

Human Chorionic Gonadotropin (hCG)

Throughout pregnancy, human chorionic gonadotropin, or hCG, is a hormone that is present in both the blood and urine. Shortly after the embryo is implanted in the uterus, or about three weeks into a four-week menstrual cycle, hCG is detected in the blood. A rise in hCG levels alerts the body to your pregnancy and prompts the womb to begin preparing a secure environment for the growing baby.

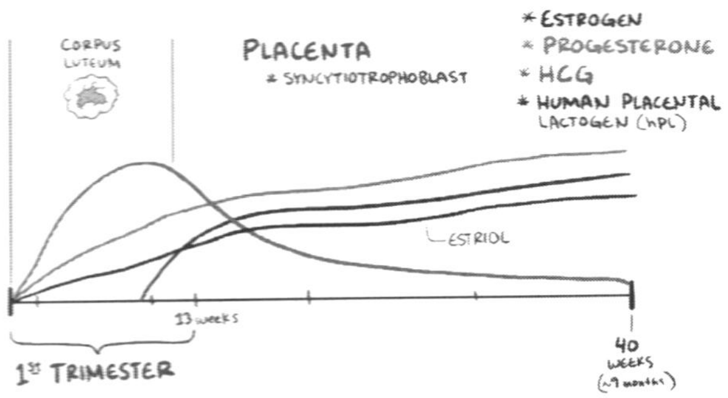

Source: https://en.m.wikipedia.org/wiki/File:Pregnancy_hormone_graph.png.

An embryo starts producing hCG when it forms, and this helps other crucial pregnancy hormones like progesterone and estrogen to be produced. In order for the uterus to receive and nourish the embryo after implantation, this thickens and increases the blood supply to its lining. A healthy pregnancy and the development of your unborn child depend on the proper balance of these vital hormones.

Detecting hCG in the urine is how home pregnancy tests operate. The detectable levels of hCG in the early stages of pregnancy should approximately double every two days. Around the first day of a missed menstrual cycle, the hormone can be found in the urine. It is best to wait a few days after missing a period before taking a pregnancy test for maximum accuracy. The amount of hCG in the body cannot be determined by a urine test; it can only determine whether it exists.

To measure hCG levels in the early stages of pregnancy, physicians may employ one of two blood test types. The most popular one measures the amount of hCG in the blood and is a quantitative hCG blood test. Milli-international units of hCG per milliliter of blood (mIU/mL) are the units used to report the result. HCG levels can differ significantly between individuals and between pregnancies. But generally speaking, anything over 25 mIU/mL indicates pregnancy, and less than 5 mIU/mL indicates not to be pregnant.

When it comes to warning doctors about potential pregnancy complications, such as miscarriage, HCG levels are helpful. It is commonly advised that women whose first-trimester hCG levels drop over the course of two to three days in two quantitative hCG blood tests are on the verge of miscarriage. This is particularly valid for those who also experience other miscarriage symptoms, like vaginal bleeding.

Later in pregnancy, such as the second and third trimesters, declining hCG levels are most likely not a reason for alarm. When assessing a pregnancy's progress beyond the first trimester, most doctors do not measure quantitative hCG levels; however, single hCG levels may be measured as part of the alpha-fetoprotein (AFP) prenatal screening test, which screens for potential birth defects

Summary

- Antenatal care is the systemic supervision of women during pregnancy to monitor the progress of foetal growth and to ascertain the well-being of the mother and the foetus.
- The simplest way for you to confirm pregnancy in the first trimester is to conduct a urine examination using a pregnancy test kit. The pregnancy test should be offered to any woman in the reproductive age group who comes to you with a history of amenorrhoea or symptoms of pregnancy.
- Registering every pregnancy within 12 weeks is primarily the responsibility of the ANM. Opportunities such as the Village Health and Nutrition Day (VHND) should be optimally utilized for ensuring early registration and antenatal check-ups.
- Most pregnancies progress without incident. But approximately 8 percent of all pregnancies involve complications that, if left untreated, may harm the mother or the baby.
- Gestational diabetes occurs when a woman who didn't have diabetes before pregnancy develops the condition during pregnancy.
- Infections, including some sexually transmitted infections (STIs), may occur during pregnancy and/or delivery and may lead to complications for the pregnant woman, the pregnancy, and the baby after delivery.
- Miscarriage is the term used to describe a pregnancy loss from natural causes before 20 weeks. Signs can include vaginal spotting or bleeding, cramping, or fluid or tissue passing from the vagina.
- Attendance of antenatal preparation classes presents an opportunity whereby psychological problems experienced during pregnancy can be confronted.
- Women's health, their response to and their utilization of prenatal care, are affected by their social circumstances. In general, women with disadvantaged sociodemographic characteristics have less adequate prenatal care.
- Prenatal diagnosis refers to those testing modalities used during pregnancy to screen and diagnose fetal aneuploidies and anomalies.
- Fetal lung maturity testing is recommended when considering delivery at <39 weeks unless clinically indicated for maternal/fetal reasons.

References

1. Alfirevic, Z., Stampalija, T., & Medley, N. (2015). Fetal and umbilical Doppler ultrasound in normal pregnancy. *The Cochrane Database of Systematic Reviews, 4*(4), CD001450. doi:10.1002/14651858.CD001450.pub4. PMID: 25874722.
2. Allen, L. H. (2000). Anemia and iron deficiency: effects on pregnancy outcome. *American Journal of Clinical Nutrition, 71*(5), 1280s–1284s. Retrieved November 9, 2016, from https://academic.oup.com/ajcn/article/71/5/1280S/4729385.
3. Bricker, L., Medley, N., & Pratt, J. J. (2015). Routine ultrasound in late pregnancy (after 24 weeks' gestation). *The Cochrane Database of Systematic Reviews,* 6(6), CD001451. doi:10.1002/14651858.CD001451.pub4. PMID: 26121659.

4. Brown, H. C., Smith, H. J., Mori, R., & Noma, H. (2015). Giving women their own case notes to carry during pregnancy. *The Cochrane Database of Systematic Reviews, 2015*(10), CD002856. doi:10.1002/14651858.CD002856.pub3. PMID: 26465209.

5. Carberry, A. E., Gordon, A., Bond, D. M., Hyett, J., Raynes-Greenow, C. H., & Jeffery, H. E. (2014). Customised versus population-based growth charts as a screening tool for detecting small for gestational age infants in low-risk pregnant women. *The Cochrane Database of Systematic Reviews, 5*(5), CD008549. doi:10.1002/14651858.CD008549.pub3. PMID: 24830409.

6. Catling, C. J., Medley, N., Foureur, M., Ryan, C., Leap, N., Teate, A., & Homer, C. S. (2015). Group versus conventional antenatal care for women. *The Cochrane Database of Systematic Reviews, 2*(2), CD007622. doi:10.1002/14651858.CD007622.pub3. PMID: 25922865.

7. David, R., Evans, R., & Fraser, H. S. F. (2021). Modelling prenatal care pathways at a central hospital in zimbabwe. *Health Services Insights, 14*, 11786329211062742. doi:10.1177/11786329211062742. PMID: 34880627.

8. Dowswell, T., Carroli, G., Duley, L., Gates, S., Gülmezoglu, A. M., Khan-Neelofur, D., & Piaggio, G. (2015). Alternative versus standard packages of antenatal care for low-risk pregnancy. *The Cochrane Database of Systematic Reviews, 2015*(7), CD000934. doi:10.1002/14651858. CD000934.pub3. PMID: 26184394.

9. Hernandez-Diaz, S., Toh, S., & Cnattinguis, S. (2009). Risk of pre-eclampsia in first and subsequent pregnancies: prospective cohort study. *British Medical Journal, 338*, b2255. Retrieved July 31, 2012, from http://www.ncbi.nlm.nih.gov/pmc/articles/PMC3269902/?tool=pubmed (accessed on 17 May 2024).

10. Le Strat, Y., Dubertret, C., & Le Foll, B. (2011). Prevalence and correlates of major depressive episode in pregnant and postpartum women in the United States. *Journal of Affective Disorders, 135*(1–3), 128–138. doi:10.1016/j.jad.2011.07.004.

11. Leeman, L., & Fontaine, P. (2008). Hypertensive disorders of pregnancy. *American Family Physician, 78*, 93–100. PMID: 18649616.

12. Mbuagbaw, L., Medley, N., Darzi, A. J., Richardson, M., Habiba Garga, K., & Ongolo-Zogo, P. (2015). Health system and community level interventions for improving antenatal care coverage and health outcomes. *The Cochrane Database of Systematic Reviews, 12*(12), CD010994. doi:10.1002/14651858.CD010994.pub2. PMID: 26621223.

13. Meis, P. J., Klebanoff, M., Thom E., Dombrowski, M. P., Sibai, B., Moawad, A. H., et al. (2003). Prevention of recurrent preterm delivery by 17 alpha-hydroxyprogesterone caproate. *New England Journal of Medicine, 348*, 2379–2385. PMID: 12802023.

14. Nabhan, A. F., & Aflaifel, N. (2015). High feedback versus low feedback of prenatal ultrasound for reducing maternal anxiety and improving maternal health behaviour in pregnancy. *The Cochrane Database of Systematic Reviews, 2015*(8), CD007208. doi:10.1002/14651858. CD007208.pub3. PMID: 26241793.

15. Robert Peter, J., Ho, J. J., Valliapan, J., & Sivasangari, S. (2015). Symphysial fundal height (SFH) measurement in pregnancy for detecting abnormal fetal growth. *The Cochrane Database of Systematic Reviews, 2015*(9), CD008136. doi:10.1002/14651858.CD008136.pub3. PMID: 26346107.

16. Sandall, J., Soltani, H., Gates, S., Shennan, A., & Devane, D. (2016). Midwife-led continuity models versus other models of care for childbearing women. *The Cochrane Database of Systematic Reviews, 2016*(4), CD004667. doi:10.1002/14651858.CD004667.pub5. PMID: 27121907.

17. Whitworth, M., Bricker, L., & Mullan, C. (2015). Ultrasound for fetal assessment in early pregnancy. *The Cochrane Database of Systematic Reviews, 2015*(7), CD007058. doi:10.1002/14651858.CD007058.pub3. PMID: 26171896.

Chapter

CHILDBIRTH AND POSTPARTUM CARE

4

Contents

Unit Introduction 122
4.1. Overview of Childbirth 124
4.2. Vaginal Birth 125
4.3. Labor Induction and Caesarean Section 131
4.4. Management 132
4.5. Complications 136
4.6. Postpartum Care 141
Summary 147
References 147

Unit Introduction

An intense event, childbirth carries emotional, cognitive, social, and cultural significance in addition to extreme physical stress. When the uterus contracts, the cervix dilates, and the baby and placenta are delivered, women must adjust to sudden physical changes. Laboring women have been shown to exhibit general stress responses, including increases in blood pressure and cardiac output, as well as the release of endorphins, epinephrine, and catecholamines. Both intense positive and negative emotions are typically experienced during labor and the baby's birth. The woman must also meet cognitive demands as she adjusts to the birth's events. If birth attendants are seen as unhelpful or dismissive, the woman's partner and the medical staff may have less supportive interpersonal dynamics, or the woman may experience higher levels of stress. Last but not least, becoming a mother and giving birth are linked to numerous societal norms and expectations. For instance, childbirth is heavily medicalized in Western societies, but women are frequently encouraged to attempt a "natural" birth with little assistance or painkillers.

Therefore, giving birth is a severe and acute stressor that many women experience. Additionally, it makes it possible to investigate how pre-event and event factors interact to create perceived stress and how this affects psychological and physical consequences. This is in line with the diathesis stress approach to health outcomes, which takes into account the interaction between event characteristics and pre-existing vulnerability (social, psychological, and physical) to determine outcomes. The designation of childbirth as an acute stressor, though, is a bit artificial; the effects of childbirth need to be viewed in the context of prenatal and postnatal adjustments to motherhood and a new baby, both of which can be challenging and stressful.

Psychosocial factors have a significant impact on both psychological and physical outcomes, including psychopathology and maternal satisfaction, as well as physical outcomes like morbidity and mortality, according to research on their role in birth outcomes. The postnatal period is linked to several psychological issues that are thought to be unique to childbirth, such as puerperal psychosis, postnatal depression, and the baby blues. Whether childbirth has particular effects that set postnatal psychopathology apart from psychopathology that manifests at other times is still up for debate. Postpartum depression has also been connected to childbirth in more recent times.

Thus, a variety of psychosocial factors impact both the experience and result of childbirth. These factors' relative importance varies depending on the outcome and the person. The postpartum phase typically lasts six to eight weeks after the baby is delivered and ends when the mother's body has almost fully recovered from being pregnant. The weeks immediately after delivery set the stage for both the mother and her child's long-term health and wellbeing. Establishing a trustworthy postpartum (afterbirth) period is therefore essential and should be integrated into ongoing, continuous, all-encompassing care. The first month after delivery is when most deaths of mothers and babies take place. Effective postpartum care is therefore essential to enhancing the mother's and the baby's short- and long-term health outcomes.

Orientation and Directional Terms

Term	Definition	Illustration
Psychosocial	The psychosocial approach looks at individuals in the context of the combined influence that psychological factors and the surrounding social environment have on their physical and mental wellness and their ability to function.	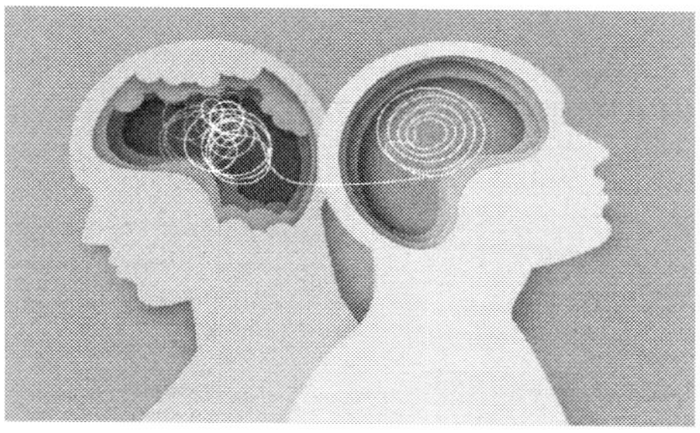
Cesarean sections	A cesarean section, also known as a C-section, is a surgical procedure that involves delivering a baby through incisions in the mother's abdomen and uterus.	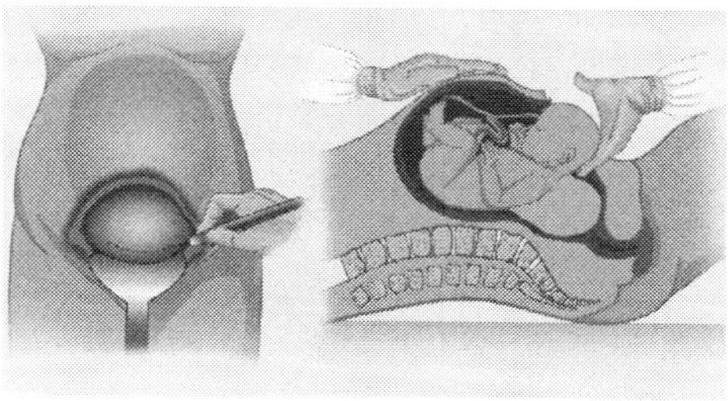
Uterus	The uterus is a hollow muscular organ located in the female pelvis between the bladder and rectum.	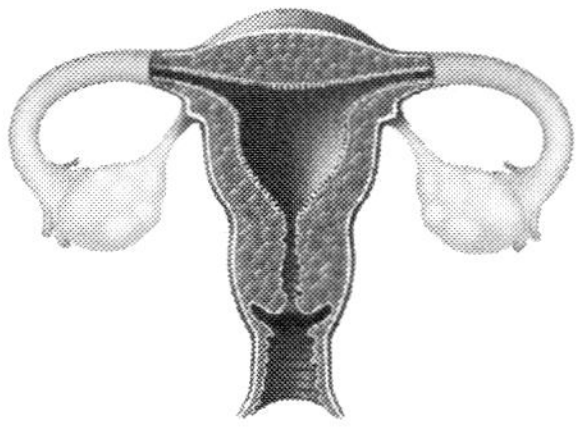
Postnatal psychopathology	Postpartum psychosis (PPP) is a rare but severe mental health emergency that can occur after childbirth.	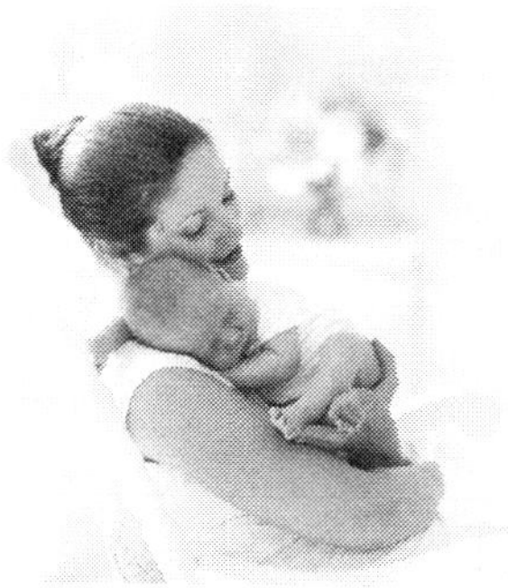

4.1. Overview of Childbirth

The term "childbirth," which is another name for "labor and delivery," refers to the end of a pregnancy when one or more babies are delivered by vaginal delivery or cesarean section. Worldwide, there were roughly 140.11 million births in 2019. The majority of births take place at home in developing nations, whereas most deliveries in developed nations take place in hospitals.

Vaginal delivery is the most commonly used method of childbirth globally. It consists of four stages: the cervix shortens and opens during the first stage, the baby descends and is born in the second, the placenta is delivered in the third, and the mother and infant recover during the fourth stage, known as postpartum. In the first stage, the mother may experience abdominal cramping or back pain lasting around 30 seconds every 10 to 30 minutes, with contractions becoming stronger and closer together over time. The second stage concludes when the baby is completely born, followed by the delivery of the placenta in the third stage. The fourth stage involves the mother's recovery, delayed clamping of the umbilical cord, and monitoring of the baby. Major health organizations recommend skin-to-skin contact immediately after birth, regardless of the delivery method, and suggest delaying procedures on the newborn for at least one to two hours or until after the first breastfeeding.

Given the higher risk of complications from a cesarean section and the inherent advantages of a vaginal delivery for both mother and child, a vaginal delivery is advised over a cesarean section. Opioids, spinal blocks, and relaxation techniques are a few ways that can help with pain. Limiting the number of interventions during labor and delivery, such as elective cesarean sections, is best practice; however, in certain situations, a scheduled cesarean section needs to be planned for the mother to recover and have a successful delivery. If unanticipated problems arise or there is little to no progression through the birthing canal during a vaginal delivery, an emergency cesarean section may be advised.

Every year, complications arising from pregnancy and childbirth lead to approximately 500,000 maternal deaths, 7 million severe long-term issues, and 50 million adverse health outcomes for postpartum women, the majority of whom are in developing nations. Obstructed labor, postpartum hemorrhage, eclampsia, and postpartum infection are among the mother's complications. Prematurity, birth trauma, and low oxygen levels at birth are among the complications that the baby faces.

4.1.1. Signs and Symptoms

The most prominent sign of labor is strong repetitive uterine contractions. Pain in contractions has been described as feeling similar to very strong menstrual cramps. Crowning may be experienced as an intense stretching and burning. The Lamaze method of childbirth teaches that making noises such as moaning, groaning, grunting, repeating words over and over, and any sound that one's body may wish to naturally make may help to relieve pain and help labor to progress. According to Lamaze, "While the media would have you believe that all birthing women scream, in reality, it's not the most common noise." They say that screaming may be a sign that the laboring woman is beginning to panic and the support team should help her back to regulated breathing.

A specific type of pain that women experience during childbirth in the lower back, just above the tailbone, is referred to as back labor. Another prominent sign of labor is the rupture of membranes, commonly known as "water breaking."

A fluid-filled sac surrounds and cushions a developing baby during pregnancy. The sac typically bursts at the start of or during labor. It could result in a woman's vagina leaking tiny amounts of fluid either continuously or sporadically. The liquid is either pale yellow or clear. The medical professional may perform an amniotomy to break the amniotic sac if it hasn't already during labor. During an amniotomy, a tiny hole in the sac is created by a thin plastic hook, which breaks the water. Prelabor rupture of the membranes is the term used to describe when the sac bursts before labor begins.

Contractions will typically start within 24 hours after the water breaks. If not, the care provider will generally begin labor induction within 24 to 48 hours. If the baby is preterm (less than 37 weeks of pregnancy), the healthcare provider may use a medication to delay delivery.

4.1.1.1. Psychological

Oxytocin, a hormone that is known to induce feelings of contentment, decreases in anxiety, and feelings of calmness and security around the mate, is abundant during the later stages of gestation. It is thought that oxytocin, which is released more frequently during labor when the fetus stimulates the cervix and vagina, is crucial for the development of maternal behavior and the bonding of a mother to her child. Research indicates that after interacting with the baby, the father of the child also experiences an increase in oxytocin levels. Additionally, parents exhibiting higher levels of oxytocin demonstrated greater responsiveness and synchronization in their interactions with their children. Oxytocin is released when a child is nursed, which facilitates the baby's easier access to the nipple.

4.2. Vaginal Birth

The term "station" describes how the level of the ischial spines and the fetal presenting portion relate to one another. The station is zero, which is synonymous with engagement, when the presenting portion is at the ischial spines. When a fetal segment is visible above the spines, the distance is expressed in terms of minus stations, which vary in value from −1 to −4 cm. Plus stations (+1 to +4 cm) are used to indicate the distance if the presenting portion is below the ischial spines. The presenting portion is visible at +3 and +4, where it is at the perineum.

As the fetal head passes through the birth canal, it may momentarily change shape, becoming more elongated or cone-shaped. This is known as molding, and it occurs more frequently in women giving birth vaginally for the first time.

The physical and chemical alterations in the cervix that occur in preparation for the fetus's eventual stretching as it exits the uterus and enters the birth canal are known as cervical ripening. For women who are at risk of preterm labor, a Bishop score scoring system can be used to assess the degree of cervical ripening to predict when the baby will be born and when labor will begin. It is also used to predict how a woman will react to being put into labor for a medical reason or a postdate pregnancy. Cervical ripening can be induced in a few different ways, enabling the uterine contractions to dilate the cervix.

Four phases of labor occur during vaginal delivery: the first is the contraction and opening of the cervix; the second is the baby's descent and birth; the third is the placenta's delivery; and the fourth is the recovery phase, which lasts for two hours following the delivery. Abdominal cramps or back pain, lasting approximately 30 minutes, are the hallmark of the first stage. These cramps usually occur every 10 to 30 minutes. The pain and the contractions get closer together and stronger over time. The infant's complete ejection marks the end of the second stage. The placenta is delivered during the third stage. Recovery, the uterus starts to contract to a pre-pregnancy state, delaying the clamping of the umbilical cord, and monitoring the neonatal vitals and tone are all part of the fourth stage of labor. As of 2014, all major health organizations recommend that the infant be placed on the mother's chest as soon as possible after a live birth, regardless of the method of delivery. This is known as skin-to-skin contact, and routine procedures should be postponed for at least one to two hours, or until the baby has had its first breastfeeding experience (Figure 4.1).

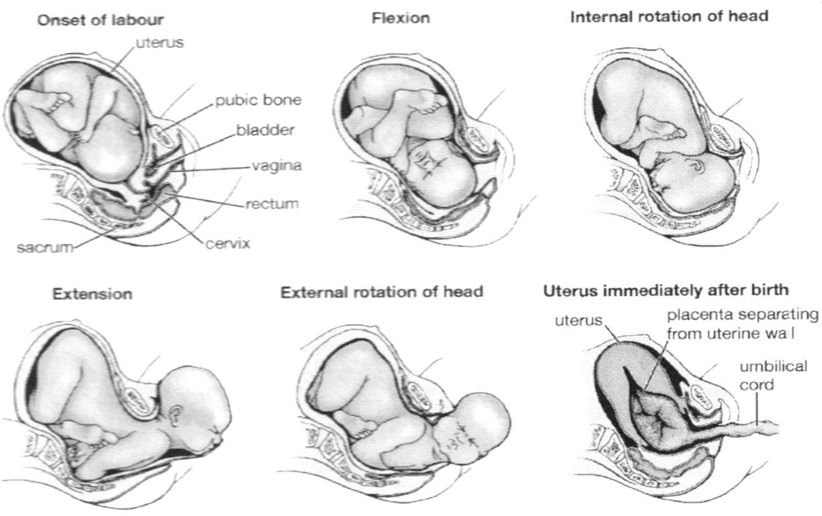

Figure 4.1. *The core stages associated with labor.*

Source: *Nsugbe, E., Samuel, O. W., Sanusi, I., Vishwakarma, S., & Adams, D., (2021). Pregnancy labor prediction using magnetomyography sensing and a self-sorting cybernetic model. Engineering Proceedings, 10(1), 60. https://doi.org/10.3390/ecsa-8-11312.*

4.2.1. Onset of Labor

Definitions of the onset of labor include:

- Frequent uterine contractions occurring at least every six minutes, accompanied by a change in cervical effacement or dilation between digital exams.
- Regular contractions occurring less than 10 minutes apart and progressive cervical dilation or cervical effacement.
- At least three painful regular uterine contractions during 10 minutes, each lasting more than 45 seconds.

Many women are known to experience what has been termed the "nesting instinct." Women report a spurt of energy shortly before going into labor. The phenomenon known as "lightening," in which the baby moves down from the rib cage with its head engaging deeply in the pelvis, is a common indicator that labor is about to start. Because her lungs have more space to expand, the pregnant woman may then find breathing easier, but pressure on her bladder may result in a greater need to void (urinate) more frequently. Lightening can happen several weeks, several hours, or even before labor starts. Some women also experience an increase in vaginal discharge several days before labor begins when the "mucus plug," a thick plug of mucus that blocks the opening to the uterus, is pushed out into the vagina. The mucus plug may become dislodged days before labor begins or not until the start of labor.

While inside the uterus the baby is enclosed in a fluid-filled membrane called the amniotic sac. Shortly before, at the beginning of, or during labor the sac ruptures. Once the sac ruptures, termed "the water breaks," the baby is at risk for infection and the mother's medical team will assess the need to induce labor if it has not started within the time they believe to be safe for the infant.

4.2.2. Stages of Labor

4.2.2.1. First Stage

The first stage of labor is divided into latent and active phases, where the latent phase is sometimes included in the definition of labor, and sometimes not.

Generally speaking, the latent phase starts when the woman starts to feel regular uterine contractions. On the other hand, Braxton Hicks contractions, also known as false labor and beginning around 26 weeks of pregnancy, are rare, erratic, and only cause mild cramping. The uterine muscles contracting before a baby is born are called Braxton Hicks contractions. During the final weeks of pregnancy, cervical dilation and cervical effacement, or the thinning and stretching of the cervix, happen. By the time the latent phase ends, effacement is typically complete or almost complete, and dilation is roughly 5 cm. During a vaginal exam, one can feel the extent of cervical dilation and effacement.

The definitions of the active phase of labor vary geographically. According to the World Health Organization, the active first stage is a time frame during which there are frequent, excruciating contractions in the uterus, a significant degree of cervical effacement, and a faster rate of cervical dilatation, starting at 5 cm and continuing until full dilatation for the first and subsequent labors. The criteria for what constitutes active labor was modified in the United States from 3 to 4 cm to 5 cm of cervical dilation for multiparous mothers who had previously given birth and to 6 cm for nulliparous women who had not previously given birth. The goal of this was to raise the percentage of vaginal deliveries.

A cervical exam can be used by medical professionals to determine the mother's progress in labor by assessing the cervical dilation, effacement, and station. These components make up the *Bishop score*. It is also possible to forecast the outcome of an induction of labor using the Bishop score. The cervix integrates into the lower segment of the uterus during effacement. Uterine muscles shorten the upper segment and draw the lower segment upward during a contraction, producing a gradual expulsive motion. After that, the presenting fetal portion is allowed to descend. When the cervix widens to the point where the baby's head can pass through, full dilation occurs, which for a term baby is about 10 cm.

The length of the latent first stage varies greatly from woman to woman and has not been found to be standard. But in the first labor (primiparae), the active first stage (from 5 cm to full cervical dilatation) typically lasts no more than 12 hours, and in subsequent labors (multiparae), it typically lasts no more than 10 hours. Dystocia of labor, also known as dysfunctional labor or failure to progress, is characterized by a difficult or unusually slow labor that involves progressive dilation of the cervical canal or non-descent of the fetus. For many years, the diagnosis of labor dystocia was made using Friedman's Curve, which was created in 1955. More recent studies in medicine, however, indicate that the Friedman curve might not be applicable right now[when?].

For Example: Compared to a woman without a history of psychological issues, a woman with a history of mental health issues may be more vulnerable to postnatal psychopathology, meaning that other factors during and after childbirth may not be as crucial. This is one of the difficulties with conducting research in this field, which leads to inconsistent results. Thus, when making conclusions, it's critical to take the methodological quality of the studies and the strength of the evidence into account.

4.2.2.2. Second Stage: Fetal Expulsion

When the cervix reaches its full dilation and the baby is born, the expulsion stage comes to an end. The urge to start pushing is felt when pelvic pressure increases due to increased pressure on the cervix. The head is fully engaged in the pelvis at the start of the normal second stage; its widest diameter has surpassed the level of the pelvic inlet. The fetal head then proceeds to descend through the vaginal opening, beneath the pubic arch, and into the pelvis. The additional maternal efforts of pushing or bearing down—akin to defecating—help with this. Crowning is the term used to describe how the fetal head appears at the vaginal opening. The mother will now experience a sharp burning or stinging feeling.

An intact amniotic sac allows for the birth of an infant in cases where it hasn't ruptured during labor or pushing. The term "delivery en caul" describes this. The successful conclusion of the second stage of labor is indicated by the baby's complete expulsion. Some newborns, particularly preterm ones, are covered in a white substance called vernix that has a waxy or cheese-like consistency. For a few hours following birth and during fetal development, it is believed to play some protective roles. The second phase differs for every woman. While births in subsequent labors typically take two hours to complete, first labors typically take three hours. Extended second-stage labors lasting more than three hours are linked to decreased rates of spontaneous vaginal birth and rising rates of infection, perineal tears, and obstetric hemorrhage, along with the requirement for the neonate to receive critical care.

4.2.2.3. Third Stage: Placental Expulsion

The third stage of labor, also known as the involution stage, lasts from immediately following the expulsion of the fetus until immediately following the expulsion of the placenta. The process of placental expulsion starts with a physiological separation from the uterine wall. Depending on whether active or expectant management is used, the estimated average time from the baby's delivery to the placenta's full expulsion is 10 to 12 minutes. Up to 3% of vaginal deliveries have a third stage that lasts more than 30 minutes, which raises the possibility of the placenta being retained.

The placenta can be expelled spontaneously with active management, or it can be expelled naturally with expectant management. Active management includes fundal massage and controlled traction of the umbilical cord after placenta delivery, as well as the administration of uterotonic medication within the first minute of fetal delivery. Uterine massage is then performed every 15 minutes for two hours. To help prevent postpartum hemorrhage, the World Health Organization, the International Federation of Gynecology and Obstetrics, and the International Confederation of Midwives have recommended in a joint statement that active management of the third stage of labor be used in all vaginal deliveries. As long as jaundice can be treated, delaying the clamping of the umbilical cord for at least one minute or until it stops pulsing—which could take several minutes—improves the situation. For a long time, it was thought that postpartum hemorrhage, or severe bleeding after giving birth, increased in mothers who had delayed cord cutting. Delayed cord cutting, however, was found in a recent review to result in early hemoglobin concentration, higher birth weight, and increased iron reserves up to six months after birth in healthy, full-term infants, without affecting the rate of postpartum bleeding.

4.2.2.4. Fourth Stage: Postpartum

Immediately following childbirth, the period that lasts for approximately six weeks is known as the fourth stage of labor. During this time, the terms postpartum and postnatal are frequently used. The newborn grows acclimated to life outside the mother's body while the woman's body, including hormone levels and uterus size, returns to a non-pregnant state. The postnatal period, when most deaths occur, is regarded by the World Health Organization (WHO) as the most crucial but also the most ignored time in a mother's and baby's lives.

If the mother had a ripped perineum or an episiotomy after giving birth, it is sutured. Additionally, this is the best time for the woman to start using long-acting reversible contraception (LARC), like an intrauterine device (IUD) or contraceptive implant, which can both be placed right away after giving birth while she is still in the delivery room. For the first 24 hours following delivery, the mother undergoes routine evaluations for temperature, heart rate, blood pressure, vaginal bleeding, and fundal height. After giving birth, some women may go into an uncontrollable shivering fit or get postpartum chills. Urine should be recorded as soon as it passes for the first six hours. After pains, which resemble menstrual cramps and are caused by the uterus contracting to stop the flow of blood too much, last for a few days. The term "lochia," or vaginal discharge, usually lasts for a few weeks. It starts out bright red and progressively turns pink, brown, yellow, or white.

In the past, newborns born in hospitals were taken from their mothers soon after birth and were only reunited with them during feeding periods. Mothers were informed that their infant would be secure in the nursery and that having more time to rest would result from being apart. As attitudes started to shift, some hospitals started to offer the option of rooming in, which allowed the baby to share the mother's room after a period of standard hospital procedures and observation. By 2020, staying in a room has progressively become the norm in maternity units.

4.2.3. Early Skin-to-Skin Contact

Skin-to-skin contact, also known as kangaroo care, is a method of caring for newborns where they are held chest-to-chest and skin-to-skin with a parent, usually their mother or father. This involves keeping both the baby and parent without shirts or undergarments on their chests. Research has shown that this practice can reduce infant crying, improve breathing and heart stability, regulate blood sugar levels, and enhance the duration of breastfeeding. Studies have also shown that skin-to-skin contact at birth increases the chances of successful breastfeeding.

As of 2014, the American Academy of Pediatrics and all other significant organizations that oversee the health of infants support early postpartum SSC. According to the World Health Organization (WHO), the baby's safe transition from placental to mammary nutrition marks the end of the birthing process. After a vaginal birth, or as soon as the mother is conscious and receptive after a Caesarean section, it is recommended that the newborn be placed skin-to-skin with the mother, delaying any routine procedures for a minimum of one to two hours. Until the mother recovers from the anesthesia, the baby may also be held SSC by the father or another support person.

Even a brief separation before the baby has had its first feed can disrupt the bonding process, according to the World Health Organization, so any initial observations of the infant should be made while the child is still close to the mother. In addition, they recommend as much skin-to-skin contact as possible in the early postpartum days, particularly if it was disrupted for any reason.

Women to have a delivery team that includes a support person who will advocate to assure that:

- The mother and her baby are not separated unnecessarily;
- The baby will receive only her milk;
- The baby will receive no supplementation without a medical reason;
- All testing, bathing or other procedures are done in the parent's room.

It has long been recognized that interactions with her infant increase a mother's level of the hormone oxytocin. A comprehensive review of oxytocin's effects in 2019 discovered that fathers who participate in SSC also have higher levels of oxytocin. According to two studies, chest-to-chest contact (i.e., elevated paternal oxytocin levels) eases parents' post-interaction stress and anxiety when the baby is dressed only in a diaper and placed between the parent's breasts.

4.2.4. Discharge

The World Health Organization advises hospital stays for births that take place in medical facilities to last at least 24 hours for an easy vaginal delivery and 96 hours for a cesarean section. An easy delivery takes an average of less than a day in Egypt and up to six days in (pre-war) Ukraine, according to data collected in 2016. In Australia, the average is 2 + 8 days, while in the UK, it is 1 + 5 days. Despite the low percentage, two-thirds of women in the UK give birth with the assistance of a midwife, and occasionally the mother opts for a hospital birth to be nearer the extensive emergency care available. But, after giving birth, a woman under a midwife's care may leave the hospital, and her midwife will continue to provide care at home. Within the U. S. The average duration of stay has decreased over time, from 4 1½ days in 1970 to 2 days now. The CDC said that people could no longer afford to stay in hospitals and blamed the decline on rising healthcare costs. Congress passed the Newborns' and Mothers' Health Protection Act in 1996 to prevent it from falling any lower. This act mandates that insurers provide at least 48 hours of coverage for simple deliveries.

4.3. Labor Induction and Caesarean Section

A cesarean section, commonly known as a C-section, or labor induction is used to induce labor in a growing number of cases. The procedure or medicine that promotes childbirth and delivery is known as labor induction. Both pharmaceutical and non-pharmaceutical methods can be used to induce labor. The two most common methods used for inductions are intravenous oxytocin therapy plus prostaglandin medication, or prostaglandin medication alone. A cesarean section involves removing the newborn via an abdominal surgical incision as opposed to a vaginal birth. While general anesthesia can also be used, epidural or spinal blocks are typically used to numb the patient during the procedure. To remove the baby, a cut is made in the patient's abdomen and then in the uterus. Prior to the 1970s, it was advised that a patient have a C-section for every child she gave birth to in the future. However, that advice has since been modified. Moms can try a trial of labor, and most can deliver their babies vaginally after a C-section, barring any other indications (VBAC). Before 39 weeks, both elective cesarean sections and induced deliveries may be dangerous or beneficial for the mother, but also for the newborn. Thus, many guidelines advise against elective cesarean sections performed before 39 weeks of pregnancy and against induced births that are not medically necessary.

4.3.1. Labor Induction

The 2012 rate of labor induction in the United States was 23.3%, and had more than doubled from 1990 to 2010. By 2022 it had climbed to 32%. When considering an elective induction of labor, the American Congress of Obstetricians and Gynecologists (ACOG) guidelines recommend a thorough evaluation of the mother-fetal status, the status of the cervix, and at least 39 completed weeks (full term) of gestation for the best possible outcome for the newborn's health.

Per these guidelines, indications for induction may include:

- Abruptio placentae;
- Chorioamnionitis;
- Fetal compromise such as isoimmunization leading to hemolytic disease of the newborn or oligohydramnios;
- Fetal demise;
- Gestational hypertension;
- Maternal conditions such as gestational diabetes or chronic kidney disease;
- Preeclampsia or eclampsia;
- Premature rupture of membranes;
- Post-term pregnancy.

Logistically, induction is also taken into consideration for factors like the distance from the hospital or psychosocial conditions; however, in these cases, confirmation of gestational age and testing are required to determine the maturity of the fetal lung. The ACOG further states that the safest delivery method in cases of vasa previa, complete placenta praevia, umbilical cord prolapse, or active genital herpes simplex infection is a cesarean section. These are the same contraindications for induced labor as they are for spontaneous vaginal delivery.

4.3.2. Cesarean Section

The World Health Organization (WHO) recommends keeping the C-section rate between 10% to 15%, as rates higher than 10% do not show a decrease in morbidity and mortality. However, in 2018, a group of medical professionals expressed concern over the alarming increase in C-section rates globally. A Lancet report revealed that C-sections had more than tripled from 6% to 21% of all births. The March of Dimes, a maternal and child health organization, attributed this rise mainly to an increase in elective C-sections rather than those that are truly necessary or indicated.

Looking at the C-section rates between 1976 and 1996, one large study done in the U.S. found that the proportion of pregnancies delivered by C-section increased from 6.7% in 1976 to 14.2% in 1996, with maternal choice the most frequent reason given. By 2018 the rate had climbed to one-third of all births.

4.4. Management

Women receiving obstetric care are frequently subjected to institutional routines, which may negatively impact the course of labor. To reduce the need for obstetric intervention, supportive care during labor may include information and advocacy, comfort measures, emotional support, and information that may enhance both the physical process of labor and women's feelings of competence and control. Doulas, nurses, midwives, and other hospital staff members, as well as the woman's preferred social network companions, can all offer ongoing support. As long as the father does not display excessive anxiety, there is growing evidence that having the father involved in the birth improves both the birth and the postpartum period. Ongoing labor support could make it easier for women to give birth naturally—that is, without the need for a vacuum, forceps, or cesarean section—with somewhat shorter labors and happier postpartum experiences. In addition to lowering the likelihood that mothers will take painkillers during labor, continuous labor support may also lower the five-minute Agpar scores of newborns.

4.4.1. Preparation

There is a continuous discussion about eating and drinking during labor. While some contend that eating during labor has no negative effects on the process, others are still concerned about the possibility of a general anesthetic in the event of an emergency cesarean, the increased relaxation of the esophagus during pregnancy, and the increased risk of aspiration events (choking on recently eaten foods) in the event of an emergency delivery. According to a 2013 Cochrane review, individuals who are unlikely to require surgery do not experience any different risks from allowing food and drink during labor when under good obstetrical anesthesia. Furthermore, they admit that skipping meals does not indicate that the stomach is empty or that its contents are less acidic. They consequently concluded that women ought to have the freedom to eat and drink during labor, or not.

Shaving the area surrounding the vagina was once common because it was thought to lower the risk of infection, facilitate instrumental deliveries, and make an episiotomy (a surgical incision to enlarge the vaginal entrance) easier. Although shaving is becoming less common, it is still a standard practice in some nations despite a systematic review that found no evidence to support its recommendation. Later side effects include redness, irritation, and several small scratches from the razor. Using providone-iodine solution or the antiseptic chlorhexidine in the vagina has been one more attempt to prevent infection. There isn't much proof that chlorhexidine is beneficial. Providone-iodine is found to reduce risk when performing a cesarean section.

4.4.2. Forceps or Vacuum Assisted Delivery

Approximately 1 in 8 births involve an assisted delivery, which may be necessary if the mother or the child seems to be in danger during a vaginal delivery. The techniques are known as vacuum extraction, also known as ventouse extraction, and obstetrical forceps extraction. When performed correctly, they are both considered safer than an unplanned C-section, with some preference for forceps over vacuum. Even though it's thought to be safe, there are some risks for the mother, such as the possibility of a more serious vaginal tear that affects the anus or rectum's muscle or wall. There is compelling evidence that prophylactic antibiotics can lower the risk of infection for women having an operative vaginal delivery using forceps or vacuum extraction. Blood clots are more likely to form in the legs or pelvis; to prevent clots, doctors may prescribe anti-clot stockings or medication. While it is not uncommon following childbirth, urinary incontinence is more prevalent following an instrument delivery. Physiotherapy and specific exercises will aid in the condition's improvement.

4.4.3. Pain Management During Childbirth

The treatment or avoidance of pain that a woman may experience during labor and delivery is known as pain management during childbirth. The size and position of the baby, the size of the woman's pelvis, her emotions, the intensity of the contractions, and her perspective all play a role in how much pain a woman experiences during labor. In labor, tension makes the pain worse. Almost all women are concerned about how they will handle the pain during labor and delivery. Every woman experiences childbirth differently, so it is impossible to predict how much pain a woman will experience during labor and delivery.

Some women manage just using natural pain relief techniques. Many women combine natural remedies for pain relief with prescription drugs and medical procedures. Some women may find that managing their fear and developing a positive mindset about childbirth help them deal with the pain. Labor pain is not the same as pain from an injury or disease. Rather, the baby is being forced down and out of the birth canal by the uterus's contractions. Stated differently, labor pain results from a purposeful process.

4.4.3.1. Pain Control

4.4.3.1.1. Non-Pharmaceutical

Some women would rather not take analgesics while giving birth. Psychological readiness could be advantageous. Pain relief methods include massage, acupuncture, relaxation techniques, and submersion in water. It has been discovered that acupuncture and relaxation reduce the need for cesarean sections. The first stage of labor pain has been found to be relieved by immersion in water, which also reduces the need for anesthesia and shortens the labor period. However, the safety and effectiveness of water birthing, or immersion during childbirth, has not been proven or linked to any benefits for the mother or fetus (Figure 4.2).

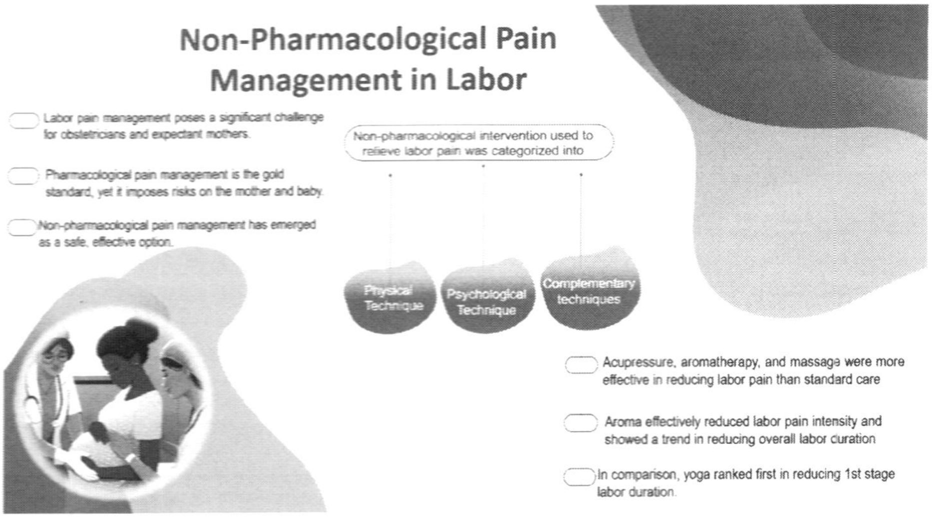

Figure 4.2. *Non-pharmacological pain management in labor.*

Source: *Nori, W., Kassim, M. A. K., Helmi, Z. R., Pantazi, A. C., Brezeanu, D., Brezeanu, A. M., Penciu, R. C., & Serbanescu, L., (2023). Non-pharmacological pain management in labor: A systematic review. Journal of Clinical Medicine, 12(23), 7203. https://doi.org/10.3390/jcm12237203.*

Most women prefer to have a support person during labor and delivery, whether it be a layperson like the baby's father, a family member, or a close friend, or a professional like a midwife, nurse, or doula. According to studies, an infant's Apgar score improves when they receive continuous support during labor and delivery, which also lessens the need for medication and may result in a vaginal or caesarean delivery.

4.4.3.1.2. Pharmaceutical

The effectiveness and side effects of various pain management techniques vary, as does the impact on the mother and her unborn child. In Europe, doctors frequently recommend inhaled nitrous oxide gas, particularly Entonox, which is a mixture of 53% nitrous oxide and 47% oxygen. In the UK, midwives are allowed to use this gas over the counter. Opioids like fentanyl can be used, but if given to a newborn too soon after birth, the baby may experience respiratory depression.

Regional anesthetics such as epidurals (EDA) and spinal anesthesia are commonly used in hospitals for medical pain management. Although epidural analgesia is a generally safe and effective way to relieve pain during labor, it has been linked to higher costs, longer labor times, and more surgical intervention (especially for the delivery of instruments). The new epidural techniques, however, may not have any impact on labor duration, the need for C-section deliveries, or the use of instruments, according to a more recent Cochrane review. When epidural analgesia is administered, pain, fear, and stress hormones decrease initially but later rise again in laboring women without epidurals. In contrast, these hormones rise during labor for these women. Epidural medications can pass through the placenta and enter the fetus's circulation. Epidural analgesia does not appear to have an immediate effect on the newborn status as assessed by Apgar scores, nor does it have a statistically significant effect on the risk of cesarean section.

4.4.4. Augmentation

After labor has started, augmentation is the process of stimulating the uterus to lengthen and intensify contractions. When uterine contractions are deemed to be too weak, slow progress of labor (dystocia) is commonly treated with a variety of augmentation techniques. The most popular strategy for raising the rate of vaginal delivery is oxytocin. The World Health Organization advises against using it unless it has been accurately confirmed that labor is not progressing normally to prevent harm. It can be used alone or in conjunction with amniotomy, or rupture of the amniotic membrane. Antispasmodic medication is not advised by the WHO to prevent labor delays.

4.4.5. Episiotomy

For a long time, it was believed that an episiotomy healed more quickly than a spontaneous tear and could help prevent more serious vaginal tears. When the baby's head passes through the vaginal opening, perineal tears may happen, particularly if the baby descends rapidly. Tears may start in the perineal skin and spread to the muscles, anus, and anal sphincter. They were once common, but are now understood to be generally unnecessary. When necessary, the obstetrician or midwife performs a surgical incision in the perineum to avoid severe tears that may be challenging to mend. The potential benefits and risks for mother and child were compared between routine episiotomy and episiotomy as needed (restrictive) in a 2017 Cochrane review. According to the review, there seem to be several advantages to using restrictive episiotomy policies as opposed to routine episiotomy. At seven days, women had less suturing, less posterior perineal trauma, less severe perineal trauma, and fewer healing complications. There was no difference in the incidence of pain, painful sex, urine incontinence, or severe vaginal/perineal trauma after delivery.

4.4.6. Multiple Births

In cases of a head first-presenting first twin, twins can often be delivered vaginally. In some cases, twin delivery is done in a larger delivery room or in an operating theatre, in the event of complication, e.g.,

- Both twins born vaginally – this can occur both presented head first or where one comes head first and the other is breech and/or helped by a forceps/ventouse delivery.
- One twin born vaginally and the other by cesarean section.
- If the twins are joined at any part of the body – called conjoined twins, delivery is mostly by cesarean section.

4.4.7. Fetal Monitoring

A Doppler fetal monitor (doptone) or a basic Pinard stethoscope can be used to monitor the fetus externally during childbirth. Cardiotocography (CTG) is a noninvasive method of external fetal monitoring (EFM) during childbirth. It uses a cardiotocograph with two sensors: the heart (cardio) sensor is an ultrasonic sensor that works similarly to a Doppler fetal monitor in that it continuously emits ultrasound and uses the characteristic of the reflected sound to detect the motion of the fetal heart. The tocodynamometer (toco), a pressure-sensitive contraction transducer, has a flat section that is secured to the skin around the abdomen by a band. An estimate of contraction can be obtained by comparing the internal pressure with the pressure needed to flatten a section of the wall. A cardiotocograph can be used for either continuous or intermittent monitoring. The World Health Organization (WHO) states that continuous cardiotocography is not advised for assessing the health of the fetus in healthy women going through spontaneous labor. According to the WHO, "all stakeholders should be made aware that continuous CTG is not evidence-based and does not improve birth outcomes in countries and settings where this practice is used defensively to protect against litigation."

Before internal (invasive) monitoring is used, a mother's water must break. An intrauterine pressure catheter (IUPC) or a fetal scalp electrode to provide an extra measure of fetal heart activity are two examples of more intrusive monitoring techniques. Testing of the fetal scalp pH may also be necessary.

4.5. Complications

There has been a 44% decrease in maternal deaths since 1990. However, data from 2015 shows that 830 women perish daily from pregnancy- or childbirth-related causes, and that 20 to 30 more suffer injuries, infections, or disabilities for every woman who passes away. The majority of these wounds and fatalities could be avoided.

4.5.1. Maternal Mortality and Adverse Health Consequences

In 2008, the World Health Organization (WHO) called for midwife training to be strengthened to improve maternal and newborn health services, citing the fact that over 100,000 women die annually from complications during pregnancy and childbirth, at least 7 million suffer from major health issues, and 50 million more experience negative health outcomes after giving birth. The World Health Organization launched Action for Safe Motherhood, a midwife training program, to assist in the improvement of midwifery skills.

It is concerning that the US has a rising rate of maternal deaths. Out of the 14 developed nations examined in 1990, the United States came in at number 12. But since then, while the US rate has sharply increased, the rates in every other nation have improved consistently. The US death rate had increased to 26.4, while the death rates of the other 14 developed nations examined in 1990 are all less than 10 deaths per 100,000 live births. Finland was the safest country at 3.8, while the United Kingdom was ranked second highest at 9 points. Additionally, out of the 700 to 900 US women who died from pregnancy-related causes, 70 suffer major complications like organ failure and hemorrhage, accounting for more than 1% of all births.

In 2022, according to the WHO, while the rates of maternal deaths in other developed countries were declining, the US had the highest rate of maternal deaths of any country. According to a 2020 CDC report, the maternal death rate for Black women was found to be 2.9 times higher than that of White women, at 55.3 deaths per 100,000 live births. The death rate for Black women has also been steadily rising. According to a 2023 study, the death rate for Native American women was even higher—3.5 times higher than that of White women. According to the report, one reason for the high rate is that Native American women receive care from a Federal Healthcare System that is underfunded and overburdened, with monthly visits typically lasting only three to seven minutes. A brief visit like this leaves little time for the patient to discuss any issues she may be having or for an appropriate health assessment to be completed.

4.5.2. Infant Mortality

The infant mortality rate in the United States is likewise high when compared to other developed countries. According to the Trust for America's Health, as of 2011, approximately one-third of births in the United States involve complications. Many of these issues are directly linked to the health of the mother, such as rising rates of type 2 diabetes, obesity, and physical inactivity. The U.S. S. The goal of the Centers for Disease Control and Prevention (CDC) is to lower the rates of maternal and newborn deaths by promoting better health for women before they become pregnant.

A 2015 Save the Children report, which examined 168 countries worldwide, discovered that approximately 8,000 newborns perish in the first month of life every day. Although 70% of infant deaths could have been avoided with the use of basic interventions like hand-held breathing masks, antibiotics, and other basic measures, more than 1 million babies worldwide pass away during their first day of life. Out of all the industrialized nations in the world, the United States had the highest infant death rate on its first day of life. Approximately 11,300 babies in the US pass away within the first 24 hours of their lives every year, which is 50% more than all other industrialized nations put together.

4.5.3. Labor and Delivery Complications

4.5.3.1. Obstructed Labor

Poor or uncoordinated uterine action, an abnormal uterine position (e.g., breech or shoulder dystocia), and cephalopelvic disproportion (a small pelvis or large infant) can all cause the second stage of labor to be delayed or prolonged. Extended labor can lead to various complications such as obstetric fistula, maternal exhaustion, and fetal distress.

4.5.3.2. Eclampsia

When seizures (convulsions) start in a woman who has pre-eclampsia, it is called eclampsia. Pre-eclampsia is a pregnancy condition characterized by elevated blood pressure and either excessive protein excretion in the urine or other organ dysfunction. Prenatal care routinely screens for pre-eclampsia. Onset can occur prior to, during, or infrequently following delivery. Around 1% or so of women who have eclampsia pass away.

4.5.4. Maternal Complications

A puerperal or postpartum disorder is a complication that typically occurs during the postpartum period. This period can be divided into three stages: the initial phase occurring within six to 12 hours after childbirth, the subacute period lasting two to six weeks, and the delayed period lasting up to six months. During the subacute period, 87% to 94% of women experience at least one health issue, while 31% report long-term health problems persisting beyond the delayed period.

4.5.4.1. Postpartum Bleeding

The World Health Organization states that hemorrhage is the primary cause of maternal deaths globally, accounting for roughly 27.1% of maternal fatalities. Postpartum hemorrhage accounts for two-thirds of maternal deaths from bleeding. There are four primary categories into which postpartum hemorrhage causes can be divided: tissue, thrombin, trauma, and tone. Tone is a symbol of uterine atony, or the uterus's inability to contract sufficiently after delivery. Ruptures of the uterus or cuts are examples of trauma. Conditions that can result in a retained placenta are included in tissue. Thrombin is a molecule implicated in the blood clotting system of humans and is indicative of all coagulopathies.

4.5.4.2. Postpartum Infections

Any bacterial infections of the reproductive tract that occur after childbirth or miscarriage are referred to as postpartum infections, medically known as puerperal fever and known historically as childbed fever. A fever higher than 38.0°C (100.04 °F), chills, lower abdominal pain, and possibly foul-smelling vaginal discharge are the typical signs and symptoms. After the first 24 hours and during the first 10 days after delivery, the infection typically manifests. In the developing world, infection continues to be a leading cause of morbidity and mortality among mothers. Many lives were saved by Ignaz Semmelweis's groundbreaking research on the pathophysiology and treatment of childbed fever.

4.5.4.3. Psychological Complications

Positive and negative emotions may surface during childbirth because it can be a powerful experience. Tokophobia is the abnormal and enduring fear of childbirth. Around the world, 4–25% of women report having a fear of giving birth, with 3–6% of pregnant women reporting a clinical fear. After giving birth, most new mothers may feel a little unhappy and worried. Given the amount of care that babies require, it is common for mothers to feel anxious or worn out from giving it. Up to 80% of moms experience the emotions, which are sometimes referred to as the "baby blues." They usually go away on their own, are fairly mild, and last for a week or two.

The baby blues and postpartum depression are not the same thing. Extreme sadness and anxiety are common symptoms of postpartum depression, which can make it difficult for a woman to take care of her family or herself. Treatment is typically necessary for postpartum depression due to the severity of its symptoms. The illness, which affects about 15% of babies born, can start any time after or just before childbirth, but it usually does so a week or two after delivery.

A psychological condition known as childbirth-related posttraumatic stress disorder can arise in women who have recently given birth. Among the causes are conditions like an emergency Caesarean section, premature labor, poor care during labor, a lack of social support after delivery, and more. Invasion symptoms, nightmares, flashbacks, avoidance symptoms (such as forgetting all or some of the event), difficulties forming a mother-child attachment, and other symptoms resembling those frequently seen in posttraumatic stress disorder (PTSD) are a few examples of symptoms. Many times, postpartum depression or adjustment disorders are mistakenly diagnosed as the cause of PTSD symptoms in women who have recently given birth. These diagnoses may result in insufficient care. Postpartum psychosis is an uncommon mental health emergency characterized by sudden onset in the first two weeks following childbirth and symptoms of mania (high mood and racing thoughts), depression, severe confusion, loss of inhibition, paranoia, hallucinations, and delusions. The symptoms can shift rapidly and vary. Usually, hospitalization is necessary. The most severe symptoms can linger for 2 to 12 weeks, and it can take up to a year to recover.

4.5.5. Fetal Complications

Five causes make up about 80% of newborn deaths globally: prematurity, low-birth-weight, infections, lack of oxygen at birth, and trauma during birth.

4.5.5.1. Stillbirth

Fetal death occurring at or after 20 to 28 weeks of pregnancy is the standard definition of stillbirth. As a result, the newborn exhibits no signs of life. With better health systems, most stillbirths can be prevented globally. The majority of stillbirths—roughly half—occur during childbirth, and they are more prevalent in developing nations than in developed ones. Other options include using drugs to induce labor or performing a dilation and evacuation procedure, depending on how far along the pregnancy is. Women are more likely to experience another stillbirth after one, but most subsequent pregnancies do not present with the same issues.

Approximately 2 million stillbirths occurred after 28 weeks of pregnancy worldwide in 2019; this is equivalent to 1 in 72 total births or one every 16 seconds. In Sub-Saharan Africa and South Asia, stillbirths are more frequent. Though more slowly, stillbirth rates have decreased since the 2000s.

4.5.5.2. Preterm Birth

Preterm birth occurs when an infant is born before reaching 37 weeks of gestational age. Approximately 15 million infants worldwide are born prematurely. Premature birth is the primary cause of mortality in children under the age of five, with survivors often facing learning disabilities, visual/hearing impairments, and other health issues. The reasons for early birth may vary, ranging from unknown factors to chronic conditions like diabetes and infections. The World Health Organization has created guidelines aimed at enhancing the survival and overall health of preterm infants.

If a pregnant woman goes into preterm labor, medications called tocolytics can be given to delay delivery. Tocolytics work by stopping contractions of the uterus that would otherwise cause labor to progress. The most commonly used tocolytics are beta-agonists, calcium channel blockers, and magnesium sulfate. The purpose of using tocolytics is not to prolong the pregnancy until full term, but rather to postpone delivery so that glucocorticoids can be administered. These medications help the baby's lungs to mature, reducing the risk of morbidity and mortality from infant respiratory distress syndrome (Figure 4.3).

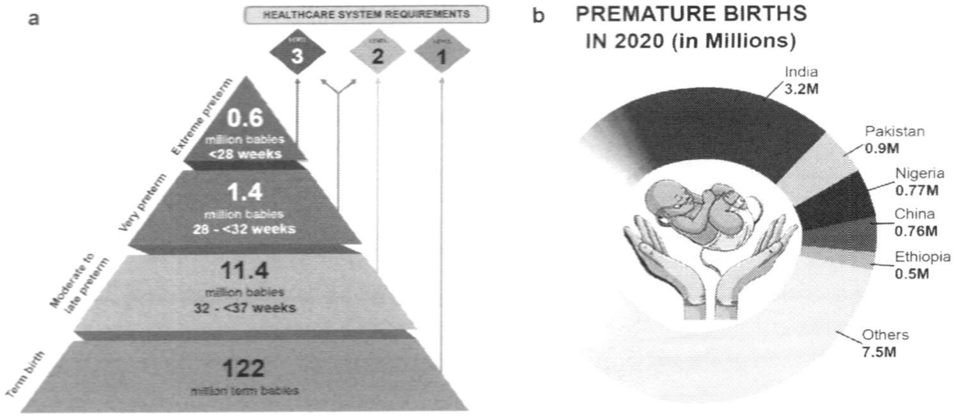

Figure 4.3. *Preterm births.*

Source: *Gondane, P., Kumbhakarn, S., Maity, P., & Kapat, K., (2024). Recent advances and challenges in the early diagnosis and treatment of preterm labor. Bioengineering, 11(2),161. https://doi.org/10.3390/bioengineering11020161.*

4.5.5.3. Post-Term Birth

When a woman reaches 42 weeks of gestation—two weeks past the typical 40-week mark—and has not yet given birth, the condition is referred to as post-term pregnancy. Risks associated with premature births include stillbirths, fetal malnutrition, and meconium aspiration syndrome, which can affect both the mother and the child. After the 42nd week of pregnancy, the placenta, which provides the baby with oxygen and nourishment, starts to deteriorate and will finally fail. When a pregnancy is post-term, induced labor is recommended.

4.5.5.4. Neonatal Infection

During the first month of life, newborns are at risk of infection. The pathogenic bacterium Streptococcus agalactiae, commonly known as group B streptococcus, is typically responsible for these sometimes deadly infections. The baby acquires the infection from the mother during labor. In 2014, approximately one in 2000 newborns were estimated to develop a group B streptococcus infection within the first week of life, often presenting as respiratory issues, sepsis, or meningitis.

If left untreated, sexually transmitted infections (STIs) can lead to birth defects and infections in newborns, especially in regions with high rates of infection. Many STIs show no symptoms or only mild symptoms that may go unnoticed. Mortality rates from certain infections can be significant, such as the 30% perinatal mortality rate linked to untreated syphilis.

4.5.5.5. Perinatal Asphyxia

The medical condition known as perinatal asphyxia is caused by a newborn baby not getting enough oxygen during the birthing process, which can be harmful to the baby physically. The majority of an infant's organs, including the heart, lungs, liver, gut, and kidneys, can also sustain hypoxic damage; however, brain damage is the most serious and may not recover fully or rapidly. Lack of oxygen can cause a child to become permanently disabled, such as developing cerebral palsy.

4.5.5.6. Mechanical Fetal Injury

Fetal macrosomia (big baby), maternal obesity, the need for an instrumental delivery, and an inexperienced attendant are risk factors for fetal birth injury. Breech presentation and shoulder dystocia are two particular circumstances that can lead to birth injuries. The majority of birth injuries heal without causing long-term damage, but injuries to the brachial plexus can result in Klumpke's paralysis or Erb's palsy.

4.6. Postpartum Care

The first six weeks after giving birth is known as the postpartum period. While it is a happy time, it also involves mothers adjusting and healing. It is a time to bond with your baby and to have a follow-up appointment with your doctor to ensure your health post-delivery.

4.6.1. Adjusting to Motherhood

After a baby is born, adjusting to daily life can be difficult, particularly for new mothers. Taking care of your baby is important, but you also need to take care of yourself. For the first six weeks following delivery, the majority of new mothers do not go back to work. This gives people time to adjust and establish a new normal. A baby requires frequent feedings and changes, which can cause insomnia. It can be exhausting and frustrating.

The good news is that you'll eventually fall into a routine. In the meantime, here's what you can do for an easier transition:

1. **Get Plenty of Rest:** Get as much sleep as possible to cope with tiredness and fatigue. Your baby may wake up every two to three hours for feeding. To make sure you're getting enough rest, sleep when your baby sleeps.
2. **Seek Help:** Don't hesitate to accept help from family and friends during the postpartum period, as well as after this period. Your body needs to heal, and practical help around the home can help you get much-needed rest. Friends or family can prepare meals, run errands, or help care for other children in the home.
3. **Eat Healthy Meals:** Maintain a healthy diet to promote healing. Increase your intake of whole grains, vegetables, fruits, and protein. You should also increase your fluid intake, especially if you are breast-feeding.
4. **Exercise:** Your doctor will let you know when it's OK to exercise. The activity should not be strenuous. Try taking a walk near your house. The change of scenery is refreshing and can increase your energy level.

A new baby can alter your dynamic with your partner and cause adjustments for the entire family. It can be problematic if you and your partner don't spend as much quality time together during the postpartum period. Though it's a difficult and stressful time, there are strategies to help you get through it. Firstly, exercise patience. Recognize that changes occur in every couple following the birth of a child. You'll get used to it eventually, but adjustment takes time. Taking care of a newborn becomes easier every day. Communicate as a family as well. Discuss the issue and show understanding if a spouse or other children feel excluded from the family. Don't feel bad about spending time alone together as a couple during the postpartum period, even though you and your partner will be tending to your baby's needs for most of the day.

4.6.2. Baby Blues vs. Postpartum Depression

Having the baby blues during the postpartum period is normal. This can last up to two weeks and usually occurs a few days after giving birth. Most of the time, your symptoms will fluctuate and you won't always have them.

About 70 to 80% of new mothers experience mood swings or negative feelings after giving birth. Baby blues are caused by hormonal changes and symptoms may include:

- Unexplained crying;
- Irritability;
- Insomnia;
- Sadness;
- Mood changes;
- Restlessness.

4.6.3. Function

4.6.3.1. Timing of Postnatal Visits

The American College of Obstetrics and Gynecology (ACOG) changed its recommendation in April 2018 from one six-week postpartum visit to 12 weeks of support. Additionally, according to ACOG, a thorough postpartum visit should be scheduled no later than 12 weeks after delivery. Postpartum (Bauman, B. L., Ko, J. Y., et al. 2020) evaluation should also be completed within the first three weeks following delivery, either in person or over the phone.

4.6.3.2. Components of Postpartum Care

1. **Vaginal Pain:** When a vaginal delivery occurs spontaneously, genital tract trauma is evident. While large tears may take longer to heal, minor tears that happen during childbirth usually heal in a few weeks. Encourage women to sit on a padded ring, apply an ice pack to the area to reduce pain, or take over-the-counter painkillers like acetaminophen or ibuprofen. Healthcare professionals should advise women to seek medical attention for severe, persistent pain and educate them about infection symptoms like fever.
2. **Vaginal Bleeding/Discharge:** Bloody vaginal discharge (lochia rubra) is heavy for the first 3–4 days, and slowly it becomes watery in consistency and color changes to pinkish-brown (lochia serosa). After the next 10–12 days, it changes to yellowish-white (lochia alba). Advise women to seek medical attention if heavy vaginal bleeding persists (soaking a pad or more in less than an hour). Women with heavy, persistent postpartum bleeding should be evaluated for complications such as retained placenta, uterine atony, rarely invasive placenta, or coagulation disorders. Endometritis may also occur, presenting as fever with no source, and maybe accompanied by uterine tenderness and vaginal discharge. This usually requires intravenous antibiotics. This also should be explained and advise the mother to seek immediate medical attention.
3. **Breastfeeding:** It is beneficial for the mother and the newborn. Breastfeeding women are less likely to get breast cancer, ovarian cancer, and type 2 DM. Providers should evaluate latch, swallow, nipple type and condition, and hold of infants for any problems. Interventions include professional support, peer support, and formal education. Healthcare providers should strongly encourage women to breastfeed the newborn unless it is contraindicated. The World Health Organization (WHO) recommends at

least four to six months, every three to four hours daily. Breastfeeding reduces the newborn's risk for gastrointestinal tract infections, pediatric cancers, and atopic eczema. Breastfeeding should be evaluated at each postnatal visit. (Berens, P., Labbok, et all 2015)

4. **Nutrition and Exercise:** Women at higher risk for postpartum weight retention are those with higher gestational weight gain, black race, and lower socioeconomic status, which at the same time increase their risk of future obesity and type 2 diabetes. Advise women to take a variety of healthy balanced diets and resume their normal dietary habits. All breast-feeding mothers need to take an extra 500 calories per day. Avoid strenuous activities in the early postpartum period and take plenty of rest for the first 2–3 weeks and slowly start with non-impact activities such as walking and a gradual return to previous activities is recommended.

5. **Breast Engorgement:** Women may experience full, firm, and tender breasts after the delivery. Frequent breastfeeding on both breasts is recommended to avoid engorgement. Advise women to use warm washcloths or warm showers or place cold washcloths between feedings to relieve the pain. For women who are not going to breastfeed, encourage them to use cold packs, using firm support of the breasts, take analgesics as needed, and mechanical extraction of milk.

6. **Bladder and Bowel Function:** Voiding must be encouraged and monitored to prevent asymptomatic bladder overfilling. Women are encouraged to use mild laxatives such as docusate, psyllium, bisacodyl if defecation has not occurred within 3 days of delivery. Another consideration is osmotic laxatives such as polyethylene glycol and lactulose.

7. **Sexual Relations:** Libido may decrease after the delivery because of decreased estrogen levels. This may not return for as long as one year postpartum, particularly in women who are breastfeeding. Reassurance is usually appropriate. Advise women to wait for their perineal area to heal before resuming sexual activity, and it may take 4–6 weeks for the perineal tears to heal completely.

8. **Contraception:** The ideal time to talk about postpartum contraception is during pregnancy. Start motivational interviewing with teenagers and talk about long-acting, reversible contraception when getting pregnant. Nonhormonal modalities are typically preferred for nursing women. Progestin-only contraceptives are advised by the American College of Obstetrics and Gynecologists (ACOG) to be the most effective hormonal contraceptive method for nursing mothers. Combination estrogen-progestin contraceptives should not be used by nursing mothers since they may affect the production of breast milk. After four weeks postpartum, combined estrogen-progestin vaginal rings can be used as one hormonal method. Because they don't impact milk production, hormonal methods like progestin-only oral contraceptives, depot medroxyprogesterone acetate injections, and progestin implants are preferred. A cervical cap and vaginal diaphragm should only be fitted six to eight weeks after delivery when the uterus has fully invected. The ideal time to implant intrauterine devices is usually four to six weeks after delivery. Breastfeeding is not a reliable method of birth control. The failure rate of other forms of contraception or the lactational amenorrhea method is 2%; however, certain requirements must be met. The woman needs to be amenorrheic (i.e., exclusively breastfeed on demand)., stop vaginal

bleeding eight weeks after giving birth, and have a baby under six months old. The more the baby eats solid foods, the less trustworthy this becomes. Intrauterine devices (IUDs; copper-releasing and hormone-releasing), progestin-only contraception, and barrier contraceptives are available to breastfeeding and nonbreastfeeding women alike. The WHO advises breastfeeding mothers to hold off on starting progestin-only contraceptives for six weeks after giving birth. ACOG advises against using combination hormonal contraceptives until three weeks after giving birth due to the elevated risk of thromboembolism. It is recommended that women wait a minimum of 6–18 months before attempting to conceive again.

9. **Education:** Healthcare providers should provide essential education regarding newborn care, such as umbilical cord care, bathing, breastfeeding, and the importance of immunizations.
10. **Miscarriage, Stillbirth, or Neonatal Death:** For mothers who experience any pregnancy loss, it is essential to ensure follow-up. Key elements are to provide emotional support and bereavement counseling; and referral, if appropriate, to counselor and support groups. Also, review of any laboratory or pathology studies related to the loss and counseling regarding recurrent risk and future pregnancy planning.

4.6.4. Issues of Concern

4.6.4.1. Common Postpartum Concerns

1. **Postpartum Blues:** The first week following childbirth is a common time for women to experience transient depression, also known as the "baby blues." During this time, they may experience mood swings, anxiety, crying fits, irritability, and trouble sleeping. The postpartum blues usually pass after two weeks. If depressive symptoms persist for more than two weeks, they are having trouble caring for themselves or the newborn, or they are having thoughts of hurting themselves or the baby, medical professionals should counsel them to see a doctor. Every woman should undergo screening for anxiety and mood disorders using the Edinburgh Postnatal Depression Scale, a validated tool. Screening should be done during the one-, two-, four-, and six-month well visit, according to the American Academy of Pediatrics. Encourage the partner and family to care for the newborn and offer emotional support during the first week of the postpartum period, at the very least. After giving birth, all postpartum women should be screened for resolution of the postpartum blues 10 to 14 days later, according to the National Institute for Health and Care Excellence.
2. **Intimate Partner Violence:** Use HARK (humiliation, afraid, rape, kick) or HITS (hurt, insult, threaten, scream) tools to evaluate for intimate partner violence. Prioritize patient safety, and consider referral to intimate partner violence prevention organizations.
3. **Incontinence:** Stress incontinence occurs due to extensive stretch or injury to pelvic floor muscles during labor. Risk factors for urinary incontinence three months postpartum include obesity, parity, smoking, longer duration of breastfeeding, and use of forceps during vaginal delivery.

Advise women to do Kegel's exercises regularly to strengthen pelvic floor muscles. Other considerations also are bladder training and weight loss as part of first-line treatment. It is important to let the new mother know that more than ¼ of women experience moderate or severe urinary incontinence in the first year postpartum.

4. **Hemorrhoids:** Caused by constipation and/or by pushing during the second stage of labor. The first line of treatment includes an increase in water and fiber intake and stool softeners. Some may need excision or ligation of refractory hemorrhoids or grade III or higher.

4.6.5. Clinical Significance

At least 40% of women do not seek postpartum care, according to ACOG. This trend is influenced by several factors, including racial disparities, inadequate anticipatory guidance, low socioeconomic status, lack of insurance, inadequate family support, inadequate home visitation, and poor transitional care management. The highest maternal mortality rate is among non-Hispanic blacks, according to the Pregnancy Mortality Surveillance System (PMSS).

Severe hypertension, severe bleeding, and infection are the most common causes of maternal deaths during the first week of the postnatal period; on the other hand, the most common cause of late death is cardiovascular. The US has substantially fallen behind other developed nations, like Norway and New Zealand, in providing appropriate prenatal care, and the country's mortality and morbidity rates are noticeably higher (17.4% vs. 1. 7%), and there are a lot fewer midwives and obstetricians in the US (19 vs. 65 live births per 1000. To improve maternal and neonatal mortality and morbidity, as well as to assess whether the postpartum blues and other chronic medical conditions like diabetes and hypertension can be resolved, earlier postpartum visits are required.

4.6.6. Other Issues

4.6.6.1. Health Issues That Arise During Pregnancy

1. **Pregnancy-Induced Hypertension:** Hypertensive disorder risk is higher < 48 hrs after delivery. An office visit is recommended within the first 7 days after delivery. Blood Pressure (BP) ≥150/100 mmHg can be treated with oral medication such as nifedipine or labetalol. Hospitalize if signs of end-organ (liver injury or pulmonary edema) or BP ≥ 160/110. Recommend lifestyle modification and annual BP and bodyweight monitoring follow-ups.
2. **Gestational Diabetes Mellitus (GDM):** Women with GDM are at a very high risk of developing diabetes. ACOG recommends women with GDM should have a 75-g, 2-hour fasting oral glucose tolerance test 4 to 12 weeks postpartum to screen for type 2 DM.
3. **Thyroid Disorders:** The mother can experience symptoms of hypo- or hyperthyroidism. The diagnosis of postpartum thyroiditis depends on clinical presentation and elevated free T4 and low TSH. Hyperthyroidism is transient and usually not treated. Beta-blockers can be used if needed for symptoms. Hypothyroidism is treated with levothyroxine. The American Thyroid Association recommends annual testing in women with hypothyroidism with a history of postpartum thyroiditis.

A Closer Look

Abdominal Cramping

There are many different possible reasons for abdominal cramps, which can be a very upsetting symptom. The intensity and duration of these cramps, which are characterized by an abrupt, severe pain or discomfort in the abdomen, can vary. Constipation, diarrhea, gas, and bloating are gastrointestinal problems that are frequently the cause of cramping in the abdomen. Dietary errors, food intolerances, infections, or underlying digestive disorders such as inflammatory bowel disease (IBD) or irritable bowel syndrome (IBS) can all cause these symptoms. Another common cause of abdominal pain in women is dysmenorrhea, or cramping during menstruation. These cramps usually happen right before or during the menstrual cycle, and they're frequently accompanied by headaches, exhaustion, and lower back pain.

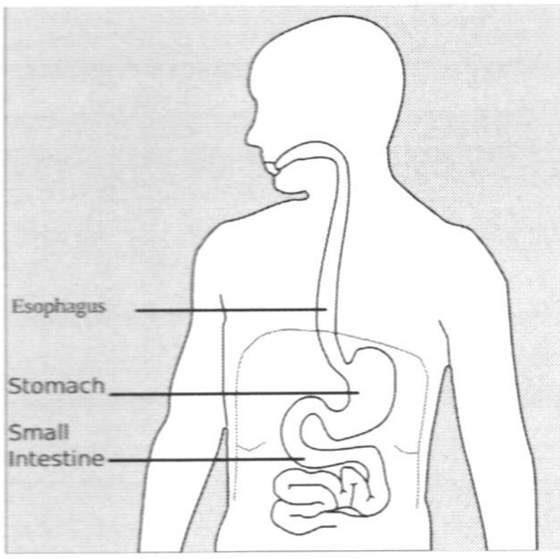

Source: By Indolences at English Wikipedia - Transferred from en.wikipedia to Commons., Public Domain, https://commons.wikimedia.org/w/index.php?curid=1582168.

More serious illnesses like kidney stones, appendicitis, UTIs, or gynecological problems like endometriosis or ovarian cysts can also be indicated by abdominal cramps. Abdominal cramps can sometimes even be a sign of a medical emergency, like a bowel obstruction or an ectopic pregnancy that has ruptured. A medical professional may conduct a physical examination, go over the patient's medical history, and prescribe diagnostic tests like blood work, imaging studies (like CT or ultrasound scans), or endoscopic procedures to identify the cause of abdominal cramps.

The underlying cause of abdominal cramps determines how to treat them. It could involve dietary adjustments, lifestyle adjustments, over-the-counter (like antacids or antidiarrheals) or prescription (like antibiotics or antispasmodics) drugs, as well as, in extreme situations, surgery. Given the wide variety of possible causes, people with severe or persistent abdominal cramps must seek medical attention as soon as possible to ensure appropriate diagnosis and treatment.

Summary

- Childbirth is an intense event that involves extreme physical stress and carries emotional, cognitive, social, and cultural significance. Physically, women have to cope with acute changes as the uterus contracts, the cervix dilates, and the baby and placenta are delivered.
- The most prominent sign of labor is strong repetitive uterine contractions. Pain in contractions has been described as feeling similar to very strong menstrual cramps. Crowning may be experienced as an intense stretching and burning.
- Skin-to-skin contact (SSC), sometimes also called kangaroo care, is a technique of newborn care where babies are kept chest-to-chest and skin-to-skin with a parent, typically their mother, though more recently their father as well.
- Obstetric care frequently subjects women to institutional routines, which may have adverse effects on the progress of labor.
- Pain management during childbirth is the treatment or prevention of pain that a woman may experience during labor and delivery.
- Augmentation is the process of stimulating the uterus to increase the intensity and duration of contractions after labor has begun. Several methods of augmentation are commonly been used to treat slow progress of labor (dystocia) when uterine contractions are assessed to be too weak.
- A puerperal disorder or postpartum disorder is a complication which presents primarily during the puerperium, or postpartum period.

References

1. Bauman, B. L., Ko, J. Y., Cox, S., D'Angelo, M. D. V., Warner, L., Folger, S., Tevendale, H. D., Coy, K. C., Harrison, L., & Barfield, W. D. (2020). Vital signs: Postpartum depressive symptoms and provider discussions about perinatal depression – United States, 2018. *MMWR Morbidity and Mortality Weekly Report*, *69*(19), 575–581.
2. Berens, P., Labbok, M., & Academy of Breastfeeding Medicine. (2015). ABM clinical protocol #13: Contraception during breastfeeding, Revised 2015. *Breastfeeding Medicine*, *10*(1), 3–12.
3. Bugental, D. B., & Johnston, C. (2000). Parental and child cognitions in the context of the family. *Annual Review of Psychology, 51*, 315–344.
4. Chepkirui, D., Nzinga, J., Jemutai, J., Tsofa, B., Jones, C., & Mwangome, M. (2020). A scoping review of breastfeeding peer support models applied in hospital settings. *International Breastfeeding Journal*, *15*(1), 95.
5. Conde, A. A., Figueiredo, B., Costa, R., Pacheco, A., & Pais, A. (2008). Perception of the childbirth experience: Continuity and changes over the postpartum period. *Journal of Reproductive and Infant Psychology*, *26*(2), 139–154.
6. Cook, A., & Stype, A. (2021). Medicaid expansion and infant mortality: the (questionable) impact of the Affordable Care Act. *Journal of Epidemiology and Community Health*, *75*(1), 10–15.
7. Declercq, E., Cunningham, D. K., Johnson, C., & Sakala, C. (2008). Mothers' reports of postpartum

pain associated with vaginal and cesarean deliveries: Results of a national survey. *Birth, 35*(1), 16–24.

8. Durik, A. M., Hyde, J. S., & Clark, R. (2000). Sequelae of cesarean and vaginal deliveries: Psychosocial outcomes for mothers and infants. *Developmental Psychology, 36*(2), 251–260.
9. Farrow, C., & Blissett, J. (2007). The development of maternal self-esteem. *Infant Mental Health Journal, 28*(5), 517–535.
10. Feltner, C., Wallace, I., Berkman, N., Kistler, C. E., Middleton, J. C., Barclay, C., Higginbotham, L., Green, J. T., & Jonas, D. E. (2018). Screening for intimate partner violence, elder abuse, and abuse of vulnerable adults: Evidence report and systematic review for the US preventive services task force. *JAMA, 320*(16), 1688–1701.
11. Florio, K. L., DeZorzi, C., Williams, E., Swearingen, K., & Magalski, A. (2021). Cardiovascular medications in pregnancy: A primer. *Cardiology Clinics, 39*(1), 33–54.
12. Gabbe, S. G., Gregory, R. P., Power, M. L., Williams, S. B., & Schulkin, J. (2004). Management of diabetes mellitus by obstetrician-gynecologists. *Obstetrics & Gynecology, 103*(6), 1229–1234.
13. George, C., & Solomon, J. (2008). The caregiving system: A behavioral systems approach to parenting. In J. Cassidy & P. Shaver (Eds.), *Handbook of attachment: Theory, research, and clinical application* (2nd ed., pp. 383–417). New York: Guilford Press.
14. Gertosio, C., Meazza, C., Pagani, S., & Bozzola, M. (2016). Breastfeeding and its gamut of benefits. *Minerva Pediatrica, 68*(3), 201–212.
15. Green, J. M., & Baston, H. A. (2003). Feeling in control during labor: Concepts, correlates, and consequences. *Birth, 30*(4), 235–247.
16. Haran, C., van Driel, M., Mitchell, B. L., & Brodribb, W. E. (2014). Clinical guidelines for postpartum women and infants in primary care-a systematic review. *BMC Pregnancy and Childbirth, 14*, 51.
17. Kalra, B., Sawhney, K., & Kalra, S. (2017). Management of thyroid disorders in pregnancy: Recommendations made simple. *Journal of the Pakistan Medical Association, 67*(9), 1452–1455
18. Lorenz, T. K., Ramsdell, E. L., & Brock, R. L. (2022). Communication changes the effects of sexual pain on sexual frequency in the pregnancy to postpartum transition. *Journal of Psychosomatic Obstetrics & Gynecology, 43*(2), 91–98.
19. Marchi, K. S., Dove, M. S., Heck, K. E., & Fan, C. (2021). The affordable care act and changes in women's health insurance coverage before, during, and after pregnancy in California. *Public Health Reports, 136*(1), 70–78.
20. McKinney, J., Keyser, L., Clinton, S., & Pagliano, C. (2018). ACOG committee opinion No. 736: Optimizing postpartum care. *Obstetrics & Gynecology, 132*(3), 784–785.
21. Monvillers, S., Tchaconas, A., Li, R., Adesman, A., & Keim, S. A. (2020). Characteristics of and sources of support for women who breastfed multiples for more than 12 months. *Breastfeeding Medicine, 15*(4), 213–223.
22. Paladine, H. L., Blenning, C. E., & Strangas, Y. (2019). Postpartum care: An approach to the fourth trimester. *American Family Physician, 100*(8), 485–491.
23. Stevens, J., Lutz, R., Osuagwu, N., Rotz, D., & Goesling, B. (2017). A randomized trial of motivational interviewing and facilitated contraceptive access to prevent rapid repeat pregnancy among adolescent mothers. *American Journal of Obstetrics & Gynecology, 217*(4), 423.e1–423.e9.

Chapter 5

NEWBORN CARE

Contents

Unit Introduction 150
5.1. Newborn Assessment and Care 152
5.2. Common Newborn Health Problems 155
5.3. Neonatal Resuscitation 158
5.4. Screening and Diagnostic Tests for Newborns 166
Summary 172
References 172

Unit Introduction

Every newborn, everywhere, has the right to high-quality universal newborn healthcare. Babies have the right to adequate nutrition, warmth, breathing, protection from harm, and immunity from infection. Access to essential newborn care—the critical care that every baby needs in the initial days following birth—should be available to all newborns. Immediate postpartum care as well as critical care for the duration of the newborn stage are both included in essential newborn care. It is required at home as well as in the medical facility.

Essential newborn care includes:

- Immediate care at birth (delayed cord clamping, thorough drying, assessment of breathing, skin-to-skin contact, early initiation of breastfeeding).
- Thermal care.
- Resuscitation when needed.
- Support for breast milk feeding.
- Nurturing care.
- Infection prevention.
- Assessment of health problems.
- Recognition and response to danger signs.
- Timely and safe referral when needed.

Orientation and Directional Terms

Term	Definition	Illustration
Immunity from infection	Immunity to infection is the body's ability to protect itself from harmful substances, like bacteria, viruses, parasites, and fungi, that can cause disease.	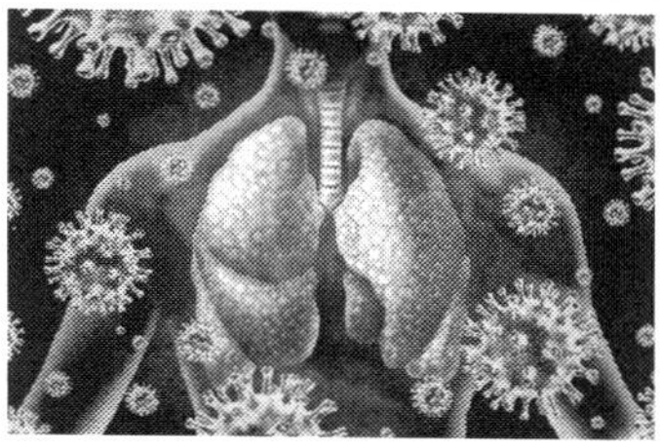
Abdominal Circumference	Abdominal circumference (AC) is a measurement used in obstetric care to assess the size of a fetus.	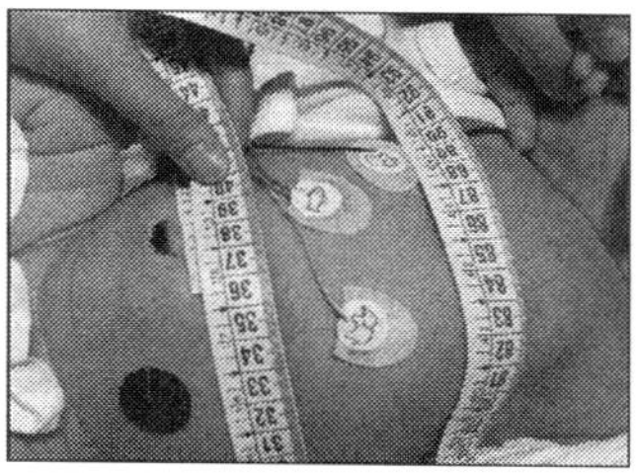
Abdomen	The abdomen is a large body cavity enclosed by the abdominal muscles, at the front and to the sides, and by part of the vertebral column at the back.	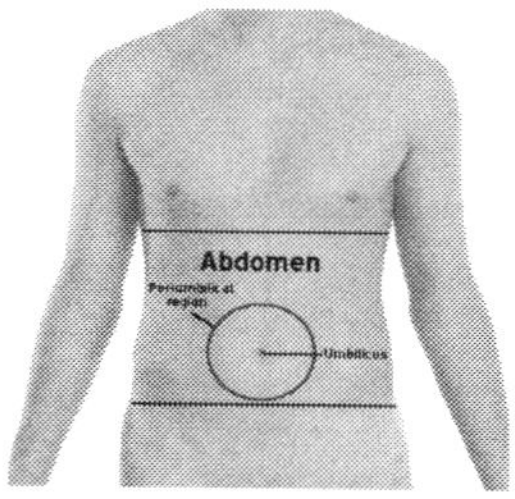
Gestational age	Gestational age is the common term used during pregnancy to describe how far along the pregnancy is.	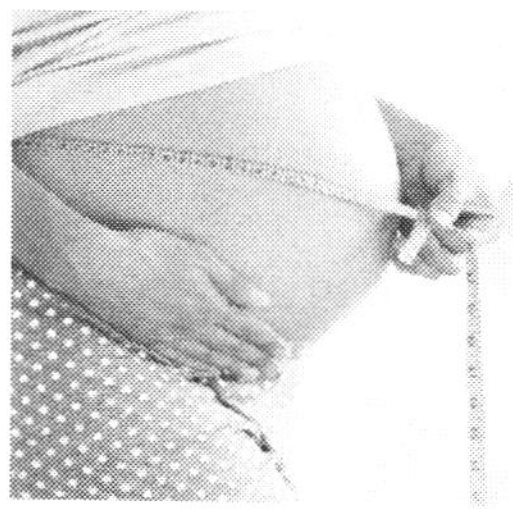
Vernix caseosa	Vernix caseosa is a white, waxy substance that covers the skin of a fetus during the third trimester of pregnancy and on a newborn after birth	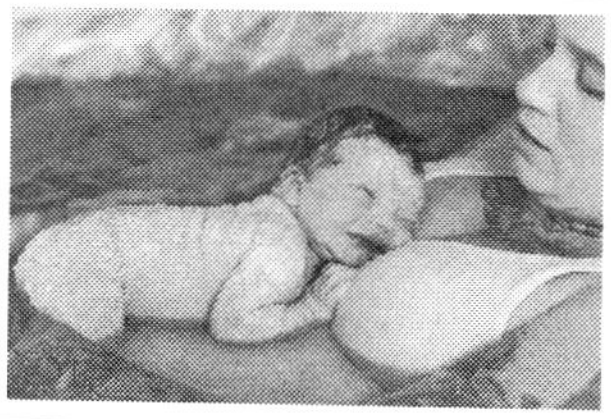

5.1. Newborn Assessment and Care

Every newborn is closely examined for indications of complications or issues at the time of birth. There will be a thorough physical examination that covers every bodily system. Doctors, nurses, and other medical professionals continuously monitor the baby's health during the hospital stay, looking for any indications of illness or problems. Assessment may include:

5.1.1. Apgar Scoring

One of the first things to determine your newborn's health is their Apgar score. Within the first few minutes of life, babies who are having trouble breathing or who require additional care are identified using the Apgar score. The baby's heart and breathing rates, muscle tone, reflexes, and color are assessed one and five minutes after birth. A score of zero, one, or two can be assigned to each area, with a maximum of 10 points. A baby is in the best possible condition if they receive a total score of 10. Most babies receive a score of eight to ten, with the immature circulation in their hands and feet deducting one or two points. A baby's Apgar score may drop if they have difficulty delivering the baby, which may also lower blood oxygen levels. When a baby receives an Apgar score of three or lower, they typically require emergency care.

5.1.2. Birthweight

The birthweight of a child is a crucial health indicator. Term babies, defined as those born between 37 and 41 weeks gestation, typically weigh around 7 pounds. (3.2 kg). Small and very large babies are generally more likely to have issues. Every day, the nursery weighs the babies to determine their nutritional, fluid, and growth requirements. It is common for newborns to lose 5% to 7% of their birthweight. This implies that a newborn weighing seven pounds, three ounces may lose up to eight ounces in the first few days of life. By the time they are two weeks old, babies usually gain this weight back. Babies that are premature or unwell might not gain weight right away. Most hospitals use the metric system for weighing babies.

Converting grams to pounds and ounces:

1 lb. = 453.59237 grams; 1 oz. = 28.349523 grams; 1000 grams = 1. Kg.

5.1.3. Measurements

Other measurements are also taken of each baby. These include the following:

- **Head Circumference:** The distance around the baby's head.
- **Abdominal Circumference:** The distance around the abdomen.
- **Length:** The measurement from the crown of the head to the heel.
- **Vital Signs:**
    - Temperature (able to maintain stable body temperature in normal room environment).
    - Pulse (normally 120 to 160 beats per minute in the newborn period).
    - Breathing rate (normally 40 to 60 breaths per minute in the newborn period).
- **General Appearance:** Physical activity, tone, posture, and level of consciousness
- **Skin:** Color, texture, nails, presence of rashes.
- **Head and Neck:**
    - Appearance, shape, presence of molding (shaping of the head from passage through the birth canal).

  - Fontanels (the open "soft spots" between the bones of the baby's skull).
- **Clavicles:** Bones across the upper chest.
- **Face:** Eyes, ears, nose, cheeks.
- **Mouth:** Palate, tongue, throat.
- **Lungs:**
  - Breath sounds, breathing pattern.
  - Heart sounds and femoral (in the groin) pulses.
- **Abdomen:** Presence of masses or hernias.
- **Genitals and Anus:** For open passage of urine and stool
- **Arms and Legs:** Movement and development.

5.1.4. Physical Examination

One of the most crucial aspects of newborn care is a thorough physical examination. Every bodily system is closely inspected for indications of sound health and regular operation. The physician searches for any indications of disease or birth abnormalities. Physical examination of a newborn often includes the assessment of the following:

5.1.4.1. Gestational Assessment

An essential component of care is determining the physical maturity of the infant. When a pregnancy's dates are unknown, a maturity assessment can be useful in providing for the needs of the unborn child. A very small baby, for instance, might be larger than it seems and require different care than a premature baby. The Dubowitz/Ballard Examination for Gestational Age is a frequently utilized assessment tool. This examination can frequently be used to estimate a baby's gestational age accurately. The Dubowitz/Ballard Exam measures a baby's reflexes, motor abilities, skin texture, and overall appearance. Within the first two hours of life, the physical maturity portion of the examination is completed. After delivery, the neuromuscular maturity assessment is finished in a day. Information often used to help estimate babies' physical and neuromuscular maturity are shown below.

5.1.4.2. Physical Maturity

The Dubowitz/Ballard Examination's physical assessment section examines physical traits that vary in appearance depending on a baby's gestational maturity stage. Physically mature babies typically score higher than premature babies.

5.1.4.3. Neuromuscular Maturity

Points are given for each area of assessment, with a low of –1 or –2 for extreme immaturity to as much as 4 or 5 for postmaturity. Areas of assessment include the following:

- Skin textures (e.g., sticky, smooth, or peeling).
- Lanugo (the soft downy hair on a baby's body). Absent in immature babies, then appears with maturity, and then disappears again with postmaturity.

- Plantar creases. These creases on the soles of the feet range from absent to covering the entire foot, depending on the maturity.
- Breast. The thickness and size of breast tissue and areola (the darkened ring around each nipple) are assessed.
- Eyes and ears. Eyes fused or open and amount of cartilage and stiffness of the ear tissue.
- Genitals, male. Presence of testes and appearance of scrotum, from smooth to wrinkled.
- Genitals, female. Appearance and size of the clitoris and the labia.

5.1.4.4. Neuromuscular Maturity

The gestational age can be estimated by adding the scores from the neuromuscular and physical assessment. For babies who are under 26 to 28 weeks old, the scores are very low; for babies who are mature and postmature, the scores are very high. These are all crucial ways to find out how your baby is doing at birth in terms of health. Your baby's doctor can plan the best possible care by identifying any issues.

5.1.5. Care of the Newborn

As healthcare providers, we have the privilege of caring for newborns, who are some of the most fascinating and inquisitive individuals you will ever come across. They bring joy to everyone they meet, and it is our responsibility to provide them with the best possible care from the moment they are born until they are ready to be handed over to their parents. (Holmes AV. 2013)

5.1.5.1. Care of the Newborn at Birth

- Newborn care is immediately done after birth in a separate space near the birthing area.
- Equipment such as a radiant heat table, warm blankets, resuscitation, eye care, suction, weighing scale and equipment for oxygen administration are already prepared and ready to use.
- Newborn identification and registration is an important step after immediate newborn care to avoid switching of babies or kidnapping in the healthcare facility.
- An identification band is placed around the newborn's arm or leg which contains the mother's hospital number, the mother's full name, sex, date, and time of the infant's birth.
- The newborn's footprints are then taken and kept for permanent identification.
- The birth registration of the infant is taken care of by the physician or nurse-midwife who supervised the delivery.
- The mother's name, the father's name, and the infant's name and birthdate, as well as the place, are recorded.
- The newborn's chart is also a mine of information when it comes to the newborn's welfare.
- Essential information such as the time of the infant's birth, the Apgar score, eye care given, immunizations, and the general condition of the infant must be reflected on the chart.

5.1.5.2. Care of the Newborn in the Postpartum Period

- Newborn care varies among cultures and in some areas in the world.
- During the initial feeding, a term newborn could be fed immediately after birth while a formula-fed one should be fed at 2 to 4 hours of age.

- Bathing is done an hour after birth to gently wash away the **vernix caseosa**, and this is done daily.
- Areas such as the newborn's face, skin folds, and diaper area are the areas that need washing regularly.
- The nurse must supervise the bathing together with the parents.
- The bath water must be pleasantly warm as well as the room to prevent chilling.
- Bathing should be before feeding and not after it to prevent aspiration and vomiting.
- Equipment needed during bathing is a basin of water, washcloth, soap, towel, diaper, a clean shirt, and comb.
- Start bathing the infant from the cleanest area (the eyes) towards the dirtiest area (the diaper area), and soap is never used for the baby's face, only for the body.
- Do not soak the cord when you wash the skin around it.
- Instruct the parents that the sleeping position of the infant must be flat on the back to prevent SIDS, but never place a pacifier on the infant during sleep.
- During a diaper change, the area must be washed and dried well to prevent diaper rash.
- Petroleum jelly or a mild ointment is applied on the buttocks to avoid accumulation of ammonia and remove meconium.
- Vaccination for Hepatitis B and Vitamin K administration is also essential in the postpartal period.

5.2. Common Newborn Health Problems

Some common health issues they face are jaundice, cough, vomiting, and fever. The many changes that accompany the arrival of a baby can make the early days of parenting seem overwhelming. Furthermore, the majority of parents lack knowledge about how to handle issues with infants and newborns, which increases anxiety. Newborns have a sensitive immune system that is still developing. They run the risk of becoming infected often as a result. These infections could result in complications if they are not treated promptly. Therefore, parents must be aware of common infant problems and how to handle them.

When it comes to health problems, the newborn stage is the most critical. Here are a few health conditions that are fairly common in newborns:

5.2.1. Abdominal Distension

Most newborns have protruding bellies. But if your baby's belly feels hard and swollen in between feeds, do some sleuthing.

5.2.2. Birth Injuries

A difficult labor can leave your newborn with some birth injuries. Most newborns recover quickly from these injuries, so don't stress about it. Some common birth injuries your infant may encounter are a broken collarbone, muscle weakness, forceps marks, skin marks, and disturbed head formation.

5.2.3. Bluish Skin

Bluish skin is one of the issues with baby skin. Blue hands and feet are quite common in newborns, so there's no need to be concerned. When they cry, newborns occasionally experience blueness around their mouth and tongue. However, the blueness fades over time.

However, you should see your doctor right away if your child's pink skin does not return (Figure 5.1). (Visscher MO, Adam R, et al. 2015)

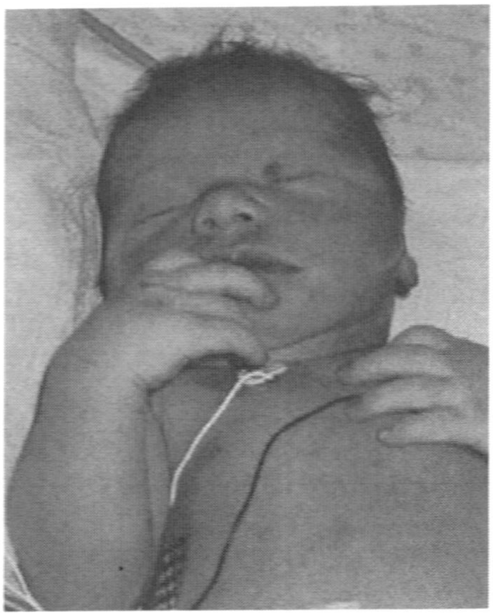

Figure 5.1. *Blue skin.*

Source: By Author: Jules Atkins, RMSupplied by: Brandi Catt - Transferred from en.wikipedia, Attribution, https://commons.wikimedia.org/w/index.php?curid=5388053.

5.2.4. Coughing

A baby may cough during feedings because the milk may occasionally flow in too quickly. However, consult a physician if your child frequently gags during feedings or if she has an intractable cough. It might point to an issue with the digestive or pulmonary systems. You must rule out whooping cough if your child is coughing uncontrollably, especially at night.

5.2.5. Jaundice

Jaundice is a common issue in infants. Many newborns have elevated bilirubin levels because of the immaturity of their livers. The majority of newborn jaundice cases go away with time. However, it can also result in major issues. Thus, *if your doctor prescribes a jaundice treatment,* follow it. An earlier theory that suggested brain damage is caused by neonatal jaundice was shown to be unfounded.

5.2.6. Respiratory Distress

A newborn needs several hours to breathe consistently. But after her body adjusts to breathing, she shouldn't experience any more problems. Babies' breathing difficulties are caused by a variety of factors. Examine your baby's nasal passages if you notice that she is having trouble breathing. Breathing problems are typically brought on by obstructions in the nasal passages. The use of saline drops can help with this issue.

But if you notice any of the following symptoms, go see your pediatrician immediately:

- Rapid breathing;
- Flaring of the nose;
- Grunting while breathing;
- Blue skin color that refuses to fade.

If you had preterm labor, your baby is at a higher risk of developing respiratory distress.

5.2.7. Vomiting

For infants, vomiting is a common health issue. After feeding, it's common for babies to spit up milk. However, frequent vomiting is not typical. Ascertain that your child is not allergic to breast milk or lactose intolerant to avoid frequent spit-ups and vomiting. To keep your baby from throwing up her entire meal, you must also burp her often. Your child may require medical attention if she is throwing up and not gaining enough weight. Be mindful of the color as well. See your doctor about treatment options and potential infections if your baby's vomit appears green. Vomiting could also be caused by digestive problems.

5.2.8. Fever

The issue is not a fever. A fever is merely a sign that the body of your child is attempting to fight off an infection. Even minor fevers don't require medical attention. However, you should take your child to the doctor if she has a high fever. A high fever (102 F) has the potential to induce seizures and be extremely concerning.

5.2.9. Colic

If your child cries all the time and you're not sure why, colic is the reason! Babies that are colicky are generally healthy and don't exhibit any other symptoms of discomfort. Make sure your child is not allergic to the formula you are using, as this can also lead to colic in infants. Fortunately, by the time your baby is three months old, the majority of colic cases have resolved.

5.2.10. Skin Problems

Infants and babies have sensitive skin. So it is common for them to experience skin problems. Some of the common skin problems your baby may encounter include:

5.2.10.1. Diaper Rash

One of the more common skin problems in babies is diaper rash. To prevent this common yet painful condition, keep the following points in mind:

- Be regular when it comes to changing your baby's diaper. Change the diaper every four hours even if it is not soiled.
- Use a diaper rash cream in case your baby develops a rash.
- If you are using a cloth diaper, use fragrance and dye-free detergents.

5.2.10.2. Cradle Cap

Cradle cap too is a common skin problem among babies. If your baby has developed a cradle cap, do not worry. Try these methods to manage it:

- Wash the baby's hair every day;
- Use a mild shampoo.

5.2.11. Cold and Flu

Babies and infants are susceptible to certain infections. Colds and the flu are examples of viral infections that are typically safe and resolve without seriously harming your baby's health. However, a common cold in babies can develop into pneumonia, which is a very dangerous illness. Therefore, it's crucial to visit your doctor even if your child just has a common cold.

5.2.12. Ear Infections

Little ones also get ear infections very frequently. Your baby may have an ear infection if she is fussier than normal and pulling at her ear. While bacterial infections may require an antibiotic dosage, viral infections resolve on their own after a certain amount of time.

5.2.13. Oral Thrush

Another infection that could strike your little child is oral thrush. It is determined that your baby has oral thrush when yeast takes over its mouth. See if your child requires a prescription for antifungal medication by speaking with your pediatrician.

5.2.14. Diarrhea

Diarrhea is also common among infants and babies. As long as you keep your baby hydrated, you need not worry about diarrhea. Continue breastfeeding and start giving an ORS solution prepared at home.

5.2.15. Constipation

Is your baby straining while passing stool? She may be suffering from constipation! Common among babies, constipation is not a big health issue unless it is causing your little one acute discomfort (Figure 5.2).

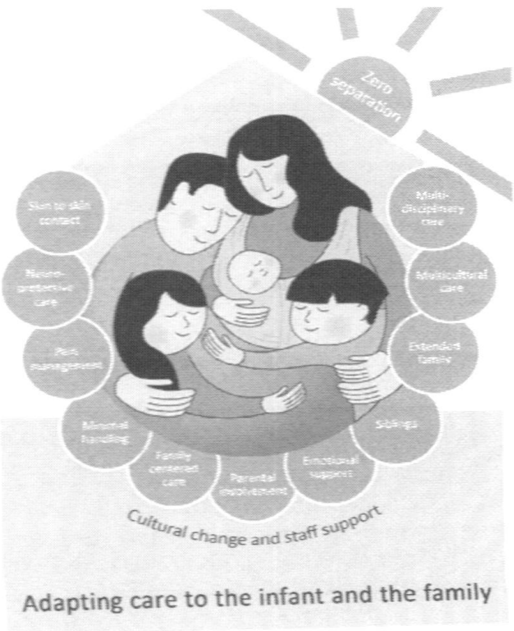

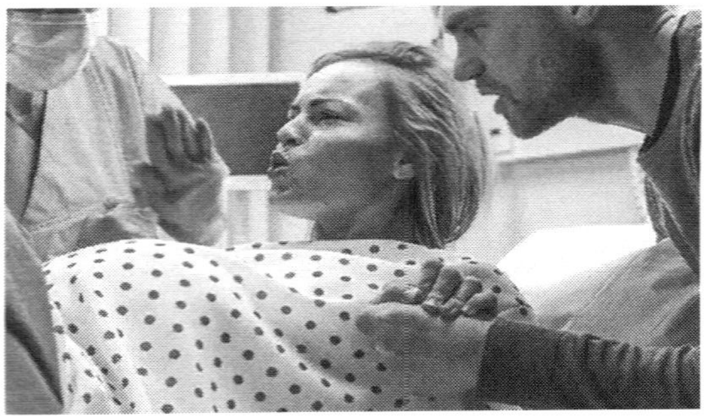

Figure 5.2. *Infant care.*

Source: *Lyngstad, L. T., Le Marechal, F., Ekeberg, B. L., Hochnowski, K., Hval, M., & Tandberg, B. S., (2022). 10 years of neonatal intensive care adaption to the infants' needs: implementation of a family-centered care model with single-family rooms in Norway. International Journal of Environmental Research and Public Health, 19(10), 5917. https://doi.org/10.3390/ijerph19105917.*

5.3. Neonatal Resuscitation

Significant physiological alterations occur concomitant with childbirth, occasionally revealing medical conditions that were not problematic during intrauterine life. Because of this, every birth requires the presence of a neonatal resuscitation specialist. The risk of neonatal pathology can be determined with the aid of growth parameters and gestational age.

A newborn that is not breathing or has other serious health issues is revived with the help of neonatal resuscitation. Roughly 10% of newborns need some kind of respiratory support. Less than 1% require prolonged resuscitation. Depression can have many different causes, some of which need resuscitation from birth. The need for resuscitation rises significantly if birthweight is < 1500 g (Table 5.1).

Table 5.1. *Resuscitation at Birth-the Terms*

Immediate Assessment and Stimulation of the Newborn Baby
Immediate assessment, warming, drying and tactile stimulation (rubbing with the drying cloth, rubbing the back or flicking the feet) of the newborn at the time of birth. This is not the same as the WHO package of essential newborn care which is more complex and includes immediate breastfeeding, resuscitation, thermal care, eye care, immunization etc.
Basic Newborn Resuscitation
Airway clearing (suctioning if required) head positioning and positive pressure ventilation via bag-and- mask.*
Advanced Newborn Resuscitation (not estimated for LiST)
Basic neonatal resuscitation (as above) *plus* endotracheal intubation, supplemental oxygen, chest compressions, and medications.

Source: Lee, A. C., Cousens, S., Wall, S. N., et al., (2011). Neonatal resuscitation and immediate newborn assessment and stimulation for the prevention of neonatal deaths: A systematic review, meta-analysis and Delphi estimation of mortality effect. BMC Public Health, 11(3), S12. https://doi.org/10.1186/1471-2458-11-S3-S12.

5.3.1. Apgar Score

The Apgar score is used to describe a neonate's cardiorespiratory and neurologic condition at birth. The score is not a tool to guide resuscitation or subsequent treatment and does not determine the prognosis of an individual patient.

The Apgar score assigns 0 to 2 points for each of the 5 measures of neonatal health. Scores depend on physiologic maturity and birthweight, maternal perinatal therapy, and fetal cardiorespiratory and neurologic conditions. A score of 7 to 10 at 5 minutes is considered normal; 4 to 6, intermediate; and 0 to 3, low. Usually, scores are assigned only at 1 and 5 minutes of life. If scores are ≤ 5 at 5 minutes of life, scores should continue to be assigned every 5 minutes until the score is > 5.

There are multiple possible causes of low (0 to 3) Apgar scores, including severe, chronic problems that have a poor prognosis and acute problems that can be quickly resolved and have a good prognosis. A low Apgar score is a clinical finding and not a diagnosis (Table 5.2).

Table 5.2. *Neonatal Deaths and Addressing Them*

Effect on Intrapartum-Related Neonatal Deaths ("Birth Asphyxia")
Cause specific effect Immediate newborn assessment, drying, and stimulation 10% (Range 0–25%, IQR 5–15%) Basic neonatal resuscitation (facility) 30% (95% CI: 16–41%) Basic neonatal resuscitation (community) 20% (Range 10–50%, IQR 15–25%) (**note that the resuscitation effect is in addition to* immediate assessment, drying, and stimulation) *Quality of input evidence:* Basic neonatal resuscitation (facility) - moderate (3 low quality before-and-after studies, upgraded for consistency) Immediate newborn assessment, drying, and stimulation – very low (based on Delphi) Basic neonatal resuscitation (community) – very low (based on Delphi) *Proximity of the data to cause specific mortality effect:* Moderate (cause specific mortality but lack of consistency in cause-of-death definitions) *Limitations of the evidence:* There is a lack of rigorous evaluation particularly for the effect of immediate newborn assessment, drying, and stimulation. Data are compromised by misclassification of live births and intrapartum stillbirths and by inconsistencies in cause-of-death attribution between term intrapartum-related neonatal deaths and preterm complications especially if a clinical case definition of "not breathing at birth" ("birth asphyxia") is applied which includes both categories. *Possible adverse effects:* Babies who survive despite severe brain injury may have long term impairments. There is a dearth of data on long term outcomes from low and middle income settings.
Effect on neonatal deaths due to preterm direct complications
Cause specific effect Immediate newborn assessment, drying, and stimulation 10% (Range 0–20%, IQR 5–15%) Basic neonatal resuscitation (facility) 10% (Range 4–30%, IQR 10–20%) Basic neonatal resuscitation (community) 5% (Range 1–40%, IQR5–10%) (**note that the resuscitation effect is in addition to* immediate assessment, drying, and stimulation) ***Quality of input evidence:*** Very low (all based on Delphi) ***Limitations of the evidence:*** As discussed above. ***Possible adverse effects:*** As discussed above.

Source: Lee, A. C., Cousens, S., Wall, S. N., et al., (2011). Neonatal resuscitation and immediate newborn assessment and stimulation for the prevention of neonatal deaths: A systematic review, meta-analysis and Delphi estimation of mortality effect. BMC Public Health, 11(3), S12. https://doi.org/10.1186/1471-2458-11-S3-S12.

5.3.2. Resuscitation

The most recent guidelines for neonatal resuscitation from the American Heart Association and the American Academy of Pediatrics should be followed.

Preparation is essential. Identify perinatal risk factors, assign roles to team members, and prepare and check equipment:

- At least 1 person skilled in the initial steps of neonatal resuscitation, including giving positive pressure ventilation (PPV), should be in attendance at every birth, and additional personnel with the ability to do a complete resuscitation should be rapidly available even in the absence of specific risk factors. A team of 4 or more members may be required for a complex resuscitation, and depending on the risk factors, it may be appropriate for the entire resuscitation team to be present before the birth.
- Before a preterm delivery, set room temperature to 23 to 25° C (74 to 77° F).
- A thermal mattress, hat, and plastic bag or wrap should be used for preterm infants < 32 weeks gestation.

Many perinatal risk factors increase the likelihood of a need for resuscitation. In addition to those noted in table Problems in the Neonate That May Require Resuscitation, some other risk factors include (Figure 5.3):

- Lack of prenatal care;
- Gestational age < 36 weeks or ≥ 41 weeks;

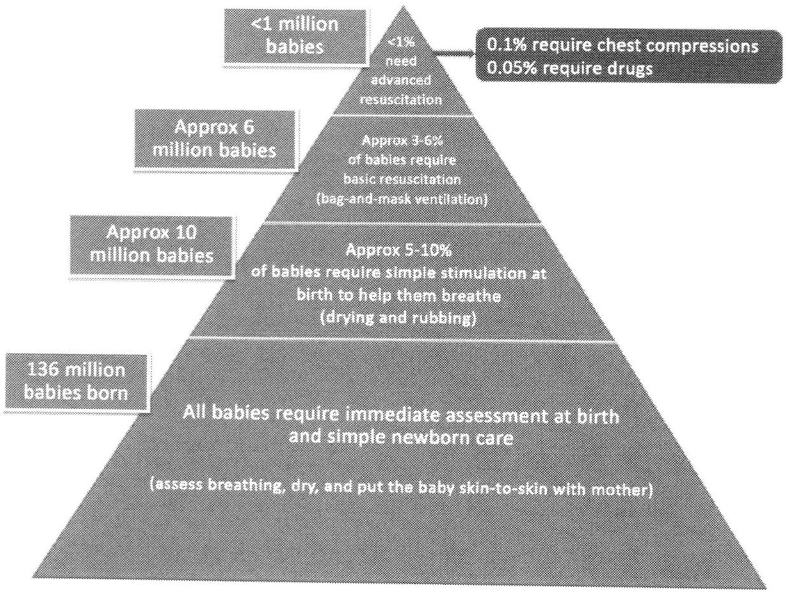

Figure 5.3. *Resuscitation of neonates.*

Source: Lee, A. C., Cousens, S., Wall, S. N., et al., (2011). Neonatal resuscitation and immediate newborn assessment and stimulation for the prevention of neonatal deaths: A systematic review, meta-analysis and Delphi estimation of mortality effect. BMC Public Health, 11(3), S12. https://doi.org/10.1186/1471-2458-11-S3-S12.

- Multiple gestations;
- Need for forceps, vacuum assistance or emergency cesarean delivery;
- Meconium-stained fluid;
- Shoulder dystocia, breech, or other abnormal presentation;
- Certain abnormal heart rate patterns in the fetus;
- Signs of infection in the infant;
- Maternal risk factors (e.g., fever, untreated or inadequately treated group B strep infection).

5.3.3. Initial Measures

Initial measures for all neonates include:

- Rapid assessment (within 60 seconds of birth) of breathing, heart rate, and color;
- Providing warmth to maintain a body temperature of 36.5 to 37.5° C;
- Drying;
- Stimulation of infant;
- Positioning to open the airway;
- Suctioning if needed.

Suctioning, including the use of a bulb syringe, is indicated only for infants who have obvious airway obstruction or who require positive pressure ventilation. It is recommended to delay clamping the umbilical cord by 30 seconds for both preterm and term infants who do not need resuscitation. However, there is insufficient evidence to support delayed cord clamping for infants who do require resuscitation. For the majority of babies who are vigorous and do not need resuscitation, it is important to establish skin-to-skin contact with the mother as soon as possible.

The decision on whether resuscitation is needed is primarily based on the baby's respiratory effort and heart rate. Using a 3-lead cardiac monitor is the preferred method to assess heart rate. Additionally, it is important to monitor oxygen saturation using pulse oximetry with a preductal probe on the right wrist, hand, or finger, considering the expected gradual increase in oxygen saturation during the first 10 minutes of life (Table 5.3).

Table 5.3. *Neonatal Oxygen Saturation Targets*

Time After Delivery	Preductal* SpO_2
1 minute	60–65%
2 minutes	65–70%
3 minutes	70–75%
4 minutes	75–80%
5 minutes	80–85%
≥10 minutes	85–95%

*The right upper extremity receives preductal blood.

SpO_2 = oxygen saturation.

5.3.4. Ventilation and Oxygenation

It may be beneficial to stimulate the newborn by rubbing their back or flicking their foot soles if their breathing effort is low. Unless necessary for airway obstruction, suctioning is not a useful stimulation technique and can trigger a vagal response that results in bradycardia and apnea. Supplemental oxygen and/or continuous positive airway pressure (CPAP) is recommended for infants with a heart rate of ≥ 100 beats per minute who exhibit respiratory distress, labored breathing, and/or persistent cyanosis.

For babies whose heart rates range from 60 to. < 100 beats/minute who have apnea, gasping, or ineffective respirations, positive pressure ventilation (PPV) using a mask is indicated. Before giving PPV, the airway should be cleared by gently suctioning the mouth first and then the nose with a bulb syringe. The infant's head and neck are supported in the neutral (sniffing) position, and the mouth is slightly opened with the jaw brought forward. Initial ventilator settings for a term infant are peak inspiratory pressure (PIP) of 20 to 25 cm H_2O, positive end-expiratory pressure (PEEP) of 5 cm H_2O, and an assist control (AC) or intermittent mandatory ventilation (IMV) rate of 40 to 60 breaths/minute. There is insufficient data to recommend a specific inspiratory time, but inflations of > 5 it is not advised to use seconds.

If the heart rate is <60 beats/minute, neonates require compressions and PPV while awaiting endotracheal intubation (Figure 5.4).

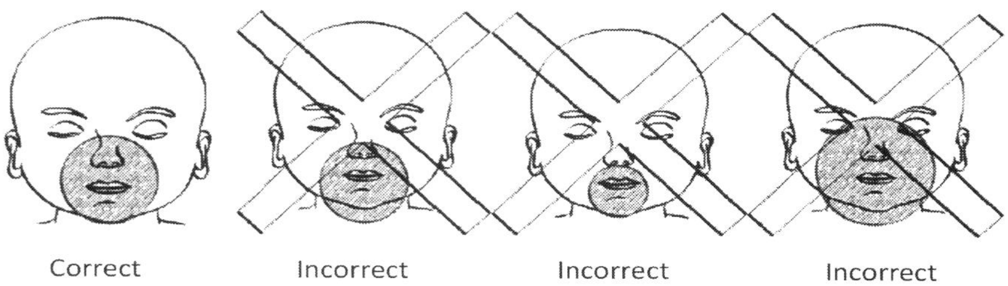

Figure 5.4. *Mask position.*

Source: *https://medicalguidelines.msf.org/sites/default/files/Figure+10-2_FR.png.*

The heart rate's quick recovery is the primary indicator of ventilation efficacy. If the heart rate doesn't rise in 15 seconds, check that the mask is securely fastened, make sure the airway is open by adjusting the head, mouth, and chin positions, suction the mouth and airway with a bulb syringe or a size 10 to 12 F catheter, and measure the rise in the chest wall. To make sure the chest wall rises sufficiently, raise the airway pressure. A term infant may require an initial peak inspiratory pressure (PIP) of 25 to 30 cm H_2O to produce adequate ventilation, even though the PIP should be adjusted to the lowest level to which the infant responds. Preterm babies typically require lower pressures to receive enough ventilation. Neonatal lungs are easily damaged by even brief exposure to high tidal volume, especially in preterm infants, so it's critical to regularly monitor and modify PIP during resuscitation. Although they have been described as potentially useful, the function of devices that measure and regulate tidal volume during resuscitation remains undetermined (Figure 5.5).

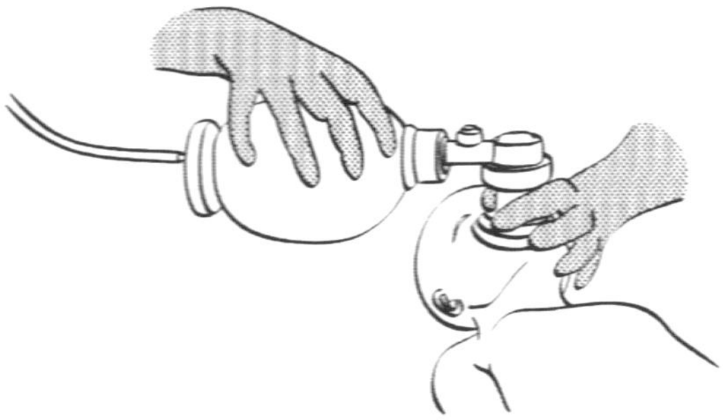

Figure 5.5. *Manual ventilation.*

Source: *https://medicalguidelines.msf.org/sites/default/files/Figure+10-3.png.*

To adjust the oxygen concentration based on the infant's clinical condition, additional oxygen should be given along with a blender. For term infants, positive pressure ventilation should start with 21% O_2 (room air); for preterm infants ≤ 35 weeks, it should start with 21% to 30% O_2 and be titrated based on pulse oximetry readings. 100% fractional inspired oxygen (FiO_2) should be administered to a baby who needs compressions or intubation, or who does not show an increase in heart rate in response to PPV. Avoiding hyperoxia (O_2 saturation >95%). Congenital heart disease may be the cause of persistent cyanotic infants who have otherwise responded well to resuscitation but show no signs of lung disease.

5.3.5. Intubation and Chest Compression

In cases where the baby is not responding to mask-administered positive pressure ventilation or if their heart rate is <60 beats per minute, endotracheal intubation should be performed. If PPV is necessary for a baby with a prenatally diagnosed or clinically suspected diaphragmatic hernia, then immediate endotracheal intubation is advised. In this case, it is best to avoid using PPV with a bag and mask to prevent colon inflation and further compromising the lungs. A cardiac monitor is the most accurate tool for determining the infant's heart rate in the event that intubation is required.

The size of the tube and depth of intubation are selected according to the infant's weight and gestational age.

For endotracheal tube diameter:

- 2.5 mm for infants < 1000 g or < 28 weeks gestation.
- 3 mm for infants 1000 to 2000 g or 28 to 34 weeks gestation.
- 3.5 mm for infants > 2000 g or > 34 weeks gestation.

For insertion depth, the marker at the lip should typically be at:

- 5.5 to 6.5 cm for infants who weigh < 1 kg.
- 7 cm for infants who weigh 1 kg.
- 8 cm for infants who weigh 2 kg.
- 9 cm for infants who weigh 3 kg.

Many endotracheal tubes have insertion markings to be positioned at the level of the vocal cords to guide the initial placement.

Clinicians should listen for bilaterally equal breath sounds as soon as the patient is intubated. If the tube is inserted too deeply, it is common to have selective intubation of the right mainstem bronchus with decreased breath sounds on the left. Using a colorimetric detector, check for exhaled CO_2 to confirm tracheal intubation. Tracheal intubation is confirmed by a positive test, which is indicated by the colorimetric indicator changing from purple/blue to yellow. Although esophageal intubation is the most common cause of a negative test result, it can also happen from inadequate ventilation or extremely low cardiac output. A constant yellow hue may be the result of direct exposure to adrenaline or it may be a sign that something is wrong with the equipment.

Proper endotracheal tube depth should result in the tip of the tube being about halfway between the clavicles and the carina on chest x-ray, coinciding roughly with vertebral level T1–T2.

For infants ≥ 34 weeks (or ≥ 2000 g), a laryngeal mask airway may be used if there is difficulty intubating the infant. Infants of any gestational age can be sustained with appropriate bag-and-mask PPV if team members are unable to place an endotracheal tube. In these infants, a nasogastric tube should be placed to allow for decompression of the stomach.

Suctioning should be performed if, following intubation, the patient's heart rate does not decrease and there is not enough chest rise with a sufficient peak inspiratory pressure, suggesting that the airway is obstructed. Catheters with thinner diameters (5 to 8 F) can effectively remove thin secretions from an endotracheal tube; however, they are not useful for thick secretions, blood, or meconium. In these situations, the trachea may occasionally be directly suctioned using a larger (10 to 12 F) catheter, or the endotracheal tube may be removed while continuous suction is applied using a meconium aspirator.

The baby is reintubated after the trachea is suctioned. Chest compressions should be administered using the 2-thumb/chest encircling technique in a coordinated ratio of 3 compressions to 1 ventilation, with 90 compressions and 30 ventilations per minute, if the infant is sufficiently ventilated and the heart rate is still < 60 beats per minute. It is no longer advised to apply the two-finger chest compression technique. Chest compressions should always be started with intubation if it hasn't already been done, and 100% oxygen should be administered. Chest compressions for 60 seconds should be followed by a new evaluation of the heart rate.

If severe bradycardia persists while the infant is adequately ventilated and chest compressions have been given for 1 minute, catheterize the umbilical vein or place an intraosseous (IO) needle to give intravascular epinephrine as soon as possible. While access is being established, a dose of epinephrine may be given via the endotracheal tube, but the efficacy of this route is unknown. The suggested dose of epinephrine is 0.02 mg/kg (0.2 mL/kg of the 0.1 mg/mL solution, previously known as 1:10,000 solution) IV/IO, repeated as needed every 3 to 5 minutes. The suggested endotracheal dose of epinephrine to be used while establishing vascular access is 0.1 mg/kg (1 mL/kg of a 0.1-mg/mL solution [1:10,000 solution]). Higher doses of epinephrine are not recommended.

5.3.6. Failure to Respond to Resuscitation

It is advised to perform volume expansion with 10 mL/kg of 0.9% saline IV over 5 to 10 minutes if the infant is not responding to resuscitation and exhibits pallor and/or poor perfusion. Given the risk of intraventricular hemorrhage, crystalloid or colloid boluses should be administered to preterm infants over longer periods (30 to 60 minutes). O-negative packed red blood cells that are not cross-matched can also be utilized to increase blood volume, particularly in cases of sudden or severe blood loss. During resuscitation, medications like aspirin and sodium bicarbonate are not advised. In the early stages of treating respiratory depression, naloxone is not advised, and a 2018 Cochrane review concluded that there is not enough data to assess the medication's safety and effectiveness in newborns.

Pneumothorax needs to be ruled out if the baby does not react to resuscitation or if they respond at first but then suddenly start to deteriorate. While the presence of bilateral diminished breath sounds on auscultation may lead to a clinical suspicion of pneumothorax, it should be noted that breath sounds are well-transmitted across the precordium. Chest transillumination is an option, although it is frequently restricted by the inability to completely darken the space and the unavailability of an instantaneous, powerful light source. Furthermore, in small infants with thin skin, a pneumothorax may be misdiagnosed, and in large infants with thick skin, it may go unnoticed. When used in resuscitation, a chest x-ray usually takes too long to be useful; however, if bedside ultrasonography is available quickly, it can provide an accurate diagnosis in a timely manner. Even in the absence of a definitive diagnosis, bilateral thoracentesis should be considered empirically because pneumothorax is a reversible cause of unresponsiveness to resuscitation. In some cases, thoracentesis is diagnostic and therapeutic for an unsuspected pleural effusion.

5.3.7. No Resuscitation

In some cases, resuscitation may not be appropriate:

- Infants with known lethal anomalies diagnosed before birth: Consult with the family well before the delivery to arrive at a mutually agreeable plan.
- Extremely preterm infants: Follow institutional guidelines, bearing in mind that prenatal gestational age estimates are often not precise.

Resuscitation should be tried in infants whose birth defects are unexpectedly severe and for which an initial diagnosis and/or prognosis may be incorrect. A neonatologist ought to be involved in decisions regarding the threshold of viability whenever feasible. To determine the estimated date of delivery and potential range of gestational age, one should independently obtain obstetric dating data from the mother directly and from her medical records. Current local and national outcomes data based on fetal sex, singleton/multifetal gestation status, expected gestational age and birthweight (if known), and prenatal corticosteroid treatment should be considered when having a conversation with the parents. When there are several appropriate methods, the parents' opinion is the most crucial in deciding whether or not to try resuscitation.

For the majority of families and medical professionals, the infant's survival with minimal morbidity is the main objective of resuscitation. It is deemed reasonable to stop resuscitation in cases where an infant is born without any discernible vital signs and does not show any signs of life after receiving appropriate resuscitation for approximately 20 minutes. This infant is unlikely to meet the goal. Nevertheless, there are no clear recommendations on how long to continue resuscitation in cases of persistent severe bradycardia or what to do if the patient's heart rate rises after resuscitation has been discontinued. In such situations, the treatment goals should be taken into consideration when determining whether the intervention is appropriate.

5.4. Screening and Diagnostic Tests for Newborns

Almost all newborns (Holmes AV, 2013) will undergo a basic blood test to screen for conditions that don't show symptoms right away. A few of these conditions are linked to hormones, blood, metabolism, or heredity. In the US, screening tests are mandated in every state, though the exact tests carried out differ from state to state. The baby is given a heel-prick to draw blood. The blood droplets are gathered onto specialized paper or in a tiny vial. After that, the blood is sent for analysis. The heel of the baby may be slightly red where it was pricked, and some babies may have bruises, but these usually go away in a few days.

Newborn screening tests may include:

1. **Phenylketonuria (PKU):** It is an inherited disease in which the body cannot metabolize a protein called phenylalanine. It is estimated that one in every 10,000 to 15,000 babies is born with PKU in the U.S. Without treatment, PKU can cause intellectual disability. Newborn screening for PKU is required in all 50 states.
2. **Congenital Hypothyroidism:** This is a condition in which the baby is born with too little thyroid hormone. Hypothyroidism is also quite common and has almost doubled in the past 20 years to approximately one in 2,500 to 3,000 babies born in the U.S. Untreated low thyroid hormone levels can lead to mental developmental problems and poor growth. All 50 states screen for hypothyroidism.
3. **Galactosemia:** This is an inherited disorder in which the baby is unable to metabolize galactose, a milk sugar. It is estimated to occur in about one baby in every 53,000 births. Without treatment (avoidance of milk), galactosemia can be life-threatening. Symptoms may begin in the first two weeks of life. All states screen for galactosemia.
4. **Sickle Cell Disease:** This inherited disorder occurs primarily in African Americans, but may also occur in Hispanics and Native Americans. The disease causes a severe form of anemia. There are different types of the disease. The disease occurs in about one out of every 365 African American births and one out of every 16,300 Hispanic American births. Early diagnosis of sickle cell disease can help lower some of the risks which include severe infections, blood clots, and stroke.
5. **Maple Syrup Urine Disease:** This is an inherited disorder that is very common in the Mennonite population. The disorder is caused by an inability of the body to properly process certain parts of protein called amino acids. The name comes from the characteristic odor of maple syrup in the baby's urine caused by the abnormal protein metabolism. If untreated, it is life-threatening as early as the first two weeks of life. Even with treatment, severe disability and paralysis can occur.
6. **Homocystinuria:** This inherited disorder affects one in 200,000 babies and causes intellectual disability, bone disease, and blood clots. It is caused by a deficiency of an enzyme necessary to digest an amino acid called methionine.
7. **Biotinidase Deficiency:** This inherited disorder is characterized by a deficiency of the biotinidase enzyme. This enzyme is important in metabolizing biotin, a B vitamin. It affects one in 60,000 to 75,000 babies in the U.S. and is most common in people of European descent. Lack of the enzyme can lead to severe acid build-up in the blood, organs, and body systems.
8. **Congenital Adrenal Hyperplasia:** Most states screen for this inherited disease of the adrenal glands. Babies born with congenital adrenal hyperplasia (CAH) cannot make enough of the hormone cortisol, which helps control energy, sugar levels, blood pressure, and how the body responds to the stress of injury or illness. The Endocrine Society estimates the incidence of CAH at one in about 15,000, depending on the severity of the disease. It is extremely common in a certain group of Eskimos

in western Alaska. CAH may also affect the development of the genitals and the hormones of puberty.

9. **Medium Chain Acyl-CoA Dehydrogenase Deficiency (MCAD):** This disorder of fatty acid oxidation can cause sudden death in infancy and serious disabilities in survivors, such as intellectual disability. MCAD affects about one baby per 15,000 births, almost exclusively in people of northwestern European descent.

Additional tests screen for lysosomal storage disorders, organic acid disorders, hemoglobin disorders, fatty acid oxidation disorders, amino acid disorders, cystic fibrosis, and severe combined immunodeficiency.

Most screenings can't be done until after a baby has been fed formula or breast milk for at least 24 hours. If you are released from the hospital before this point or the baby cannot be tested before release, then your baby might require additional testing.

Most states screen for hearing loss and critical congenital heart defects:

- **Hearing Loss:** Three in every 1,000 newborns have significant hearing loss, and nearly all states screen newborns for hearing loss.
- **Critical Congenital Heart Disease (CCHD):** It is estimated to affect two out of every 1,000 babies born each year in the US. Pulse oximetry is a non-invasive test that measures how much oxygen is in the blood and can help to identify babies that may be affected with CCHD before they leave the newborn nursery.

5.4.1. The Screening Procedures

There are three parts to newborn screening: the blood test (or heel stick); the hearing screen; and pulse oximetry.

5.4.1.1. Blood Test

An experienced member of the hospital staff, such as a nurse, midwife, or physician, will first complete a newborn screening card. The filter paper used to gather the baby's blood sample is one component of this card. The other section contains vital data that the lab running the screen needs to know, like the baby's name, sex, weight, date and time of birth, heel stick collection date and time, and first feeding date and time. For the follow-up results, it will also contain the parents' contact details and the baby's primary care physician's information.

A tiny sample of blood will be drawn from the baby's heel during the blood test, also known as a heel stick. Holding their child while the heel stick is being done is a welcome way for parents to participate in this procedure. Research indicates that when moms or medical professionals provide comfort to infants during this phase, likelihood of crying in infants decreases. The medical practitioner will create multiple "dried blood spots" on the filter paper card by applying blood droplets. After that, the state laboratory receives the newborn screening card for examination.

Requests for supplemental screening, commonly referred to as additional screening, can be made by families. Extra testing that can be carried out following enrollment in the newborn screening program in your state is referred to as additional screening. If there is a family history of a particular condition or other health issues, this may be done. There are more conditions that can be identified at birth even though every state screens for a variety of them. We advise speaking with a healthcare provider about any concerns you may have and about further screening. Be sure to enquire about the conditions that your state covers as well as any information that extra screening might yield. Since state programs do not cover additional screening or follow-up care, it is also crucial to speak with your insurance provider to find out about their policies regarding this type of coverage.

5.4.1.2. Hearing Screen

Two different tests can be used to screen for hearing loss in babies. Both tests are quick (5–10 minutes), safe and comfortable with no activity required from your child. In fact, these tests are often performed while a baby is asleep. One or both tests may be used.

1. **Otoacoustic Emissions (OAE) Test:** This test is used to determine if certain parts of the baby's ear respond to sound. During the test, a miniature earphone and microphone are placed in the ear and sounds are played. When a baby has normal hearing, an echo is reflected back into the ear canal, which can be measured by the microphone. If no echo is detected, it can indicate hearing loss.
2. **Auditory Brain Stem Response (ABR) Test:** This test is used to evaluate the auditory brain stem (the part of the nerve that carries sound from the ear to the brain) and the brain's response to sound. During this test, miniature earphones are placed in the ear and sounds are played. Band-Aid-like electrodes are placed along the baby's head to detect the brain's response to the sounds. If the baby's brain does not respond consistently to the sounds, there may be a hearing problem.

5.4.1.3. Pulse Oximetry Testing

Pulse oximetry, or pulse ox, is a non-invasive test that measures how much oxygen is in the blood. Infants with heart problems may have low blood oxygen levels, and therefore, the pulse ox test can help identify babies that may have Critical Congenital Heart Disease (CCHD). The test is done using a machine called a pulse oximeter, using a painless sensor placed on the baby's skin. The pulse ox test only takes a couple of minutes and is performed after the baby is 24 hours old and before he or she leaves the newborn nursery.

A Closer Look

Gestational Age:

The amount of time a fetus grows inside the mother's uterus is known as its gestational age. The physical and cognitive development of the fetus, along with its growth stage, are all correlated with its gestational age. When assessing the possible harm that could result from fetal exposure to toxins or infection, the gestational age of the fetus is particularly significant. It also directly affects the planning of the best course of medical care in such circumstances.

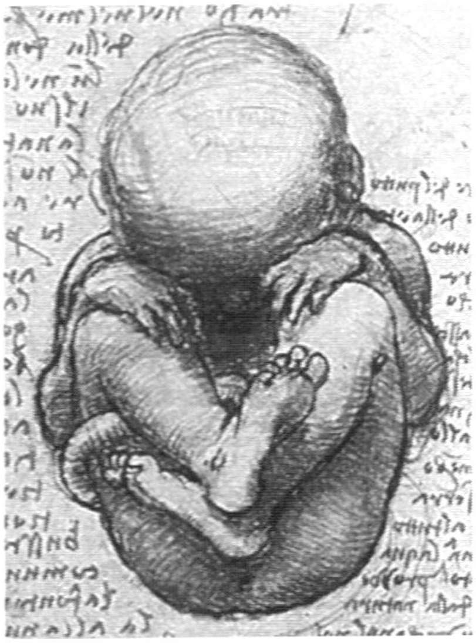

Source: By Leonardo da Vinci – http://www.drawingsofleonardo.org, Public Domain, https://commons.wikimedia.org/w/index.php?curid=628261.

The two stages of gestational age are referred to as embryonic and fetal. The embryonic period comes before the fetal period, which lasts from week 10 of pregnancy until delivery. Gestational ages are connected to benchmarks for prenatal development. For instance, the bones and cartilage, as well as all the essential organs, have started to form at the gestational age of 7 to 8 weeks. The genitalia have developed by weeks 9 to 13 of gestation, and the fetus as a whole weighs approximately one ounce (0.06 pounds). The eyes of the fetus have developed by weeks 21 to 23, and a stethoscope can pick up the sound of the fetal heartbeat. Fetal development is finished by 40 weeks. Therefore, the gestational age range for a normal pregnancy is 38 to 42 weeks, with 40 weeks typically being considered full-term. Premature babies are defined as those born before 38 weeks of pregnancy and are more vulnerable to disease and even death.

The number of weeks since the first day of the mother's most recent menstrual cycle is typically used to calculate gestational age; however, this method may not be precise due to differences in ovulation dates. Ultrasound is one of the other techniques used to precisely calculate gestational age; growth is measured by taking measurements of the head and abdomen. A modified version of the Dubowitz Scale called the Ballard Scale (or New Ballard Score) can be used to determine a newborn's gestational age after birth. Six criteria are evaluated in each area as part of the Ballard Scale examination of the newborn's neuromuscular and physical maturity. The Dubowitz Exam is a longer evaluation than the Ballard system because it covers more criteria (10 neurological and 11 physical) and is therefore focused on the newborn's neurological and physical maturity.

While gestational age can be precisely calculated, the growth and development of a fetus can differ from week to week throughout the gestational cycle. For instance, more than 25% of live births in low- and middle-income nations result in babies who are small for gestational age (SGA), meaning that their length or birthweight fell at or below the 10th percentile. SGA babies may be more susceptible to disorders like attention deficit/hyperactivity disorder (ADHD) and learning impairments.

Summary

- High-quality universal newborn health care is the right of every newborn everywhere. Babies have the right to be protected from injury and infection, to breathe normally, to be warm and to be fed.
- The Apgar score is one of the first checks of your new baby's health. The Apgar score is assigned in the first few minutes after birth to help identify babies that have difficulty breathing or have a problem that needs further care.
- A complete physical examination is an important part of newborn care. Each body system is carefully examined for signs of health and normal function.
- Vomiting is a common health problem among infants. It is normal for infants to spit up milk after feeding. But frequent vomiting is not normal. To prevent frequent vomiting and spit-ups, make sure your baby is not lactosei intolerant or allergic to breast milk.
- Extensive physiologic changes accompany the birth process, sometimes unmasking conditions that posed no problem during intrauterine life.
- A heel-prick is used to sample the baby's blood. The blood drops are collected in a small vial or on a special paper. The blood is then sent for testing.

References

1. Holmes AV. Establishing successful breastfeeding in the newborn period. Pediatr Clin North Am. 2013 Feb;60(1):147-68.
2. Lawrence RM, Lawrence RA. Breastfeeding: more than just good nutrition. Pediatr Rev. 2011 Jul;32(7):267-80.
3. McCandless, S. E., & Kripps, K. A. (2020). Genetics, inborn errors of metabolism, and newborn screening. In A. A. Fanaroff & J. M. Fanaroff (Eds.), *Klaus and Fanaroff's Care of the High-Risk Neonate* (7th ed., pp. xxx-xxx). St. Louis, MO: Elsevier.
4. Moon RY, Hauck FR, Colson ER. Safe Infant Sleep Interventions: What is the Evidence for Successful Behavior Change? Curr Pediatr Rev. 2016;12(1):67-75.
5. Sahai, I., & Levy, H. L. (2018). Newborn screening. In C. A. Gleason & S. E. Juul (Eds.), *Avery's Diseases of the Newborn* (10th ed., pp. xxx-xxx). Philadelphia, PA: Elsevier.
6. Stewart D, Benitz W., Committee On Fetus And Newborn. Umbilical Cord Care in the Newborn Infant. Pediatrics. 2016 Sep;138(3)
7. Visscher MO, Adam R, Brink S, Odio M. Newborn infant skin: physiology, development, and care. Clin Dermatol. 2015 May-Jun;33(3):271-80.
8. Warren JB, Phillipi CA. Care of the well newborn. Pediatr Rev. 2012 Jan;33(1):4-18.

Chapter 6

CHILD HEALTH AND DEVELOPMENT

Contents

Unit Introduction 174
6.1. Growth and Development Milestones 176
6.2. Health and Nutrition of Children 180
6.3. Basic Nutrition for Children 188
6.4. Common Childhood Illnesses 193
6.5. Child Abuse and Neglect 199
Summary 206
References 207

Unit Introduction

Development and child health are closely related, serving as the cornerstones of a child's future. A child's journey begins at conception and is shaped by their surroundings, their genetic makeup, and the level of care they receive. An important factor in a child's growth and well-being is nutrition. Sufficient nourishment throughout pregnancy and the early years of life is essential for healthy organ, tissue, and cognitive development. Malnutrition can affect physical growth, and cognitive function, while increasing susceptibility to diseases. These effects can persist throughout life, regardless of the cause—inadequate or low-quality food intake. Early life events influence a child's physical and mental health in addition to diet. Healthy development requires responsive caregiving, loving surroundings, and chances for play and exploration. Infancy-created secure attachment bonds establish a foundation of safety and trust that serves as a springboard for wholesome relationships and emotional fortitude in later life.

Another essential component of children's development and health is physical activity. Frequent exercise lowers the risk of obesity and associated health problems by improving cardiovascular health, motor skills, and coordination. When kids play outside and explore their environment, they not only improve their physical health but also their cognitive and creative abilities.

Despite being a crucial aspect of total wellbeing, mental health is frequently disregarded when talking about the development and health of children. Youngsters encounter stressors and a spectrum of emotions that could be harmful to their mental health. Creating a supportive atmosphere, imparting coping mechanisms, and encouraging resilience are all necessary to support their emotional development. For mental health concerns to be prevented in the long run and to encourage the best possible development, early detection and treatment are essential. Promoting children's health and taking care of any emerging health issues require access to high-quality healthcare. To prevent disease and guarantee the best possible growth and development, routine checkups, vaccinations, and prompt medical attention are essential. The social determinants of health, such as having access to resources in the community that are supportive, safe to live in, and educated, are also included in comprehensive healthcare.

Orientation and Directional Terms

Term	Definition	Illustration
Mental health	Mental health includes our emotional, psychological, and social well-being.	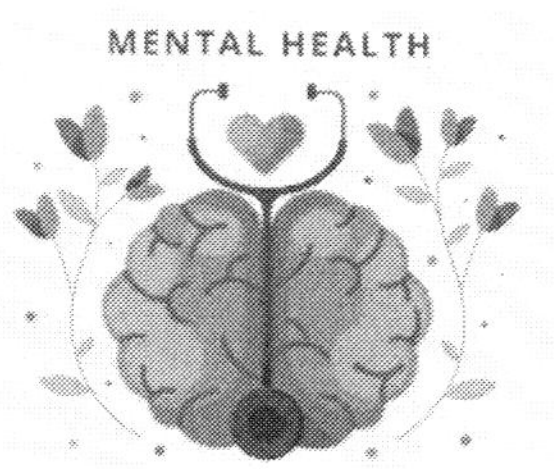
Malnutrition	Malnutrition is a condition that occurs when a person's body has too few, too many, or an imbalance of nutrients or energy.	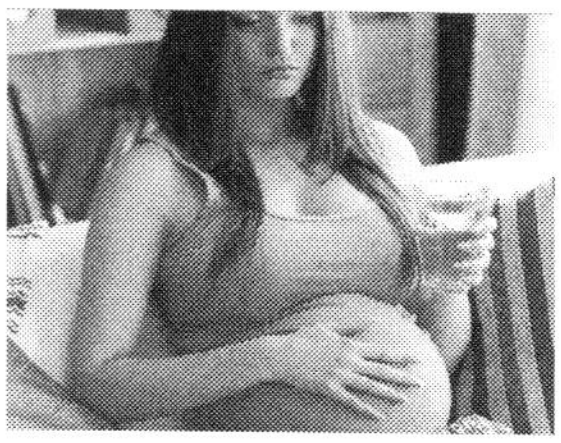
Emotional milestones	The emotional milestones that children should reach from ages birth through 6 years old.	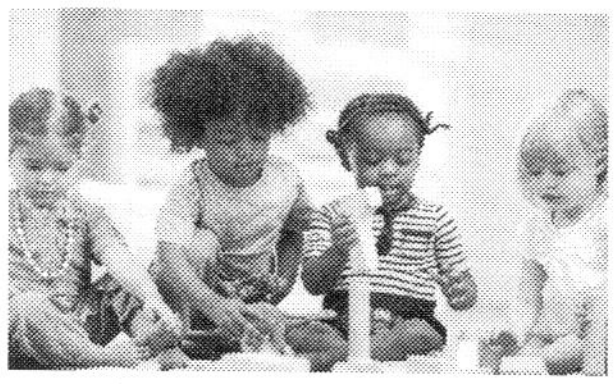
Adolescence	Adolescence is the period of transition between childhood and adulthood, typically occurring between the ages of 10 and 19.	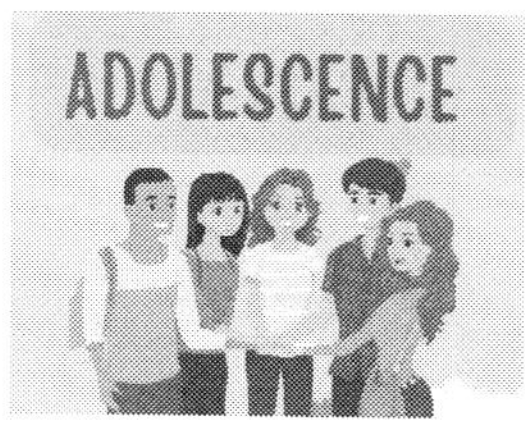

6.1. Growth and Development Milestones

A child's physical, cognitive, and emotional development can be best gauged by looking at their growth and development milestones. They offer crucial details regarding a child's development and can be used to spot any possible delays or issues with development. Parents, caregivers, and medical professionals can make sure that children receive the support and interventions they require to thrive by having a better understanding of these milestones.

6.1.1. Physical Development Milestones

The term "physical development milestones" describes how a child's size, form, and abilities change over time. These benchmarks offer crucial details regarding a child's general health and wellbeing and can be utilized to spot any developmental delays or issues.

Here are some of the key physical development milestones that occur during childhood:

1. **Infancy (0–12 Months):** During this period, infants undergo rapid physical growth, doubling their birth weight by 6 months and tripling it by 12 months. They also begin to develop muscle control, can lift their heads while lying on their stomachs, roll over, sit up with support, and eventually crawl and walk.
2. **Toddlerhood (1–3 Years):** Toddlers continue to grow rapidly during this period, although at a slower rate than during infancy. They become more coordinated and are able to walk, run, climb stairs, and kick a ball.
3. **Preschool (3–5 Years):** During this period, children's growth slows down even more, and they begin to develop more refined motor skills, such as drawing, cutting with scissors, and buttoning clothes.
4. **School-Age (6–12 Years):** Children continue to grow taller and gain weight during this period, although at a slower rate than during early childhood. They also develop more precise motor skills and can participate in sports and other physical activities.

It is crucial to remember that every child develops at their own rate and that these milestones are only broad recommendations. On the other hand, if a child falls behind in reaching these benchmarks, it could indicate a developmental delay or another underlying medical issue. It is crucial to speak with a healthcare provider in these situations to find out if more testing or treatment is required.

6.1.2. Cognitive Development Milestones

The term "cognitive development milestones" describes shifts in a child's capacity for reasoning, thinking, and comprehending their environment. These benchmarks offer valuable insights into a child's cognitive growth and can be employed to detect possible developmental lags or issues.

Here are some of the key cognitive development milestones that occur during childhood:

1. **Sensorimotor Stage (Birth to 2 Years):** During this stage, infants begin to understand the world through their senses and motor abilities. They develop object permanence (the understanding that objects continue to exist even when they are not visible), and learn to coordinate their sensory experiences with their motor skills.

2. **Preoperational Stage (2 to 7 Years):** During this stage, children become more sophisticated in their thinking, but still struggle with logic and abstract concepts. They begin to develop symbolic thought, using words and images to represent objects and ideas, and engage in pretend play. However, they may struggle with conservation (the understanding that the amount of a substance remains the same even when its shape changes).
3. **Concrete Operational Stage (7 to 11 Years):** During this stage, children begin to think more logically and understand the concept of conservation. They are able to classify objects and understand relationships between them and can use concrete operations (such as addition and subtraction) to solve problems.
4. **Formal Operational Stage (11 Years and Up):** During this stage, adolescents develop the ability to think abstractly and reason logically. They can understand hypothetical situations and engage in deductive reasoning. They may also develop a greater understanding of moral and ethical issues.

It is crucial to speak with a healthcare provider in these situations to find out if more testing or treatment is required. Furthermore, offering children an environment that is both stimulating and encouraging can support their general growth and development as well as cognitive development.

6.1.3. Emotional Development Milestones

The term "emotional development milestones" describes shifts in a child's capacity to control their emotions, comprehend and communicate their feelings, and form bonds with other people. These benchmarks can be used to spot possible developmental delays or issues and are crucial for a child's social and emotional health.

Here are some of the key emotional development milestones that occur during childhood:

1. **Infancy (0–12 Months):** During this period, infants develop the ability to recognize and respond to familiar faces, voices, and smells. They also begin to show signs of attachment to primary caregivers, such as seeking comfort and security from them.
2. **Toddlerhood (1–3 Years):** Toddlers begin to develop a sense of self, including their own emotions and preferences. They also become more aware of the emotions of others and may engage in simple forms of empathy, such as comforting someone who is crying.
3. **Preschool (3–5 Years):** During this period, children continue to develop their emotional awareness and regulation skills. They begin to understand and express more complex emotions and may develop the ability to self-soothe when upset. They also begin to form relationships with peers and develop social skills such as sharing and taking turns.
4. **School-Age (6–12 Years):** Children continue to develop their emotional regulation skills during this period, and may begin to develop a greater understanding of the emotions of others. They also become more independent and begin to form their own identities.

Please keep in mind that these milestones serve as rough guidelines and each child progresses at their own rate. If a child is severely delayed in meeting these milestones, it could indicate a developmental delay or underlying health issue. In these instances, seeking advice from a healthcare provider is crucial to determine if further assessment or assistance is needed. Creating a supportive and caring atmosphere for children can aid in fostering their emotional development and enhancing their overall health and wellness.

6.1.4. Parental Role in Supporting Child Development

Parents play a crucial role in supporting the growth and development of their children. Here are some ways in which parents can support their child's development:

1. **Provide a Safe and Nurturing Environment:** Children need a safe and supportive environment to grow and develop. This includes physical safety, emotional security, and opportunities for learning and exploration.
2. **Engage in Positive Interactions:** Positive interactions with parents and caregivers help children develop positive self-esteem, social skills, and emotional regulation. Parents can engage in positive interactions by listening to their child, responding sensitively to their needs, and praising their efforts.
3. **Provide Opportunities for Play and Exploration:** Play is an important part of child development, and parents can support this by providing opportunities for play and exploration. This can include providing toys and games that are age-appropriate, encouraging outdoor play, and participating in play with their child.
4. **Read to and with Their Child:** Reading is an important way to support language development and literacy skills. Parents can read to their children regularly, and also encourage their children to read independently.
5. **Model Positive Behaviors:** Children learn from their parents' behaviors, so it is important for parents to model positive behaviors such as kindness, empathy, and respect for others. This can help children develop these skills themselves.
6. **Support Their Child's Education:** Parents can support their child's education by being involved in their school, helping with homework, and encouraging their child to take an interest in learning.
7. **Provide a Healthy Lifestyle:** A healthy lifestyle is important for child development, and parents can support this by providing nutritious food, encouraging physical activity, and ensuring that their child gets enough sleep.

It is crucial to remember that each child is different and might have different needs. It is important for parents to be aware of each child's unique needs and to seek out resources and assistance when required. In addition, parents who are worried about the growth or well-being of their child should not be afraid to seek professional assistance.

6.1.5. Cultural Differences in Child Development Milestones

Child development milestones can vary across cultures due to differences in parenting styles, cultural values, and environmental factors. Here are some examples of cultural differences in child development milestones:

1. **Language Development:** These milestones can vary across cultures, with some languages having more complex grammatical structures than others. For example, children who grow up speaking Chinese or Japanese may take longer to reach language milestones in English, as English has a different grammatical structure.
2. **Social Development:** These milestones can also vary across cultures. For example, in some cultures, children may be expected to be more reserved

and less expressive of their emotions than in other cultures. This can affect their ability to form relationships and interact with peers.

3. **Physical Development:** These milestones can also be influenced by cultural factors. For example, in some cultures, infants are often carried on their caregivers' backs rather than in strollers or carriers. This can lead to differences in the timing of physical development milestones such as sitting up or crawling.
4. **Cognitive Development:** These milestones can also vary across cultures. For example, some cultures place a greater emphasis on rote memorization and academic achievement than on problem-solving and creativity.

It's critical to acknowledge and honor cultural variations in the developmental milestones of children. When assisting a child's development, parents and other adults should be conscious of their unique needs as well as the cultural background of the child. It is imperative for healthcare providers and educators to exhibit cultural sensitivity and deliver culturally competent care and instruction.

6.1.6. Supporting Children with Developmental Disabilities

Assisting children with developmental disabilities can be difficult and intricate, but there are numerous strategies that parents, caregivers, and educators can utilize to provide support.

Here are some strategies that can be used to support children with developmental disabilities:

1. **Early Intervention:** Early intervention is critical for children with developmental disabilities. The earlier a child receives support and services, the better their outcomes are likely to be. This may include therapies such as speech therapy, occupational therapy, or physical therapy.
2. **Individualized Education Plan (IEP):** An individualized education plan (IEP) is a document that outlines the educational goals and accommodations for a child with a disability. It is developed collaboratively with the child's parents, educators, and healthcare providers. An IEP can help ensure that the child receives appropriate support and accommodations in the classroom.
3. **Assistive Technology:** These can be helpful for children with developmental disabilities. This may include devices such as communication boards or tablets with communication apps, or adaptive equipment such as specialized chairs or writing tools.
4. **Sensory Accommodations:** Many children with developmental disabilities may have sensory processing difficulties. Providing sensory accommodations such as noise-canceling headphones, weighted blankets, or fidget toys can help children regulate their sensory input and feel more comfortable in their environment.
5. **Positive Reinforcement:** It can be an effective way to encourage and motivate children with developmental disabilities. This may include rewards such as stickers or tokens for completing tasks, or verbal praise for positive behaviors.
6. **Social Skills Training:** Children

with developmental disabilities may struggle with social skills such as making friends or understanding social cues. Social skills training can help children develop these skills through structured activities and role-playing exercises.

7. **Family Support:** It is important for children with developmental disabilities. This may include access to support groups or counseling services, as well as respite care to give caregivers a break from their caregiving responsibilities.

It's critical to keep in mind that each child is different and may require different care. Collaborating with the child's educators, family, and healthcare providers is crucial in creating a customized plan that caters to their unique requirements. Furthermore, it's critical to treat kids with developmental disabilities with compassion and understanding and to concentrate on their advantages rather than their disadvantages.

6.2. Health and Nutrition of Children

To promote healthy growth and development as well as to ward off several illnesses, children and adolescents should eat a healthy diet. The period of a person's life known as childhood is linked to growth and development. Early in life, growth is rapid; by middle childhood, it slows down; during puberty, it accelerates; and finally, linear growth stops. Physical and psychomotor maturation also occurs with age, and these changes impact feeding abilities, food preferences, body composition, and level of activity. For children's growth, health, and development, adequate nutrition is crucial. The nutritional status and overall health of young children accurately indicate a nation's level of development. These health indicators are closely related to the amount of money that nations invest in early childhood education and the protection of children's rights through current policies, plans, and initiatives. The environmental and social determinants of disease, mortality, the low quality of life of underprivileged population groups, and the stark differences in inequality between and within nations should all be taken into consideration when analyzing health and nutrition indicators.

The environments that people and the population are "exposed" to and which can affect long-term developmental and health outcomes are known as social determinants of health and nutrition. Social determinants are a wide range of traits that are ingrained in interactions between people and their socio-physical environments rather than being biologically or genetically based. They act at various levels of influence, interact with one another, and represent a broad array of characteristics. The most significant social determinants of children's health, nutrition, and development include living situations, the sociodemographics of the family, the interpersonal relationships between parents and peers, the learning environments in daycare centers and schools, neighborhood safety, and the sociopolitical context.

A well-nourished population is more productive on an individual basis, has lower healthcare costs, and performs better economically, all of which have a substantial influence on economic conditions. Malnutrition has many definitions. It should be made clear, though, that malnutrition can be primary—caused by a shortage of food—or secondary—caused by illnesses that affect how well the body uses or absorbs nutrients. Malnutrition is sometimes simply defined as a nutritional deficit linked to higher rates of morbidity and mortality. There are various types of malnutrition, including marasmus, kwashiorkor, and marasmic kwashiorkor. The word "marasmus," which translates to "consumption," refers to people who have a persistent loss of muscle mass and subcutaneous fat as a result of inadequate protein and energy intake. Kwashiorkor happens when there is little to no protein in the diet but plenty of energy. In marasmic kwashiorkor, there are elements of each of the malnutrition types listed above. Pure malnutrition disorders are actually uncommon in modern medicine. From a temporal perspective, only weight and body composition are impacted by malnutrition in its early acute stages. When it gets more severe and persistent, people experience altered height and growth retardation as well as diminished mental and physical capacity. For instance, during a respiratory or diarrheal infection, there may be decompensation (weight affecting height for age and sex) or compensation (weight for normal size) in recurrent acute episodes. Food vulnerability is the probability of a sudden drop in food availability or consumption. It represents the relationship to a critical value that establishes the minimal standards of human well-being. Those who are more likely to be denied access or consumption while also having less ability to respond to that risk are the most vulnerable. Therefore, sociocultural (education, particularly for mothers, ethnicity, and immigration), environmental (rural areas, natural disasters, and basic sanitation), economic (poverty, income, access to credit, and healthcare), and biological (low maternal weight and inadequate breastfeeding) factors should all be considered in vulnerability analyses.

The state of being caught up in an almost unbreakable cycle of disease, poverty, and inadequate nutrition is known as primary malnutrition. Stunting develops at the chronic stage of poor diet and low weight at the most acute stage due to both quantitative (scarcity) and qualitative (proper balance of macronutrients, micronutrients, and safety) factors. This makes a permanent contribution to the variables brought about by poverty, squalor and environmental issues, inadequate housing, and barriers to employment and healthcare.

6.2.1. The Importance of Nutrition for Children

Everyone needs to eat healthily, but children especially need to eat well because it is directly related to their overall growth and development. Growing up with the proper nutrition in the right amounts results in a healthier life. Kids who eat a regular diet rich in high-fiber foods and healthy fats have a much higher chance of avoiding chronic illnesses—even if those illnesses run in their families. The Academy of Nutrition and Dietetics states that by the time a baby reaches the age of one, their weight should have tripled, marking the fastest stage of human growth. Early childhood is also a critical time for the development of cognitive, behavioral, and physical skills. One of the most crucial things to make sure a child develops to their full potential is to feed them a diet rich in health and nutrients.

6.2.1.1. Promotes Optimal Growth

The body grows at a startling rate in early childhood. This rate may happen in spurts during childhood, adolescence, and puberty, but it slows down after the age of one. A child must consume a sufficient amount of food to give him the energy and nutrients he needs to grow without compromising the health of his body. Furthermore, adolescence is when almost half of the adult skeletal mass is developed. For the best skeletal and physical growth, a diet high in calcium and other vital vitamins and minerals is recommended.

6.2.1.2. Enhances Brain Development

The sufficiency and quality of your child's diet can have an impact on their brain development. Inadequate nourishment throughout fetal development and early life has been linked to learning disorders and decreased IQs. Moreover, behavioral and social problems, along with attentional problems, may arise. To support brain development, the body must receive enough energy, vitamins, minerals, and macronutrients while still allowing the rest of the body to grow and mature.

6.2.1.3. Prevents Childhood Obesity

In addition to making sure kids receive enough nourishment, it's critical to determine what and how much they're eating. According to HealthyChildren.org, nearly one in three children are overweight or obese, putting them at a higher risk of becoming obese adults and developing other chronic diseases. The amount of calories and nutrients your child consumes will vary based on his age, size, level of activity, and general health. One crucial strategy to keep your child from becoming a statistic is to give them healthy food options and to set an example of good eating habits.

6.2.1.4. Encourages Healthy Choices for Life

You can teach your child how to lead a healthier lifestyle that will promote appropriate growth and development for the rest of his life by exposing him to a range of nutritious food options. Get in touch with your child's pediatrician if you have concerns about their growth and development.

6.2.2. Nutrition and Health in Pre-School- and School-Age Children

Given that young children grow quickly, it would seem imperative to give them enough energy during this period of life. Specifically, fats, carbs, and proteins are the macronutrients found in foods that can give kids energy. Human cells depend on proteins for survival. Animal liver, meat, fish, cheese, milk, eggs, and some vegetable-based products like those made from soybeans, green beans, and legumes are excellent sources of high-quality proteins. Wheat-based products are also a source of protein, but most fruits and vegetables only have a small amount in them.

Another crucial macronutrient for maintaining a proper and balanced energy level in children is fats. Fats in the diet serve as a source of energy and essential fatty acids for children. Structural fats are vital for the cell membrane, neural fabric, and overall cellular structure, while stored fats, found primarily in adipose tissue and made up of triglycerides, act as a long-term energy reserve for the body. Carbohydrates, including sugars, starches, and fiber, are the third and most abundant source of energy for the body. Carbohydrates provide energy to all tissues in the human body, with the brain and red blood cells relying on glucose as their primary source of "fuel" for cellular activity.

In addition to the primary macronutrients, vitamins and minerals are also necessary components of a healthy diet for children in preschool and school. For proper development of vision in small children, as well as to ensure the integrity of epithelial tissue and the development of tissue differentiation, an adequate supply of vitamin A is required. Liver, dairy products, eggs, fish, margarine, and some fruits and vegetables (like carrots and yellow/orange fruit) are the main sources of vitamin A. Similar to vitamin A, B vitamins are essential for children's healthy growth, development, and sustenance. Vitamin C is essential for collagen synthesis and the immune system's optimal operation. Furthermore, vitamin C is an important supporter of the iron absorption process and has antioxidant qualities.

6.2.3. Nutrition and Health in Adolescents

Adolescents experience a growing need for independence and freedom as a result of their fast psychological and behavioral development and somatic growth, which also has a big impact on their eating habits. Puberty causes significant physical changes that are linked to fast growth and modifications. These changes are accompanied by an increase in both the quantity and quality of nutrients that a person needs, including water, fiber, vitamins, minerals, proteins, and fats.

At this age, iron and calcium deficiency are the most common nutritional deficiencies. One of the most prevalent conditions linked to dietary deficiencies is anemia brought on by an iron deficiency. Therefore, it's critical to increase consumption of iron-rich foods in adolescence, including dark green vegetables, walnuts, legumes, lean meat and fish, and iron-enriched grains. Since calcium is a component of both bone and teeth, it plays a crucial role in the rapidly developing adolescent body. For this reason, eating foods high in calcium is crucial for both boys and girls, as the latter will be more susceptible to osteoporosis as menopause sets in.

Adolescent health is linked to physical activity in addition to eating a balanced and healthful diet. Engaging in motor activity helps burn calories, relieve stress and tension, and enhance mood and psychological health. Frequent exercise and sports have a major positive impact on metabolism, and the skeletal and cardiovascular systems. Frequent movement helps adolescents maintain a healthy body weight and level of fitness, builds their strength, and prepares them for a healthier lifestyle in the future.

6.2.4. Dietary Guidelines for Children and Adolescents

In terms of how meals are divided over the course of the day, it should be noted that nutritionists recommend that children should eat five times per day.

A recommended weekly breakdown could be:

- **Grains (Bread and Pasta):** Every day.
- **Fruit and Vegetables:** Every day.
- **Milk and Dairy Products:** Every day.
- **Meat:** 2–3 times per week.
- **Fish:** At least three times per week.
- **Cheese:** Twice a week.
- **Eggs:** Once or twice a week.
- **Legumes:** At least twice a week.

Apart from recommendations pertaining solely to nutrition, it is noteworthy that consistent physical activity, primarily outdoors, is regarded as a critical component of children's and teenagers' overall health. *Variety is one of the essential components of a healthy diet.* Adolescents and children can easily get the nutrients they need for growth from a varied diet.

Briefly, the guidelines to be followed in adopting eating habits and a lifestyle which promote healthy growth in adolescents are:

- Adopt a healthy, balanced diet, which, through alternating on a daily basis all primary foods, provides all the nutrients and micronutrients (calcium, iron, vitamins, etc.) Required by adolescents;
- Avoid excessive calorie intake by avoiding consumption of high-calorie foods or those rich in fats;
- Divide nutrients in a balanced way throughout the day to assure proper equilibrium between animal and vegetable proteins which should be 1, between simple and complex sugars (through consumption of fewer sweets, more bread, potatoes, pasta or rice), and between animal and vegetable fats (using less lard and butter and more olive oil);
- Reduce added salt to a minimum to lower risk factors of developing high blood pressure, especially in adult years;
- Divide food consumption into 5 periods during the day—breakfast, mid-morning snack, lunch, afternoon snack and supper; and avoid consuming food outside the five moments of the day identified above;
- Engage in physical activity for at least one hour per day, both as sports activity and recreation;
- Reduce sedentary activity as much as possible especially that spent in front of the television or computer screen.

6.2.5. Childhood Obesity and Its Impact on Health

A serious health, social, and economic issue that is becoming more and more pressing in Western nations is childhood obesity. It arises from sustained positive energy intake, or, to put it another way, from consuming more calories than burning them off. Actually, an excess of fat mass is the definition of obesity. Both subcutaneously and viscerally, the amount and proportions of adipose mass change during the growth years. Furthermore, it is challenging to measure fat mass, and diagnoses are only based on indirect assessments. Since total fat mass is closely correlated with subcutaneous fat and the body weight-to-height relationship (BMI), BMI is the parameter most frequently used to estimate adiposity.

Experts agree on the following points:

- Overweight children have a BMI in the 85th and 95th percentile in terms of sex and age;
- Obese children have a BMI above the 95th percentile.

Overweight and obese children can result in several physical and psychological issues that can be so severe that they show up early in childhood (known as precocious consequences) as well as more serious issues that are frequently encountered later in life (known as late consequences). Childhood obesity is associated with many precocious consequences, including metabolic (insulin resistance, dyslipidemia, glucose intolerance, high blood pressure) and non-metabolic (stretch marks, Acanthosis nigricans), hepatic (fatty liver), respiratory (desaturation and nocturnal apnea), and psychological pathologies (poor body image, eating disorders, depression).

There are important emotional, social, and psychosocial repercussions of obesity for kids and teenagers. One of these is school bullying, which is linked to an increased risk of anxiety and depression. Furthermore, overweight kids are less likely to feel good about themselves and to be shunned by classmates and playmates, which is detrimental to their social and psychological growth. Lastly, because they have lower self-esteem, they are more likely to engage in unhealthy behaviors like drinking and smoking. Obesity is a condition of risk because, during the developing years, pathological anatomical alterations of metabolic origin may also manifest. These alterations include an increase in the thickness of artery walls, atherosclerotic plaques on coronary arteries, and the aorta. These plaques are linked to insulin resistance, fasting LDL cholesterol levels, and BMI from an early age. The most frequent late effect of childhood obesity is obesity persisting into adulthood: approximately. Around 70% of teenagers who are obese as adults stay that way.

Furthermore, those who were overweight or obese as children are at a higher risk of developing metabolic diseases such as mellitus diabetes, hypercholesterolemia, hypertriglyceridemia, etc., as well as cardio-circulatory conditions such as high blood pressure and heart disease, muscular skeletal conditions such as early onset arthritis resulting from static-dynamic stress on the spine and lower limb joints that bear the brunt of supporting weight. including eating disorders, gastric cancer, and other conditions.

6.2.6. Food Safety for Children

Youngsters under the age of five are more susceptible to foodborne illness and its associated health problems. Young children's food safety is influenced by the actions of their parents and other adult caregivers. It is easier for young children to get sick because their immune systems are still developing and they cannot fight off infections as well as adults can. They also produce less stomach acid, which is necessary to kill harmful bacteria.

6.2.6.1. Why Only Safe Food Should Be Eaten?

- Protects health.
- Prevents infections that cause diarrhea, stomach upset, dysentery, etc.
- Makes you feel healthy, alert, active and energetic.
- You do better in everything to do like studies, games, activities, etc. (Figure 6.1).

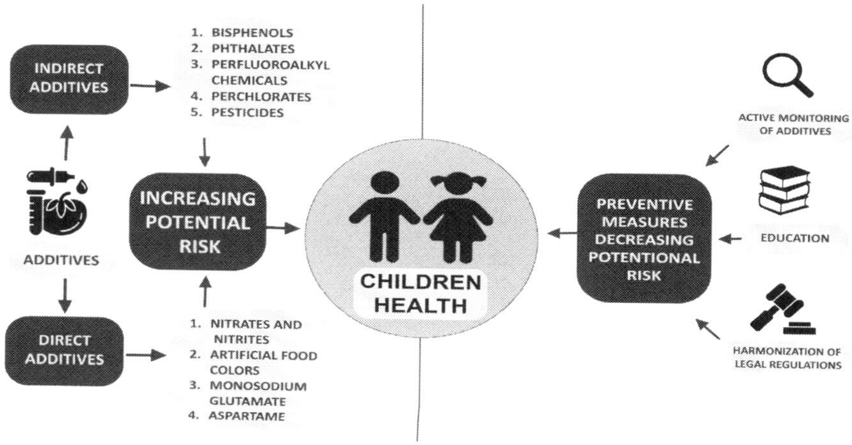

Figure 6.1. *Food safety in children.*

Source: Savin, M., Vrkatić, A., Dedić, D., Vlaški, T., Vorgučin, I., Bjelanović, J., & Jevtic, M., (2022). Additives in children's nutrition – A review of current events. International Journal of Environmental Research and Public Health, 19(20), 13452. https://doi.org/10.3390/ijerph192013452.

6.2.6.2. *Your Very Own Safety Codes!*

- Wash your hands vigorously with soap and clean water for 20 seconds before and after eating, after placing refuse in dustbins, using bathrooms, touching animals, coughing, sneezing etc.
- Throw garbage right into a covered garbage bin.
- Keep raw foods physically separated from cooked foods.
- Cover food during dusting and sweeping.
- Refrigerate food promptly.
- Wash all fruits properly under running water before use.
- Do not eat if the food does not look, taste, smell or feel fresh and normal.
- Do not touch body parts while having food.
- Do not pick up food from the ground.
- Wipe your shoes on a doormat before coming to the food serving area.
- Do not touch money, mobile, etc. after washing hands, before eating.
- Do not keep your school bags, pets, etc. in food-handling areas.
- Do not keep your spoon or fork or your hand on the desk or the floor while eating.
- Discard any packaged food if you find it tampered with.
- Do not keep food directly on your desk.
- Do not eat leftover food.
- Do not eat uncovered food.

6.2.6.3. *Safe Food – What Should You Look For?*

1. The Food Handler:

- Looks healthy and pleasant not sneezing, coughing, etc.
- Wears clean clothes.
- Has clean hands and trimmed nails.
- Has neat and tidy hair.
- No jewelry on fingers or wrist.
- Serves using a clean spatula/spoon.
- Do not touch or scratch the body, mobile or money before touching food.
- He has no cuts, open sores or skin infections. If he wears gloves, it should be changed often.
- Does not smoke or chew tobacco while handling food.

2. The Food:

- Covered.
- Properly heated before use.
- Not kept at room temperature for more than 2 hours.

- Not touched without washing hands properly.
- Look, feel, smell and taste fresh and normal.
- Frozen food like ice cream is properly frozen.
- Free from all physical impurities.
- Pack seals are intact for packaged food.
- Products are marked under 'best before,' 'expiry' or 'use by' date.
- Avoid mixing leftovers with freshly prepared food.
- Nutritious.

3. The Water:

- Running potable water used.
- Covered container with a side tap for drawing water.

4. The Ice:

- Prepared using potable water.
- Stored hygienically in clean and leak-proof containers.
- Handled hygienically using clean spoons.
- Ice for storage not to be added to beverages for consumption.

5. The Utensils for Storing and Serving:

- Clean and intact utensils are used.
- Reusable serving utensils/items are washed, cleaned and disinfected after each use.
- Single-use/disposable items are not reused.
- Clean and nontoxic material is used for packing food.
- Printed paper is not used for wrapping/storing/serving food.
- Tables and food serving counters are kept clean.

6. Environment:

- Clean-no open drain, garbage dump or toilets nearby.
- Airy, well lighted, not crowded and comfortable.
- Properly disinfected.

6.2.6.4. *Washing Hands Often Is the Key to Keeping Food Safe*

Foodborne pathogens are widely found in soil, water, animals and people. These pathogens are carried on hands, wiping cloth, and utensils, which can transfer them to food during preparation and handling:

When to Wash Hands?

- Hands should be washed before, during and after preparing a meal.
- Wash hands before eating.
- Wash hands after using the restroom.

- Wash your hands after blowing your nose, coughing or sneezing.
- Hands should be washed after handling poultry, raw meat or seafood.
- Wash hands after touching garbage, pets or any other animals.

6.2.6.5. Healthy Tiffin, Healthy Children

- The key to a child's healthy day is a balanced, healthy tiffin.
- A balanced tiffin keeps children energetic the whole day helping them concentrate on studies.
- Involve children in deciding their tiffin menu. This will encourage them to finish their meal and enable you to keep track of their nutrition.
- Fruits are an important part of a child's meal. Fruits provide adequate nutrition and vitamins.
- Sugar content in a child's tiffin should be low.

6.3. Basic Nutrition for Children

Feeding children with care will help them meet their energy needs and maintain healthy growth. It is important to encourage both physical activity and drinking lots of plain water side by side. If at all possible, the child should play and run outside for at least an hour each day.

Maintaining appropriate food intake and physical growth can be facilitated by routine growth assessment. Young children eat little at a time despite being very active. A lot of high-energy foods should be given to them, including whole-grain cereals as a source of carbohydrates, full-fat dairy or soy milk, vegetable oils, fruits (two servings), and vegetables (boiled, baked, steamed, or sautéed) (three servings). A small amount of butter can also help them get the extra energy they need. Children between 5–10 years need about 1,500 to 2,000 kilocalories a day from their food.

6.3.1. Choosing Foods for Children

Foods for children should contain some from each of the five food groups, the amount depending on the age, physical growth and level of activity of the child.

- Vegetables: plenty of colored vegetables of different types, leafy and non-leafy – one serving is half a cup of cooked vegetables or legumes, and one cup of raw salad vegetables: 5–6 servings of fruits and vegetables should be offered every day.
- Fruits of a variety of types – one serving is one medium piece or one cup of diced/canned fruit without sugar, two small fruits, such as plums, or an ounce of dry fruits.
- Whole grains, as grains or flour, such as breads, pasta, oats and cereals – a serving being a bread slice/scone/muffin or half a cup of cooked cereal, pasta or rice: 4–6 servings a day.
- Proteins, such as lean meat, poultry, eggs and fish, tofu, nuts and seeds, and legumes (peas, beans and pulses) – a serving is about 100 g raw meats/fish, two eggs, 170 g tofu, ¾ cup cooked legumes: 1–2 servings a day.
- Milk/milk products including curds and cheese are excellent sources of healthy fat and protein – a single serving is 40 g cheese, a cup of milk or soy milk (the latter with added calcium), 200 g yogurt: 2–4 servings a day.
- Fiber is excellent in helping to avoid constipation and promote a feeling of fullness, but too much is counterproductive.

Every child should be given an ample amount of water. Milk can be added to both afternoon and morning teas. Healthy and enticing snacks include little portions of recently cut, vibrantly colored vegetable sticks with delectable tomato ketchup or hummus (without added sugar or salt). Food intended for children should always be prepared and stored with the utmost care, flavor, and minimal heat or spice. Adding discretionary foods to the diet should only be done occasionally and in moderation. These include processed foods, cakes, and desserts—unnecessary sources of sugar, salt, and saturated fats.

6.3.2. How to Encourage Healthy Eating Habits?

- Eating together as a family.
- Enjoying foods from all these groups as often as possible to help children imitate the example of older siblings and parents.
- Encouraging them to help select healthy colored fruits, vegetables, and healthy meats or other foods during grocery shopping.
- Letting them help with food preparation, especially from the vegetable and pulses group.
- Preparing tasty soups and broths, which pack a lot of fiber and nutrition into a form that is easily edible and looks appealing.
- Stocking fruits rather than fruit juice and chews, and cold water rather than soda or other sweetened drinks.
- Starting the day off with a good breakfast.
- Sharing interesting information about how foods are grown and how they reach the local market.
- Encourage active outdoor play or work before or between meals for at least an hour a day.

6.3.3. Vegetarian Diets for Children

Vegetarian families should be careful to ensure that their children's diets are sufficient to promote their physical and mental development. For the purpose of fostering healthy bone and brain development, it must supply enough energy, iron, and other vital minerals and vitamins. To facilitate the absorption of fat-soluble nutrients, like vitamins A, E, and D, healthy fats must be present in the diet. Legumes and milk or soy milk and products should be consumed regularly.

A serving of lentils, nuts, or another type of leguminous protein, such as baked beans, chickpeas, hummus, nut butters, or curries, should be a part of every meal. Pulses should be cooked through to promote healthy digestion and minimize the production of gas in the intestines.

6.3.4. What Nutrients Do Children Need?

Not sure exactly what your family should be eating? We'll walk you through some of the most crucial nutrients that children should be getting daily below (remembering that each child is unique in terms of what they require depending on their age, weight, height, and other characteristics).

6.3.4.1. Protein

Protein helps a child's body build cells, break down food into energy, fight infection, and carry oxygen. According to the Cleveland Clinic, kids between the ages of 4 and 9 need about 19 grams (g) of protein daily. Those ages 9 to 13 need 34 g each day.

Foods that are good sources of protein include:

- Meat;
- Poultry;
- Fish;
- Eggs;
- Nuts;
- Beans;
- Dairy products.

If your kids are hesitant to eat the foods listed above, they can try the following items, which offer lesser amounts of the important nutrients.

- Crab cakes;
- Parmesan cheese;
- Quinoa;
- Cottage cheese;
- Green peas;
- Edamame;
- Brussels sprouts.

6.3.4.2. Carbohydrates

The main source of energy is carbohydrate energy. They facilitate the body of a child in utilizing protein and fat for tissue growth and repair. The U.S. The Department of Health and Human Services advises children over one year old to consume roughly 130 grams of carbohydrates daily. This is typically not too difficult because carbohydrates can be found in a variety of forms, including sugars, starches, and fiber. Since eating a lot of bad carbohydrates, such as soda, candy, and processed foods, is linked to obesity, diabetes, and other health issues, kids should be eating more starches and fiber and less sugar.

Foods that contain high levels of carbohydrates include:

- Breads;
- Oatmeal;
- Cereals;
- Rice;
- Crackers;
- Pasta;
- Potatoes.

6.3.4.3. Healthy Fats

Fats are easily stored in the body and provide children with a great source of energy. They also facilitate the body's correct utilization of other vital nutrients. According to the American Heart Association, children and adolescents aged 4 to 18 should consume between 25 and 35% of their total calories from fat, with the majority of fats coming from sources of polyunsaturated and monounsaturated fatty acids like fish, nuts, and vegetable oils.

Foods that contain high levels of healthy fats include:

- Whole-milk dairy products;
- Cooking oils;
- Meat;
- Fish;
- Nuts.

6.3.4.4. Calcium

Building a child's healthy bones and teeth requires calcium. It is also necessary for the heart, muscles, nerves, and blood clotting process. The FDA advises adults over four years old to aim for 1,300 mg of calcium daily, while children ages 1 to 3 should take 700 mg.

Foods that contain calcium include:

- Milk;
- Cheeses;
- Yogurt;
- Ice cream;
- Egg yolks;

- Broccoli;
- Spinach;
- Tofu;
- Calcium-fortified orange juice;
- Fortified plant-based "milks;"
- Fortified cereals.

6.3.4.5. Iron

To create healthy blood, which supplies oxygen to every cell in the body, iron is required. According to the FDA, it's also essential for immunological response, wound healing, growth and development, and reproduction. Additionally, having enough iron stores lowers the chance of developing anemia. Children from 1 to 3 years old should take 7 mg of iron per day, and older children should take increasingly more. Teenage girls who have begun menstruating might want to monitor their iron consumption more carefully.

Foods that contain high levels of iron include:

- Red meats;
- Poultry (especially dark meat);
- Shellfish;
- Whole grains;
- Beans;
- Nuts;
- Iron-fortified cereals.

6.3.4.6. Folate

One of the B vitamins, folate, is essential for expectant mothers and fathers as well as for the proper growth and development of a child's cells. Folate-deficiency anemia may result from a vitamin B12 deficiency. Children under the age of six months require 65 micrograms (mcg) of folate daily, children aged four to eight need 200 mcg, and teenagers ages 14 to 18 need 400 mcg.

Foods that contain folate include:

- Lentils;
- Chickpeas;
- Berries;
- Orange juice;
- Asparagus;
- Spinach;
- Black or kidney beans;
- Brussels sprouts.

6.3.4.7. Fiber

Fiber promotes bowel regularity in a child, and it may also reduce the chances of cardiovascular disease and cancer later in life. Fiber also lowers "bad" cholesterol and controls blood sugar. For kids up to age 3, the FDA recommends 14 g of dietary fiber per day; those ages 4 and older need about 28 g.

Foods that contain high levels of fiber include:

- Whole-grain cereals;
- Whole-grain breads;
- Chickpeas;
- Kidney beans;
- Seeds;
- Nuts.

6.3.4.8. Vitamin A

Both children and adults benefit from vitamin A in different ways. In addition to promoting growth and helping the eyes adjust to bright and dim light, it also maintains skin health and fights infection. The recommended dosages of preformed vitamin A and provitamin A carotenoids, two sources of vitamin A, are listed by the National Institutes of Health (NIH) in micrograms of retinol activity equivalents (RAE). Age and gender-specific acceptable levels vary widely; infants under six months old should receive 400 mcg RAE of vitamin A daily, whereas children between the ages of 9 and 13 should receive 600 mcg RAE.

Foods that contain high levels of vitamin A include:

- Carrots;
- Sweet potatoes;
- Squash;
- Apricots;
- Spinach;
- Broccoli;
- Fish oils;
- Eggs.
- Milk;
- Salmon.

6.3.4.9. Vitamin C

There are other uses for vitamin C besides warding off colds. In addition, it promotes strong bones and teeth, heals wounds, fortifies blood vessel walls, and holds the body's cells together. Children require roughly 25 mg of vitamin C per day, or half of a small orange, between the ages of 4 and 8. When your child reaches adolescence, they should be consuming 45 mg to 75 mg of vitamin C per day, up from the recommended 45 mg for ages 9 to 13.

Foods that contain high levels of vitamin C include:

- Citrus fruits (such as oranges and grapefruit);
- Orange juice;
- Strawberries;
- Tomatoes;
- Potatoes;
- Bell peppers;
- Broccoli;
- Cauliflower;
- Cantaloupe.

6.3.4.10. Vitamin D

Vitamin D not only helps with calcium absorption but also promotes strong bones and teeth. In addition, vitamin D is essential for various body processes like regulating blood pressure, producing hormones, and supporting immune and nervous system functions, according to the FDA. Children aged 1 to 3 should consume around 15 mcg (600 IU) of vitamin D daily, while adults need approximately 20 mcg (800 IU) per day.

Foods that contain vitamin D include the following:

- Fortified dairy products (like milk and some yogurts);
- Fortified cereals;
- Fish and fish oil;
- Eggs;
- Fortified orange juice;
- Mushrooms;
- Pork.

6.3.4.11. Potassium

Potassium regulates several body functions including heart rhythm, the nervous system, and muscle contraction. Low levels of potassium can lead to muscle weakness and abnormal heart rate. The recommended daily intake is 3,000 mg through age 3 and 4,700 mg for older children and adults, says the FDA.

Foods that contain potassium include:

- Sweet potatoes;
- Orange juice;
- Spinach;
- Beans;
- Prune juice;
- Milk;
- Yogurt;
- Salmon;
- Bananas.

6.4. Common Childhood Illnesses

It is essential for all children to receive top-notch medical care. As a parent, staying informed about the latest treatment guidelines is crucial in ensuring your child receives the best possible care. The American Academy of Pediatrics (AAP) provides information on common childhood illnesses and their prescribed treatments, which are based on scientific research and industry standards. However, your pediatrician may have different recommendations for your child depending on their individual medical history or allergies. Your pediatrician will address any variations in treatment with you. Should you have any inquiries regarding the appropriate care for your child, do not hesitate to talk to your pediatrician.

1. Sore Throat:

- Sore throats are common in children and can be painful. However, a sore throat that is caused by a virus does not need antibiotics. In those cases, no specific medicine is required, and your child should get better in seven to 10 days. In other cases, a sore throat could be caused by an infection called streptococcal (strep throat).
- Strep cannot be accurately diagnosed by simply looking at the throat. A lab test or in-office rapid strep test, which includes a quick swab of the throat, is necessary to confirm the diagnosis of strep. If positive for strep, your pediatrician will prescribe an **antibiotic**. It's very important that your child take the antibiotic for the full course, as prescribed, even if the symptoms get better or go away. Steroid medicines (such as prednisone) are not an appropriate treatment for most cases of sore throat.
- Babies and toddlers rarely get it strep throat, but they are more likely to become infected by streptococcus bacteria if they are in child care or if an older sibling has the illness. Although strep spreads mainly through coughs and sneezes, your child can also get it by touching a toy that an infected child has played with.

2. Ear Pain:

- Ear pain is common in children and can have many causes—including ear infection (otitis media), swimmer's ear (infection of the skin in the ear canal), pressure from a cold or sinus infection, teeth pain radiating up the jaw to the ear, and others.To tell the difference, your pediatrician will need to examine your child's ear. In fact, an in-office exam is still the best way for your pediatrician to make an accurate diagnosis. If your child's ear pain is accompanied by a high fever, involves both ears, or if your child has other signs of illness, your pediatrician may decide that an antibiotic is the best treatment.
- Amoxicillin is the preferred antibiotic for middle ear infections—except when there is an allergy to penicillin or chronic or recurrent infections.
- Many true ear infections are caused by viruses and do not require antibiotics. If your pediatrician suspects your child's ear infection may be from a virus, he or she will talk with you about the best ways to help relieve your child's ear pain until the virus runs its course.

3. Urinary Tract Infection:

- Bladder infections, also called urinary tract infections or UTIs, occur when bacteria build up in the urinary tract. A UTI can be found in children from infancy through the teen years and into adulthood. Symptoms of a UTI include pain or burning during urination, the need to urinate frequently or urgently, bedwetting or accidents by a child who knows to use the toilet, abdominal pain, or side or back pain.

- Your child's doctor will need a urine sample to test for a UTI before determining treatment. Your doctor may adjust the treatment depending on which bacteria is found in your child's urine.

4. Skin Infection:

- In most children with skin infections, a skin test (culture or swab) may be needed to determine the most-appropriate treatment. Tell your doctor if your child has a history of MRSA, staph infection, or other resistant bacteria or if he or she has been exposed to other family members or contacts with resistant bacteria.

5. Bronchitis:

- Chronic bronchitis is an infection of the larger, more central airways in the lungs and is more often seen in adults. Often the word "bronchitis" is used to describe a chest virus and does not require antibiotics.

6. Bronchiolitis:

- Bronchiolitis is common in infants and young children during the cold and flu season. Your doctor may hear "wheezing" when your child breathes.
- Bronchiolitis is most often caused by a virus, which does not require antibiotics. Instead, most treatment recommendations are geared toward making your child comfortable with close monitoring for any difficulty in breathing, eating, or signs of dehydration. Medicines used for patients with asthma (such as albuterol or steroids) are not recommended for most infants and young children with bronchiolitis. Children who were born prematurely or have underlying health problems may need different treatment plans.

7. Pain:

- The best medicines for pain relief for children are acetaminophen or ibuprofen. Talk to your pediatrician about how much to give your child, as it should be based on your child's weight.
- Narcotic pain medications are not appropriate for children with common injuries or complaints such as sprained ankle, ear pain, or sore throats. Codeine should never be used for children as it's been associated with severe respiratory problems and even death in children.

8. Common Cold:

- Colds are caused by viruses in the upper respiratory tract. Many young children—especially those in child care—can get 6 to 8 colds per year. Symptoms of a cold (including runny nose, congestion, and cough) may last for up to 10 days.
- Green mucus in the nose does not automatically mean that antibiotics are needed; common colds never need antibiotics. However, if a sinus infection is suspected, your doctor will carefully decide whether antibiotics are the best choice based on your child's symptoms and a physical exam.

9. Bacterial Sinusitis:

- Bacterial sinusitis is caused by bacteria trapped in the sinuses. Sinusitis is suspected when cold-like symptoms such as nasal discharge, daytime cough, or both last over 10 days without improvement.
- Antibiotics may be needed if this condition is accompanied by thick yellow nasal discharge and a fever for at least 3 or 4 days in a row.

10. Cough:

- Coughs are usually caused by viruses and do not often require antibiotics.
- Cough medicine is not recommended for children four years of age and younger, or for children 4 to 6 years of age unless advised by your doctor. Studies have consistently shown that cough medicines do not work in the 4-years-and-younger age group and have the potential for serious side effects. Cough medicines with narcotics—such as codeine—should not be used in children.

6.4.1. The Integrated Management of Childhood Illness

The whole child's health is the main focus of the Integrated Management of Childhood Illness (IMCI), an integrated approach to child health. The objectives of IMCI are to improve growth and development in infants and children under five years old, as well as to lower the rate of death, illness, and disability. IMCI consists of therapeutic and preventive components that are carried out by healthcare professionals in facilities as well as by families and communities.

The IMCI strategy, which is implemented in healthcare facilities, is centered on infants and children who present with an illness. It facilitates the precise identification of childhood illnesses in outpatient settings, guarantees the appropriate combination treatment of all major illnesses, enhances caregiver counseling, and expedites the referral of severely ill children. Developed primarily for low-resource settings, IMCI is a collection of several clinical algorithms and training materials that help clinicians and other primary health-care providers manage ill infants and children who present to medical facilities. Growth charts for infants ages 0–2 months and 2–59 months are included in IMCI. The evaluation of sick infants and children and the promotion of the health and development of well children both depend heavily on nutrition assessment. As a result, IMCI contains algorithms that medical professionals stationed at primary healthcare facilities can utilize.

6.4.1.1. Inequalities of Child Health

While there has been an almost threefold annual drop in the number of deaths among children under five since the 1970s, this decline has not been evenly distributed globally. The 1999 World Health Report states that compared to children in industrialized nations, children in low- to middle-income countries have a tenfold higher risk of dying before turning five. Over 50 countries continued to have childhood mortality rates exceeding 100 per 1,000 live births in 1998. In these countries, over 10 million children pass away before turning five each year. Malnutrition, diarrhea, measles, malaria, and acute respiratory infections (primarily pneumonia) account for seven out of 10 of these deaths, and these conditions frequently coexist.

6.4.1.2. Rationale for an Evidence-Based Syndromic Approach to Case Management

Numerous well-known preventive and treatment techniques have already shown to be successful in saving the lives of young people. Measles deaths have been successfully decreased as a result of childhood vaccinations. Diarrhea-related deaths have significantly decreased as a result of oral rehydration therapy. Antibiotics that are effective have prevented pneumonia in millions of children. More children are now able to recover from malaria and lead healthy lives thanks to prompt treatment. The number of child fatalities has decreased even with small improvements in breastfeeding habits. A comprehensive summary of these interventions consists of 16 essential family practices. Even though each of these interventions has demonstrated remarkable results, mounting data indicates that better results may be obtained by managing sick children through a more integrated approach. Programs for children's health must go beyond treating specific illnesses to include a child's general health and wellbeing. Since many diseases' signs and symptoms overlap in children, it can be challenging to make a single diagnosis and may not be practical or appropriate. This is particularly true for first-class medical facilities, where X-rays, minimal or no laboratory testing, and few instruments are used during examinations. The need for curative care was the primary driving force behind the development of the IMCI strategy, but it also takes into account critical components of disease prevention and health promotion such as nutrition and immunization. The strategy aims to decrease mortality as well as the incidence and severity of disease and disability, while also promoting better growth and development. The age group that experiences the greatest number of deaths from common childhood diseases is children under five, and this is the target audience for the IMCI clinical guidelines.

6.4.2. Daily Health Check

A staff member will welcome every family to the child care center and spend a few minutes getting to know the parent and child while doing a daily health check. The adult should be sitting down on the child's level.

Here is a list of possible visual signs and symptoms to check:

- Face and head (cuts, bruises, sore spots).
- Eyes, ears, nose (redness, discharge, swelling, pain).
- Hair (clean; check for lice or ringworm).
- Arms and legs (cuts, bruises, burns, sores or wounds, pain).
- Hands (sores, wounds, burns, unusual scars).
- Feet (limping, pain, wounds, burns).
- Skin (rashes, irritation, insect bites).
- General appearance (body, hair and clothing clean; energy level; extreme hunger).
- Obvious signs of illness (droopy appearance; listless; upset stomach).
- "Hidden" areas (check for obvious signs of physical or sexual abuse during first bathroom break – bruising, pain during urination or bowel movement, bleeding).
- Other.

The tactile (touch) health check involves gently rubbing your hand on the child's back, shoulder, or head as you greet him or her. This is one way to observe signs of possible illness or injury on areas of the body which are covered by clothing or hair.

- General feeling of warmth, indicating possible fever.
- Possible bruising or soreness; the child may flinch or pull away from your touch.

Verbal communication as you greet each child may provide clues to possible illness or injury. Talk to the child and ask questions such as:

- Did you get a good night's sleep?
- If an injury or apparent sore is observed, ask the child "How did you get hurt?"

Also, communicate with the parent:

- Did child sleep normally?
- Is child eating and drinking normally? When was the last time child ate or drank?
- How did child seem to feel and act at home?
- Have any unusual events taken place?
- Have bowel movements and urine been normal? When was the last time child used toilet or diaper was changed?

6.4.3. Recommendations for Exclusion

Mild illness is common among children. Most children will not need to be excluded from their usual source of care for mild illnesses. Examples include common cold, diarrhea, HIV infections, etc.

After a child has attended school for a full year, the rate of illness starts to decline. The germs found in community outbreaks are the same ones found in early childhood programs. Most infections are minor, self-limiting, and heal on their own. During their kindergarten year, children who participate in early education or child care programs experience a reduction in infections.

6.4.4. Preparing for Managing Illness

Caregivers should:

1. Encourage all families to have a backup plan for child care in the event of short or long term exclusion.
2. Review the inclusion and exclusion policies with families before enrollment. Clarify that the program staff, (not the families), will make the final decision about whether children who are ill may stay based on the program's inclusion and exclusion criteria and their ability to care for the child without compromising the care of other children in the program.
3. Develop procedures for handling children's illnesses, including care plans and inclusion and exclusion policies. Consider asking a health professional (such as a public health nurse) to help you.
4. Request a healthcare provider's note to readmit a child if needed to determine whether the child is a health risk to others, or if the healthcare provider's guidance is needed about any special care the child requires.
5. Rely on the family's description of the child's behavior to determine whether the child is well enough to return, unless the child's status is unclear from the family's report.

6.4.5. Key Criteria for Exclusion of Children Who Are Ill

When a kid gets sick but doesn't need to go to the doctor right away, it has to be decided if they can stay in the care system or if they should be sent home and "excluded" from it for a while. For the most part, diseases can be excluded.

The caregiver should determine if the illness:

1. Prevents the child from participating comfortably in activities.
2. Results in a need for care that is greater than the staff can provide without compromising the health and safety of other children.
3. Poses a risk of spreading harmful diseases to others.

If any of the above criteria are met, the child should be excluded, regardless of the type of illness.

After the sick child has left and the surfaces and toys have been cleaned and disinfected, the child should be kept away from other children and cared for in a location where no other children or adults will use the toys, equipment, or surfaces. Until the parent comes to pick up the child, the child will be looked after by a staff member that they know well.

When a child requires exclusion the caregiver will:

- Provide care for the child in a place where the child will be comfortable and supervised by someone who knows the child well and who will continue to observe the child for new or worsening symptoms.
- Document all signs and symptoms of illness including time and circumstances when symptoms appeared, temperature (if taken), and any changes in the child's condition. A potentially contagious child should be separated from other children by at least three feet. Each facility should have a predetermined physical location(s) where an ill child(ren) could be placed until care can be transferred to a parent or family member.
- Contact the family and ask that someone pick the child up as soon as possible once it is determined the child needs to be excluded.
- Discuss the signs and symptoms of illness with the parent who is assuming care. Review guidelines for returning to child care. If necessary, provide the family with written notes that may be given to the healthcare provider. The communication should include onset time of symptoms, observations about the child, vital signs and times (e.g., temperature 101.5°F at 10:30 AM) and any actions taken and the time actions were taken (e.g., one children's acetaminophen given at 11:00 AM). The nature and severity of symptoms and or requirements of the local or state health department will determine the necessity of medical consultation. Telephone advice, electronic transmissions of instructions are acceptable without an office visit.
- Follow the advice of the child's healthcare provider.

If you have any concerns about a child or staff member in the program having a reportable (harmful) infectious disease, get in touch with the local health department. The health department is legally able to make the final decision regarding the care of a child with a reportable infectious disease in the event that multiple medical professionals have divergent views.

- Document actions in the child's file with date, time, symptoms, and actions taken (and by whom); sign and date the document.
- In collaboration with the local health department, notify the parents of contacts to the child or staff member with presumed or confirmed reportable infectious disease.

The final say on whether a child satisfies the exclusion criteria for participation and whether the child needs care in relation to the staff's capacity to provide it is made by the caregiver or the director of the early childhood program.

6.5. Child Abuse and Neglect

Any action or inaction on the part of a parent, caregiver, or other adult that causes harm, potential harm, or the fear of harm to a child is referred to as child abuse or neglect. There are many different types of child abuse and neglect, such as exploitation, physical, sexual, and emotional abuse. Any deliberate physical harm or injury inflicted on a child by a caregiver or parent, such as striking, kicking, or burning a child, is referred to as physical abuse. Any sexual activity involving a child, such as fondling, oral sex, having sex, or exposing them to sexual materials or activities, is considered sexual abuse. Any behavior that harms a child's emotions or psyche—such as ridiculing, insulting, or isolating them—is considered emotional abuse. Failure to meet a child's basic needs—such as clothing, food, shelter, medical attention, or supervision—is referred to as neglect. The use of a child for one's own or another's financial benefit, such as child prostitution or forced labor, is known as exploitation.

Long-term consequences of child abuse and neglect can include harm to a child's physical and mental well-being, capacity to build positive relationships, and ability to participate in society. It is critical that community members, educators, and healthcare professionals recognize the warning signs of child abuse and neglect and report any suspicions to the proper authorities. Reporting suspected cases of child abuse and neglect is required in many countries. A multifaceted strategy including early intervention, family support, and education is needed to prevent child abuse and neglect. Programs for home visits, parent education, and assistance for families dealing with mental health, drug misuse, or poverty are a few examples of this. Collaborating as a community is crucial in guaranteeing the security and welfare of every child.

6.5.1. The Types of Child Abuse and Neglect

Child abuse and neglect are serious problems that can have significant long-term effects on a child's physical and mental health, as well as their social and emotional development. There are several different types of child abuse and neglect:

1. **Physical Abuse:** It is any act of violence or harm inflicted on a child, including hitting, kicking, shaking, burning, or otherwise physically injuring a child. Physical abuse can result in bruises, broken bones, and other physical injuries.
2. **Sexual Abuse:** It involves any sexual activity or contact between an adult or older child and a child, including touching, fondling, oral sex, or penetration. Sexual abuse can have long-term emotional and psychological effects on children, including feelings of shame, guilt, and low self-esteem.
3. **Emotional Abuse:** It involves any behavior that undermines a child's emotional or psychological well-being, including verbal abuse, threats, rejection, and isolation. Emotional

abuse can have long-term effects on a child's mental health, including anxiety, depression, and other emotional and behavioral problems.

4. **Neglect:** It is the failure to provide for a child's basic needs, including food, clothing, shelter, medical care, and education. Neglect can have serious long-term effects on a child's physical and mental health, including malnutrition, illness, and developmental delays.
5. **Exploitation:** This involves any form of using a child for personal gain or profit, including forced labor, trafficking, and child pornography. Exploitation can have long-term effects on a child's physical, emotional, and psychological well-being, including trauma, depression, and anxiety.

It is crucial to remember that child abuse and neglect can happen in any family, regardless of socioeconomic background, race, or ethnicity, and that they frequently combine various forms of abuse. To protect the child's safety and wellbeing, it is crucial to identify the warning signs of child abuse and neglect and to report any suspected cases to the relevant authorities.

6.5.2. The Effects of Child Abuse and Neglect

The physical, emotional, and psychological health of a child can suffer greatly over time from abuse and neglect. The ramifications of maltreatment and disregard may persist well into adulthood, affecting an individual's capacity to establish sound interpersonal bonds, sustain employment, and lead a satisfying life.

Some of the most common effects of child abuse and neglect include:

1. **Physical Health Problems:** Physical abuse and neglect can result in a wide range of health problems, including malnutrition, poor growth and development, chronic pain, and long-term medical conditions such as heart disease and diabetes.
2. **Mental Health Problems:** Child abuse and neglect can have long-term effects on a child's mental health, including anxiety, depression, post-traumatic stress disorder (PTSD), and other emotional and behavioral problems.
3. **Social Problems:** Children who experience abuse and neglect may struggle to form healthy relationships with others and may have difficulty trusting others. They may also have problems with social skills and may struggle to connect with peers.
4. **Cognitive Problems:** Child abuse and neglect can also impact a child's cognitive development, including their ability to learn, problem-solve, and make decisions.
5. **Substance Abuse:** Adults who experienced abuse or neglect as children are at increased risk of developing substance abuse problems, including alcohol and drug addiction.
6. **Self-Harm and Suicide:** Child abuse and neglect can lead to feelings of hopelessness, despair, and worthlessness, which can contribute to self-harm and suicidal thoughts and behaviors.
7. **Criminal Behavior:** Individuals who experienced abuse or neglect as children may be at increased risk of engaging in criminal behavior later in life.

It is significant to remember that the consequences of child abuse and neglect can differ based on the degree of the abuse or neglect, how long it lasts, and the age and developmental stage of the child at the time of the abuse or neglect. For children who have been through these traumatic experiences, early intervention and treatment can help lessen the long-term effects of abuse and neglect and enhance their outcomes.

6.5.3. The Risk Factors for Child Abuse and Neglect

Child abuse and neglect can occur in any family, regardless of socioeconomic status, race, or ethnicity. However, certain risk factors may increase the likelihood of child abuse and neglect. Some of the most common risk factors for child abuse and neglect include:

1. **Parental Stress:** Parents who experience high levels of stress, including financial stress, job loss, or relationship problems, may be more likely to engage in abusive or neglectful behavior towards their children.
2. **Substance Abuse:** Parents who struggle with substance abuse, including alcohol or drug addiction, may be more likely to engage in abusive or neglectful behavior towards their children.
3. **Mental Health Issues:** Parents who experience mental health issues, including depression, anxiety, or post-traumatic stress disorder (PTSD), may be more likely to engage in abusive or neglectful behavior toward their children.
4. **Domestic Violence:** Children who witness domestic violence between their parents or caregivers may be at increased risk of experiencing abuse or neglect.
5. **Social Isolation:** Parents who are socially isolated or lack support from friends and family members may be more likely to engage in abusive or neglectful behavior towards their children.
6. **Poverty:** Children who live in poverty or who experience food insecurity may be at increased risk of experiencing abuse or neglect.
7. **Parental History of Abuse:** Parents who have experienced abuse or neglect in their own childhood may be more likely to engage in abusive or neglectful behavior towards their own children.

It is crucial to remember that these risk factors do not ensure that abuse or neglect will take place, and many families who have them are still able to give their kids secure and supportive environments. On the other hand, by recognizing and addressing these risk factors, child abuse and neglect can be avoided, and family and child outcomes can be enhanced (Figure 6.2).

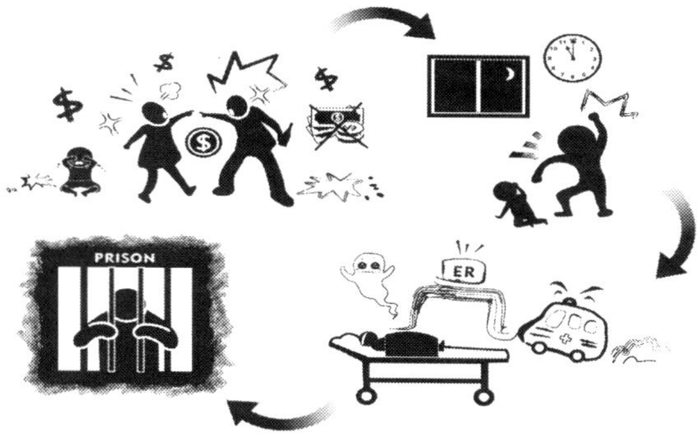

Figure 6.2. *Child abuse is serious.*

Source: *Su, H. C., & Lin, Y. H., (2023). Analyses of criminal judgments about domestic child abuse cases in Taiwan. Children, 10(7), 1237. https://doi.org/10.3390/children10071237.*

6.5.4. Recognizing and Reporting Child Abuse and Neglect

It's critical to identify and report child abuse and neglect to shield kids from additional harm. It is crucial to act and notify the proper authorities of your concerns if you believe a child is being abused or neglected.

Here are some signs of child abuse and neglect to look out for:

1. **Physical Abuse:** Unexplained bruises, welts, or marks on a child's body, or injuries that seem inconsistent with the child's explanation of what happened.
2. **Sexual Abuse:** Sexual behavior or knowledge that is inappropriate for the child's age, unexplained genital injuries or infections, or reports of sexual abuse from the child.
3. **Neglect:** A child who is consistently dirty or hungry, lacks necessary medical or dental care, or is consistently left unsupervised.
4. **Emotional Abuse:** A child who seems withdrawn, fearful, or anxious, or who exhibits extreme behavior, such as aggression or self-harm.

It's critical that you notify the proper authorities if you believe a child is being abused or neglected. Reports of child abuse and neglect in the United States should be sent to the child protective services agency in your state, which can be located online or by getting in touch with your neighborhood hospital or law enforcement office. Be ready to include as much information as you can when filing a report, such as the child's name, age, and location, the details of your concerns, and any observations or supporting documentation.

While reporting child abuse or neglect can be a challenging and emotional process, it is essential to safeguarding children from harm. In addition to helping families get the resources and support they need to address any underlying issues that may be causing the abuse or neglect, reporting your concerns can also help.

6.5.5. Prevention of Child Abuse and Neglect

Preventing child abuse and neglect is essential in promoting the health and well-being of children and families. There are several strategies that can be effective in preventing child abuse and neglect, including:

1. **Providing Parenting Education and Support:** Parenting education programs can provide parents with the knowledge and skills they need to provide safe and nurturing environments for their children. These programs can also connect families with support services, such as counseling or financial assistance, to help address underlying issues that may be contributing to stress or family conflict.
2. **Promoting Safe and Stable Housing:** Safe and stable housing can help reduce stress and provide a secure environment for children. Programs that provide affordable housing or rental assistance can be effective in promoting safe and stable housing for families.
3. **Addressing Poverty and Economic Inequality:** Poverty and economic inequality can increase the risk of child abuse and neglect. Programs that address poverty, such as job training or financial assistance, can help reduce the stress and financial strain on families.
4. **Providing Access to Mental Health Services:** Parents who struggle with mental health issues, such as depression or anxiety, may be more likely to engage in abusive or neglectful behavior towards their children. Providing access to mental health services can help parents address these issues and provide a more stable

and nurturing environment for their children.

5. **Building Social Connections and Support Networks:** Social isolation can increase the risk of child abuse and neglect. Programs that build social connections and support networks for families, such as parent support groups or mentoring programs, can be effective in reducing social isolation and promoting family well-being.

A comprehensive strategy addressing the root causes of stress and family discord is necessary to prevent child abuse and neglect. We can contribute to the prevention of child abuse and neglect as well as the promotion of the health and well-being of children and families by offering families support and resources and encouraging safe and nurturing environments for kids.

6.5.6. The Legal and Ethical Issues Related to Child Abuse and Neglect

Child abuse and neglect is not only a serious social problem, but it also raises significant legal and ethical issues. Here are some of the legal and ethical issues related to child abuse and neglect:

1. **Mandatory Reporting Laws:** In many countries, healthcare professionals, teachers, and other professionals who work with children are required by law to report suspected cases of child abuse and neglect to child protective services. Failure to report suspected abuse or neglect can result in legal and ethical consequences for the mandated reporter.
2. **Confidentiality:** Maintaining confidentiality is essential in protecting the privacy of families and children involved in cases of child abuse and neglect. However, healthcare professionals and other mandated reporters must balance the need for confidentiality with their legal and ethical obligations to report suspected abuse or neglect.
3. **Informed Consent:** In cases where child abuse or neglect is suspected, healthcare professionals and other mandated reporters must obtain informed consent from the child and/or their parents before sharing information with child protective services or other authorities.
4. **Due Process:** In cases where child abuse or neglect is suspected, the accused parties have the right to due process and fair treatment under the law. This can raise ethical issues related to balancing the rights of the accused with the need to protect the child from further harm.
5. **Cultural Sensitivity:** Cultural differences can impact the interpretation of what constitutes child abuse or neglect. Healthcare professionals and other mandated reporters must be sensitive to cultural differences and avoid making assumptions or judgments based on cultural norms that may differ from their own.
6. **Trauma-Informed Care:** Healthcare professionals and other mandated reporters must provide trauma-informed care to children who have experienced abuse or neglect. This involves recognizing the impact of trauma on a child's physical, emotional, and psychological well-being, and providing appropriate care and support to promote healing and recovery.

Social workers, medical professionals, and other professionals who work with children and families must give careful thought to the complex legal and ethical issues surrounding child abuse and neglect. We can contribute to preventing child abuse and neglect and promoting the health and safety of all children by being aware of these concerns and banding together to safeguard children's welfare.

6.5.7. The Role of Trauma-Informed Care in Addressing Child Abuse and Neglect

An approach to healthcare known as "trauma-informed care" recognizes the effects of traumatic events on a person's physical, emotional, and mental health. When it comes to treating child abuse and neglect, trauma-informed care is especially crucial because these children may have complex physical and emotional needs that call for a different kind of care.

Here are some of the ways trauma-informed care can help address child abuse and neglect:

1. **Building Trust:** Trauma-informed care focuses on building trust between the child and the healthcare provider. Children who have experienced abuse or neglect may be reluctant to trust others due to their past experiences. Trauma-informed care acknowledges this and works to build trust in a safe and supportive environment.
2. **Screening for Trauma:** Trauma-informed care involves screening for trauma and addressing the impact of trauma on the child's physical and emotional well-being. This includes assessing the child's history of abuse or neglect, as well as any other traumatic experiences they may have had.
3. **Providing Specialized Treatment:** Trauma-informed care involves providing specialized treatment for children who have experienced abuse or neglect. This may include individual or group therapy, family therapy, and medication management for conditions such as depression, anxiety, and PTSD.
4. **Collaborating with Other Providers:** Trauma-informed care involves collaborating with other healthcare providers and social service agencies to ensure that the child receives the best possible care. This may include working with child protective services, law enforcement, and other healthcare providers to develop a comprehensive treatment plan.
5. **Providing Support and Education:** Trauma-informed care involves providing ongoing support and education to the child and their family. This may include education on coping skills, stress management, and healthy communication.

One essential element of combating child abuse and neglect is trauma-informed care. Healthcare professionals can aid in the healing and recovery of children who have suffered abuse or neglect by creating a safe and encouraging environment, screening for trauma, offering specialized treatment, working with other providers, and offering continuing support and education.

A Closer Look

Child Health and Nutrition:

Food group	2 year olds	3 year olds	4 and 5 year olds	What counts as:
Fruits	1 cup	1 - 1½ cups	1 - 1½ cups	**½ cup of fruit?** ½ cup mashed, sliced, or chopped fruit ½ cup 100% fruit juice ½ medium banana 4-5 large strawberries
Vegetables	1 cup	1½ cups	1½ - 2 cups	**½ cup of veggies?** ½ cup mashed, sliced, or chopped vegetables 1 cup raw leafy greens ½ cup vegetable juice 1 small ear of corn
Grains Make half your grains whole	3 ounces	4 - 5 ounces	4 - 5 ounces	**1 ounce of grains?** 1 slice bread 1 cup ready-to-eat cereal flakes ½ cup cooked rice or pasta 1 tortilla (6" across)
Protein Foods	2 ounces	3 - 4 ounces	3 - 5 ounces	**1 ounce of protein foods?** 1 ounce cooked meat, poultry, or seafood 1 egg 1 Tablespoon peanut butter ¼ cup cooked beans or peas (kidney, pinto, lentils)
Dairy Choose low-fat or fat-free	2 cups	2 cups	2½ cups	**½ cup of dairy?** ½ cup milk 4 ounces yogurt ¾ ounce cheese 1 string cheese

Source: By US Department of Agriculture – https://choosemyplate-prod.azureedge.net/sites/default/files/audiences/HealthyEatingForPreschoolers-MiniPoster.pdf, Public Domain, https://commons.wikimedia.org/w/index.php?curid=61338010.

Supporting children's physical, cognitive, and emotional growth and development requires ensuring they have access to sufficient and nutritious food and beverages. However, in the United States, childhood food access is not always guaranteed, leading to racial and ethnic disparities. In 2020, 1 in 6 children in the US lived in food-insecure households, with Black, Latino, Native American, Asian American, and Pacific Islander children being twice as likely as white children to experience food insecurity.

In conjunction with Feeding America's Health Equity Action League (HEAL), Healthyer Generation created a spotlight issue brief for Hunger Action Month to increase awareness of the causes of this problem and possible solutions. The brief explains the relationship between nutrition, health, and child hunger and offers steps that individuals and organizations can take to promote health equity and guarantee that every child has an equal chance to lead healthy lives.

Summary

- Growth and development milestones are key indicators of a child's physical, cognitive, and emotional development. They provide important information about a child's progress and can be used to identify any potential developmental delays or concerns.
- Cognitive development milestones refer to changes in a child's ability to think, reason, and understand the world around them.
- Emotional development milestones refer to changes in a child's ability to regulate their emotions, understand and express their feelings, and develop relationships with others.
- Supporting children with developmental disabilities can be a complex and challenging task, but there are many ways that parents, caregivers, and educators can help.
- Healthy eating in childhood and adolescence is important for proper growth and development and to prevent various health conditions. Childhood is the stage in a human's life associated with growth and development.
- Proper nutrition is crucial for everybody, but it is especially important for kids because it is directly linked to their overall growth and development. The right nutrition in the right amount leads to a healthier life as they grow.
- Childhood obesity is a significant health, social and economic problem of increasing importance for Western countries. It is the result of long-term positive energy intake: in essence, more calories are ingested than are burned off.
- Children should be carefully fed so as to maintain and encourage good growth and meet their energy needs. Side by side, physical exercise should be promoted, as well as drinking plenty of plain water.
- Carbohydrates are the most important source of energy. They help a child's body use fat and protein for building and repairing tissue.
- All children deserve high-quality medical care. As a parent, it is important to be aware of the most up-to-date treatment guidelines so you can be sure your child is getting the best care possible.
- The Integrated Management of Childhood Illness (IMCI) is an integrated approach to child health that focuses on the well-being of the whole child.
- Child abuse and neglect refer to any act or failure to act by a parent, caregiver, or another adult that results in harm, potential harm, or the threat of harm to a child.
- Child abuse and neglect can have significant long-term effects on a child's physical, emotional, and psychological well-being.
- Recognizing and reporting child abuse and neglect is crucial in protecting children from further harm. If you suspect that a child is being abused or neglected, it is important to take action and report your concerns to the appropriate authorities.

References

1. American Academy of Pediatrics. (2019). *Bright Futures: Guidelines for Health Supervision of Infants, Children, and Adolescents* (4th ed.). Elk Grove Village, IL: American Academy of Pediatrics.
2. Berk, L. E. (2013). *Child Development* (9th ed.). Boston, MA: Pearson Education.
3. Shonkoff, J. P., & Garner, A. S. (2012). The lifelong effects of early childhood adversity and toxic stress. *Pediatrics, 129*(1), e232–e246. doi: 10.1542/peds.2011-2663.

Chapter 7

PROMOTING CHILDREN'S HEALTH

Contents

Unit Introduction 210
7.1. Concept of Promoting Children's Health 212
7.2. Public Health Issues Related to Maternal and Child Health 217
7.3. Relationship Between Diet and Health in Children and Adolescents 222
7.4. Healthy Diet for Child 228
Summary 240
References 240

Unit Introduction

Ensuring children's overall well-being and future success requires prioritizing their health promotion. It entails a thorough strategy that takes into account all facets of health—physical, mental, emotional, and social—building blocks for sound growth and long-term wellbeing. Good child health promotion tactics span several areas, such as public policy, education, healthcare, and community support. For children to receive early intervention, treatment for health issues, and preventive care, they must first and foremost have access to high-quality healthcare. Pediatric screenings, immunizations, and check-ups regularly can help detect health issues early and guarantee prompt interventions. Furthermore, healthcare professionals are essential in teaching parents and other caregivers about safe practices, nutrition, developmental milestones, and healthy lifestyle choices. Another essential element in advancing children's health is education. The perfect environment for teaching skills and knowledge that support healthy living is found in schools. Topics including diet, exercise, cleanliness, mental health awareness, preventing substance abuse, and sexual health education can all be included in health education curricula. Giving kids access to resources and knowledge will enable them to make lifelong healthy decisions and adopt positive habits.

Creating supportive environments in communities, schools, and families is also crucial to advancing children's health. Children's habits and attitudes toward health are greatly influenced by their parents and other caregivers. Positive parenting techniques, like building strong bonds with your children, communicating clearly, and establishing appropriate boundaries, can make a big difference in their wellbeing. Furthermore, establishing inclusive, safe areas for kids to play, work out, and interact with others encourages social development, emotional fortitude, and physical activity. Partnerships and community-based programs are essential for tackling the socioeconomic factors that affect children's health. Healthcare providers, educators, legislators, community organizations, and businesses can work together to address issues like food insecurity, housing instability, poverty, and access to healthcare services. Communities can establish settings that promote children's health and development by cooperating to identify needs, fight for resources, and carry out evidence-based interventions. Furthermore, public policies are very important in influencing the wider factors that determine children's health. Child welfare can be greatly impacted by laws pertaining to social services, healthcare, education, housing, nutrition assistance, and the environment. Children can thrive in environments that are more favorable to their needs when policies that prioritize health equity, access to care, and social support are promoted through advocacy.

Taking a comprehensive approach to promoting children's health involves considering various factors that impact their overall well-being. By dedicating resources to healthcare, education, community support, and policy changes, we can establish a supportive environment where all children can develop and succeed. Ultimately, prioritizing children's health is an investment in the future, providing them with the necessary tools to achieve their goals and live fulfilling, healthy lives.

Orientation and Directional Terms

Term	Definition	Illustration
Community organizations	Community organization is a process where people who share a common interest or live in close proximity come together to address issues that affect them.	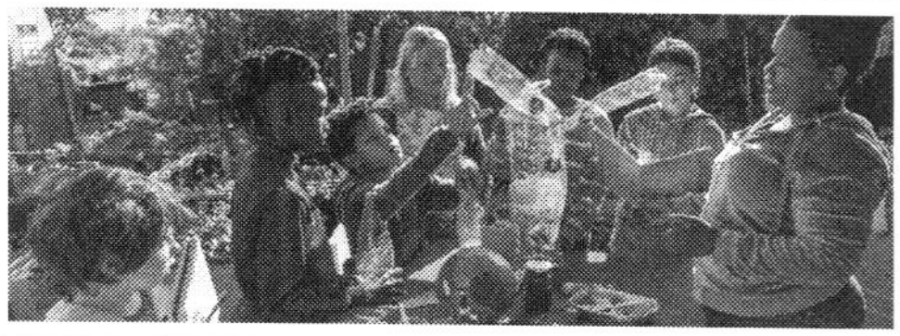
World Health Organization	The **World Health Organization** (WHO) is a specialized agency of the United Nations responsible for international public health.	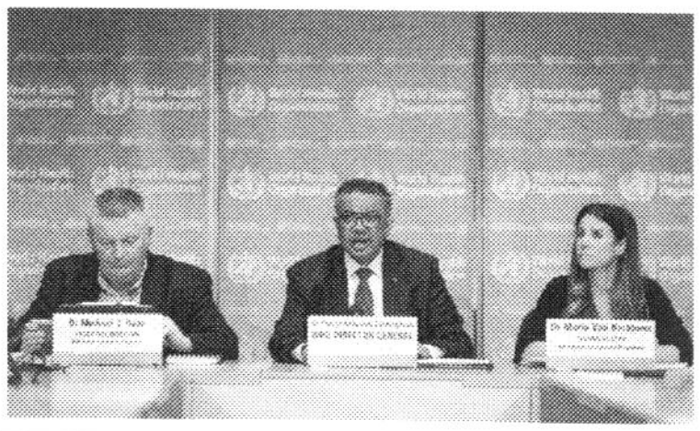
Surveillance	**Surveillance** is the monitoring of behavior, many activities, or information for the purpose of information gathering, influencing, managing, or directing.	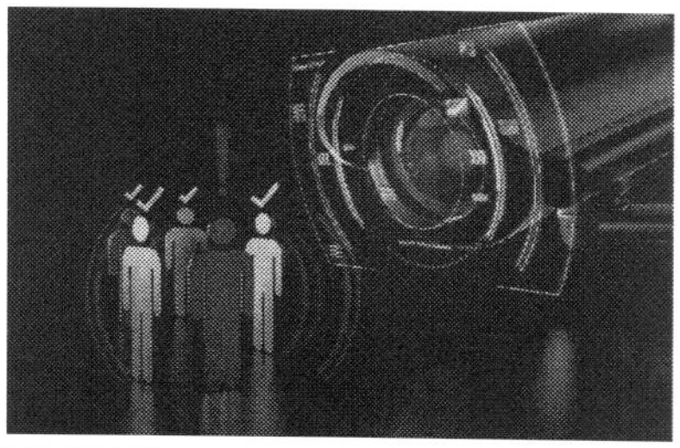
Diseases	A disease is an abnormal condition that negatively affects an organism's structure or function.	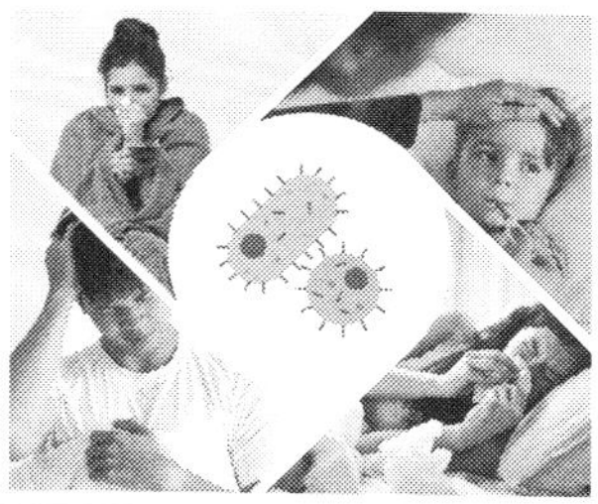
Health promotion	Health promotion is a process that helps people improve their health and take control of the factors that affect it.	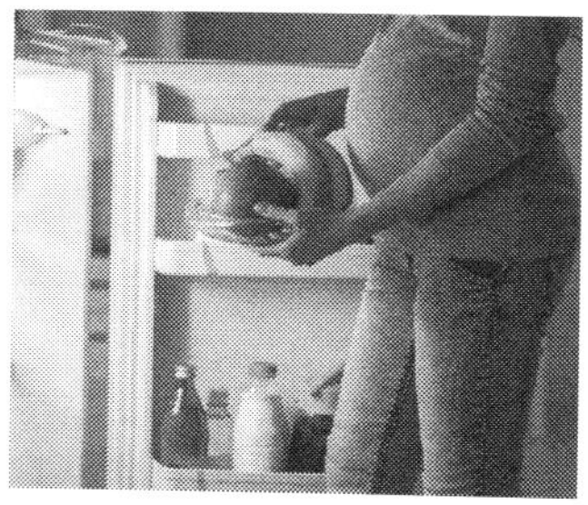

7.1. Concept of Promoting Children's Health

It's critical to first comprehend what health is to comprehend health promotion and maintenance. According to the World Health Organization, being healthy is more than just not being sick or disabled; it also involves having full physical, mental, and social well-being. It is believed that health is a dynamic, ever-evolving state that represents potential or actualization. This fundamental human right is essential to the advancement of societies.

Activities that improve wellness and well-being are referred to as health promotion. All people, even those with acute or chronic conditions, can actualize their positive health potential through these activities.

Examples include providing information and resources to:

- Enhance nutrition at each developmental stage;
- Integrate physical activity into the child's daily events;
- Provide adequate housing;
- Promote oral health;
- Foster positive personality development.

Creating sets of tactics aimed at creating environments that enable people to be healthy and make healthy decisions is the focus of health promotion. The term "health maintenance" (also called "health protection") describes actions taken to maintain a person's current level of health and to stop illness or injury from happening. Providing vaccinations to prevent illnesses, teaching about common childhood safety hazards, and developmental screening or surveillance to detect early deviations from normal development are a few examples of these activities.

Activities for maintaining and promoting health are closely related and frequently overlap, but they differ in a few ways. The goal of health maintenance is to prevent known potential health risks or to recognize them early enough to allow for intervention. The goal of health promotion is to leverage the goals and strengths of individuals, families, and communities to help them achieve greater levels of wellness.

7.1.1. Promoting Healthy Mental and Intellectual Development

Knowledge and a well-stocked toolkit for making decisions are indispensable. It is obvious that teaching your child to make healthy eating choices will provide them with a crucial foundation for a long and healthy life. However, how can sound decision-making be applied to other facets of life? The solution may seem obvious, but putting it into practice may be difficult. It is best to let your kids explore and fill their minds with as much information as they can from as many different sources as they can. Introducing your kids to a wide range of specialized subjects, such as science, language, art, sports, and many more, will help them grow healthier.

7.1.1.1. Incremental Challenges Promote Children's Mental Health and Acuity

You have to provide your kids with challenges if you want them to use their knowledge, grow as decision-makers, and become more self-sufficient. However, there is a constructive approach to challenging them that, in general, you ought to use again.

Children, regardless of their age, require appropriate challenges, which could be defined as those that:

- Allow them to take a healthy measure of risk – be careful with risks that may cause physical or emotional harm.

- Challenge them incrementally, in a way in which it is not too easy to succeed or fail.
- Compel them to use the widest range of abilities or skills that they have.

This will promote their mental health as well as their capability to develop emotionally.

7.1.2. Components of Health Promotion/Health Maintenance Visits

7.1.2.1. Growth and Developmental Surveillance in Schools

Surveillance of growth and development offers crucial hints regarding the state and surroundings of the child. At every health supervision visit, growth, child height, weight, and body mass index should be evaluated and calculated. Written copies of the information should be provided to parents, along with an interpretation. A physical examination is done to make sure the child is developing normally and that there are no unusual or mysterious physical findings. The flexible, ongoing process of skilled observations known as developmental surveillance helps to confirm that the home environment is stimulating, gives information about the child's abilities, and enables the early detection of any neurological issues. Data can be gathered from multiple sources, such as a survey filled out by the parent, interview questions, or firsthand observation of the child during the visit. To learn about any developmental worries parents may have regarding their child or adolescent, parents can also be questioned. Review the physical, social, and communicative milestones for newborns, early children, older children, and adolescents with the parents.

The delicate process of development is governed by both intrinsic factors and external factors. Since approximately 16% of children have a developmental delay or disability, it is necessary to conduct developmental screenings on all children using a consistent and structured approach.

7.1.2.2. Nutrition

Proper nutrition plays a crucial role during every health supervision check-up, as it greatly impacts overall health and supports growth and development. It is essential to assess and screen nutritional intake at each visit. Ensuring children eat age-appropriate foods that match their level of physical activity can provide the necessary energy for healthy growth, physical activity, cognitive development, and immune function. Nutrition is closely connected to both promoting good health and maintaining it.

7.1.2.3. Physical Activity

Numerous advantages for both physical and mental health come from physical activity. But for the majority of our kids, there is a growing gap between expectations and reality. Using data from the Youth Media Campaign Longitudinal Survey (YMCLS) of parents and kids, the Centers for Disease Control and Prevention (CDC) discovered that 61.5% of children aged 9 to 13 say they don't engage in any organized physical activity after school. Even though structured activities are reliable and significant forms of exercise, not all kids can or want to participate. Nevertheless, 22.6% of these kids said they don't do ANY physical activity at all outside of school. Parents reported that issues with transportation, a lack of opportunities nearby, costs, a lack of parental time, and a lack of safety in the neighborhood were among the obstacles to engaging in physical activity. Ask the child about sedentary habits as they get older, such as how many hours they spend playing video games on the computer or watching television. Check if the child participates in sports in the community or at school. To gauge the amount of activity, inquire about daily activities.

7.1.2.4. Oral Health

Although oral health may appear to be a topic that requires specialized knowledge, its implications are closely linked to general healthcare. Maintaining good oral health is vital because teeth play a significant role in language development, impacted or infected teeth can lead to overall illness, and having good teeth is related to forming a positive self-image. Tooth decay and pain in children can disrupt their daily activities such as eating, sleeping, attending school, and speaking. It is important to promote good dental health by educating about oral care and ensuring access to regular dental check-ups. Health maintenance efforts should focus on preventing cavities and other dental diseases.

7.1.2.5. Eye and Vision

Eye exams in children are very important because 25% of school-aged children and 5 to 10% of preschoolers have vision problems. Early diagnosis of a child's vision issue can be very important, as children respond better to treatment when issues are discovered early on. At six months of age, infants should have their first thorough eye examination. After that, children should have further eye exams at age three and right before they start first grade, which is around age five or six. It is advised that school-age children have an eye exam every two years if vision correction is not needed. Children who require contact lenses or eyeglasses should have an annual examination, or as suggested by the optometrist.

7.1.3. Mental and Spiritual Health

When it comes to health promotion and maintenance visits, mental and spiritual health are crucial topics to discuss. It is recommended that parents maintain a record of mental health concerns for use in health supervision visits. This aids in their comprehension that the medical expert is prepared to collaborate with them to support mental health management. Make suggestions about subjects like the mood of the child and the parent, the temperament of the child, stress and the family's coping mechanisms, or sleeping habits. Keep an eye out for indications of child abuse or neglect, stress, depression, and anxiety. Goals for the mental health of children and families should be established for both health promotion and health maintenance. The objectives of health promotion are related to protective factors like community and extended family involvement, as well as sufficient resources to address family challenges. It is beneficial to teach stress-reduction methods like visualization, relaxation, and meditation in addition to offering resources for yoga and other methods. The prevention of mental health issues is a goal of health maintenance. The spiritual dimension is a link to a force outside of oneself that inspires, respects, and directs one's search for meaning, inspiration, and purpose in life. In a broad sense, spiritual health is defined as the presence of things that give life purpose.

7.1.4. Disease Prevention Strategies

Strategies for preventing disease primarily concentrate on maintaining health or preventing illness. Certain health problems are early detectable, allowing for the start of treatment. The process of screening is intended to identify potential health conditions before symptoms manifest. It is the secondary level of prevention and is typically carried out on sizable cohorts of people who are susceptible to a condition. Developmental screening, blood pressure screening, and vision/hearing screening are a few examples. They don't consider most screening tests to be diagnostic; however, if a screening result is positive, additional diagnostic testing is ordered. Early intervention can start with the aim of lessening the condition's severity or complications once a screening test confirms the condition's existence.

7.1.4.1. Vaccination

The cornerstones of a healthy lifestyle include getting immunized and leading an active lifestyle. Vaccinations are a safe and essential component of maintaining your family's health. The reason vaccinations are so crucial is that they protect not only you but also those around you. Getting vaccinated against an illness strengthens your immune system and increases your resistance to that illness. No matter how healthy you are, if you have not received the vaccination, you will never have the antibodies to defend yourself in the event that you come into contact with the illness.

Because vaccination lowers the risk to oneself and others by keeping many people from contracting a communicable disease, it is a crucial part of public health. Vaccination is an additional means of protecting kids from common infectious diseases. Immunizations not only keep kids healthy but also lower the risk for others who are less immune, such as young children or those with long-term medical conditions.

7.1.4.2. Encourage Health Promotion Activities

To encourage healthy behaviors in their own children, families frequently require health education and counseling. Information on controlling the environment to reduce sedentary behavior, dietary adjustments to increase fruit and vegetable intake, and switching to low-fat dairy products are a few examples of targeted health education and counseling. When the family is aware of the connection between a behavior change and the subsequent health outcome, patient education and counseling are most successful. When determining whether a family would benefit from a change in health behavior, take into account the views of the family members regarding the change in health, the advantages and disadvantages of the change, and the planning of interventions to increase the likelihood of change.

Steps in promoting patient education and counseling include:

- Clarifying learning needs of child and family;
- Setting a limited agenda;
- Prioritizing needs with family;
- Selecting-teaching strategy (explaining, showing, providing resources, questioning, practicing, giving feedback);
- Evaluating effectiveness.

7.1.5. Promoting Optimal Health and Development of Children

It is possible for parents to assist their children in achieving optimal health. Early childhood lays the groundwork for a body and mind in good health. Early life experiences are critical for a child's physical, mental, and social/emotional development as well as overall health. When a baby's physical needs are regularly and consistently met, they develop a strong sense of trust and attachment to their caregiver as a source of satisfaction. Healthy infants develop into children and teenagers.

7.1.5.1. Childhood Health

Well-child visits, also known as *preventive* healthcare visits, are crucial for promoting and maintaining healthy health in newborns, kids, and teenagers. These visits give doctors the chance to physically examine the child to detect disorders and treat them early, as well as provide guidance to parents on how to support their child's physical, emotional, and mental development.

Regular vaccinations and education also help prevent disease. Doctors can watch parents interact with their children during preventive care visits and can offer guidance and answer inquiries. Promoting early childhood health focuses on early interventions and developing programs for the youngest children to maintain children's health. According to Healthy People 2020, early childhood is defined as the eight years between birth and age eight. It is noted that during this crucial time, a person experiences some of their most significant growth and development. A child's early years set the stage for their later social, emotional, cognitive, and physical growth.

Numerous factors, such as family dynamics, community dynamics, and other social determinants of health (SDOH), have an impact on children's health and well-being. These comprise the structures, guidelines, and surroundings in which kids are born and raised. Programs that aim to influence and modify specific health behaviors and outcomes from an early age can have a significant impact on health outcomes later in life, according to the Centers for Disease Control and Prevention.

Some of these programs include a focus on:

- Childhood obesity, especially programs in early childhood education settings;
- Healthy food options and nutrition;
- Physical activity;
- Chronic disease in childhood;
- Oral health;
- Healthy sleep habits;
- Access to age-appropriate screening tests for development, hearing, and vision;
- Childhood trauma and adverse childhood experiences (ACEs) prevention.

7.1.5.2. Child Development

Babies require affection and stimulation to develop emotionally and intellectually. Some parents use a range of toys and technology to give their babies an extremely structured, orderly environment. However, the presence of a happy, pleasant interaction that is enjoyed by parent and child is more significant than the specific contents of the environment. A baby's development is not hampered by parents who show them affection, smiles, frequent amicable speech, physical contact, and love but who do not purchase an array of toys and technology.

It is best to approach the goal of promoting a child's optimal development with flexibility, taking into consideration the age, temperament, developmental stage, and learning style of each individual child. It usually works best when parents, teachers, and the child take a coordinated approach. Children require an environment that fosters learning and curiosity throughout their formative years. Books and music should be given to the child. Daily interactive reading sessions with parents asking and responding to questions improve children's comprehension and attention spans while piquing their curiosity in educational pursuits. Playing video games and watching television for no more than two hours a day promotes more interactive play.

Preschool and playgroups are beneficial for a lot of young kids. Youngsters can pick up crucial social skills like sharing. They might also start to identify colors, letters, and numbers. Acquiring these abilities facilitates the adjustment to school. It's crucial to remember that possible developmental issues can be recognized and resolved early in a structured preschool environment. When their child needs care, parents often wonder what kind of environment is best and whether their child will be harmed by the care they receive from others. Research indicates that young children can thrive in both in-home and out-of-home care settings, provided that they are raised in a loving and supportive environment. Parents can choose the best environment for their child by closely observing how the child responds to a particular child care setting. Certain children do better in large group child care settings, while others might do better at home or in smaller groups.

When the child begins to receive homework assignments, parents can help by:

- Showing interest in the child's work;
- Being available to sort through questions but not finishing the work themselves;
- Providing a quiet work environment at home for the child;
- Communicating with the teacher about any concerns.

Parents should think about their child's needs as the school year goes on when choosing extracurricular activities. When given the chance to play an instrument or take part in team sports, many kids flourish. These pursuits might also offer a setting for enhancing social skills. However, if kids are overscheduled and expected to participate in too many activities, some of them may experience stress. It is important to support and encourage children in their extracurricular activities without putting undue pressure on them.

7.2. Public Health Issues Related to Maternal and Child Health

Public health issues related to maternal and child health encompass a complex interplay of factors that influence the well-being of mothers and children globally. Maternal mortality, the death of mothers during pregnancy, childbirth, or within 42 days postpartum, remains a significant concern despite progress in recent decades. In many parts of the world, particularly in low and middle income countries, maternal mortality rates remain high due to various factors, including limited access to quality healthcare, inadequate prenatal care, complications during childbirth, and socio-economic disparities.

One of the most pressing issues in maternal and child health is maternal mortality. While maternal mortality rates have declined globally, significant disparities persist between high-income and low and middle income countries. In low and middle income countries, women often lack access to skilled birth attendants, emergency obstetric care, and essential healthcare services, leading to preventable maternal deaths. Complications such as hemorrhage, sepsis, hypertensive disorders, and obstructed labor contribute to maternal mortality, highlighting the need for improved access to maternal healthcare services and skilled birth attendance.

Child mortality, defined as the death of children under the age of five, is another critical public health issue. Despite significant progress in reducing child mortality rates, millions of children die each year from preventable causes such as pneumonia, diarrhea, malaria, malnutrition, and neonatal complications. Access to essential healthcare services, including immunizations, prenatal care, postnatal care, and treatment for childhood illnesses, is crucial for reducing child mortality and improving child health outcomes (Figure 7.1).

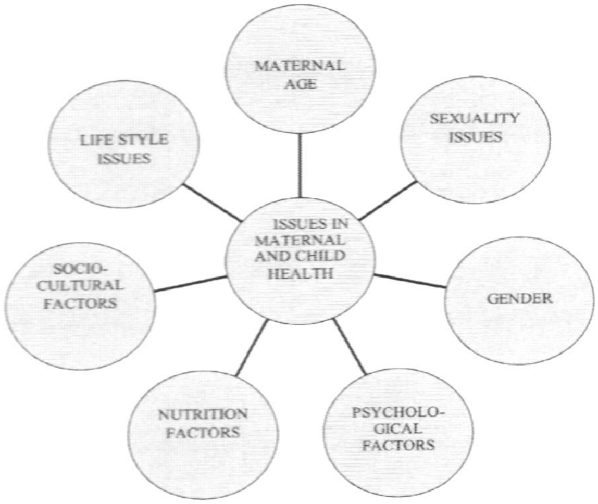

Figure 7.1. *Issues of maternal and child health.*

Source: https://image.slidesharecdn.com/issuesofmaternalandchildhealth-191120080923/75/issues-of-maternal-and-child-health-2-2048.jpg.

Nutrition plays a crucial role in maternal and child health, yet malnutrition remains a significant challenge in many parts of the world. Inadequate maternal nutrition during pregnancy can lead to adverse outcomes such as low birth weight, preterm birth, and intrauterine growth restriction, increasing the risk of neonatal mortality and long-term health problems. Similarly, childhood malnutrition contributes to stunted growth, developmental delays, and increased susceptibility to infections, perpetuating the cycle of poverty and poor health.

Access to healthcare services is a fundamental determinant of maternal and child health outcomes. In many low-income and rural areas, women and children face barriers such as geographic isolation, lack of transportation, financial constraints, and cultural beliefs that hinder access to healthcare. Improving healthcare infrastructure, training healthcare workers, and implementing community-based interventions are essential strategies for expanding access to maternal and child healthcare services.

Family planning and reproductive health are integral components of maternal and child health. Access to contraceptives and family planning services enables women to plan pregnancies, space childbirths, and prevent unintended pregnancies, reducing the risk of maternal and child mortality. Comprehensive reproductive health services, including screening for sexually transmitted infections (STIs), cervical cancer prevention, and maternal health counseling, are essential for promoting women's health and well-being throughout the reproductive lifecycle.

Addressing public health issues related to maternal and child health requires a multifaceted approach that addresses the social, economic, cultural, and political determinants of health. Empowering women, promoting gender equality, strengthening healthcare systems, improving access to education and healthcare services, and addressing socio-economic disparities are essential strategies for improving maternal and child health outcomes globally. By prioritizing maternal and child health and investing in evidence-based interventions, governments, policymakers, healthcare providers, and communities can work together to ensure that every woman and child has the opportunity to thrive.

7.2.1. Epidemiology and Disease Control

Epidemiology and disease control are fundamental aspects of public health aimed at understanding the distribution and determinants of diseases within populations and implementing strategies to prevent and control their spread. Epidemiology involves the study of the patterns, causes, and effects of health and disease conditions in populations, while disease control focuses on the implementation of interventions to reduce the burden of disease and improve public health outcomes.

One of the primary goals of epidemiology is to identify the factors that contribute to the occurrence of diseases and determine their distribution across different populations. Epidemiologists use various study designs and statistical methods to analyze data and identify risk factors associated with disease transmission and progression. This information is crucial for developing effective disease control strategies and targeting interventions where they are most needed.

Disease surveillance is a key component of epidemiology and disease control, involving the systematic collection, analysis, and interpretation of health data to monitor the occurrence of diseases and detect outbreaks in real-time. Surveillance systems enable public health authorities to track disease trends, identify emerging threats, and implement timely interventions to prevent further spread. Advanced surveillance technologies, including electronic health records, syndromic surveillance, and digital disease detection tools, have enhanced the capacity to monitor and respond to disease outbreaks rapidly.

Once disease outbreaks are detected, rapid and effective response efforts are essential to contain the spread of infection and minimize the impact on public health. Disease control strategies may include implementing quarantine and isolation measures, conducting contact tracing to identify and monitor individuals exposed to the disease, providing medical treatment and preventive interventions such as vaccines or prophylactic medications, and promoting public health measures such as hand hygiene, mask-wearing, and social distancing.

Vaccination is one of the most effective strategies for disease control, preventing millions of deaths each year from vaccine-preventable diseases such as measles, polio, and influenza. Through widespread vaccination campaigns and routine immunization programs, public health authorities can achieve herd immunity, reducing the overall prevalence of infectious diseases within populations and protecting those who are unable to receive vaccines due to medical reasons.

In addition to infectious diseases, epidemiology and disease control also play a crucial role in addressing non-communicable diseases (NCDs) such as heart disease, cancer, diabetes, and respiratory illnesses. Epidemiological studies help identify risk factors for NCDs, such as tobacco use, unhealthy diet, physical inactivity, and environmental exposures, informing the development of preventive strategies and health promotion initiatives aimed at reducing the burden of these diseases.

Globalization, urbanization, climate change, and antimicrobial resistance pose ongoing challenges to epidemiology and disease control, increasing the complexity of disease transmission and requiring innovative approaches to address emerging threats. Collaborative efforts between governments, international organizations, academia, and the private sector are essential for strengthening public health infrastructure, enhancing surveillance systems, building capacity for outbreak response, and promoting research and innovation in epidemiology and disease control.

Ultimately, epidemiology and disease control are critical components of public health practice, contributing to the prevention, detection, and control of diseases and the promotion of health and well-being for individuals and communities worldwide. By applying scientific principles, leveraging data-driven approaches, and mobilizing resources effectively, public health authorities can mitigate the impact of diseases, save lives, and improve population health outcomes.

7.2.2. Disaster Management and Emergency Preparedness

Disaster management and emergency preparedness are essential components of public health and safety systems aimed at mitigating the impact of natural and human-made disasters and ensuring an effective response to emergencies. Disaster management encompasses a range of activities, including risk assessment, planning, preparedness, response, and recovery, to minimize the loss of life, property damage, and disruption to communities.

Risk assessment is a fundamental step in disaster management, involving the identification and analysis of potential hazards, vulnerabilities, and exposures that may pose a threat to individuals, communities, and infrastructure. By understanding the risks associated with different types of disasters, such as earthquakes, floods, hurricanes, pandemics, terrorist attacks, and industrial accidents, authorities can develop targeted strategies to reduce the likelihood of disasters occurring and mitigate their impact.

Emergency preparedness involves the development of plans, policies, procedures, and resources to ensure a coordinated and effective response to emergencies. This includes establishing emergency management agencies, designating emergency shelters, stockpiling essential supplies and equipment, training personnel, conducting drills and exercises, and educating the public about disaster preparedness and response measures. Collaborative partnerships between government agencies, non-governmental organizations, community groups, businesses, and other stakeholders are critical for enhancing emergency preparedness and building resilience within communities.

During a disaster or emergency, the response phase involves mobilizing resources, coordinating activities, and implementing emergency operations to address immediate threats and protect public health and safety. This may include search and rescue efforts, medical triage and treatment, evacuation of affected populations, provision of emergency shelter and basic necessities, communication with the public, and coordination with local, national, and international partners. Effective communication and information sharing are essential for ensuring timely warnings, disseminating accurate information, and facilitating coordination among response agencies and the public.

Following the response phase, disaster recovery efforts focus on restoring infrastructure, providing assistance to affected individuals and communities, and promoting long-term recovery and resilience. This may involve debris removal, rebuilding homes and businesses, providing financial assistance and social support services, addressing mental health needs, and implementing measures to prevent future disasters. Community engagement and participation are crucial for ensuring that recovery efforts are inclusive, equitable, and sustainable, empowering affected individuals and communities to rebuild and recover from adversity.

Disaster management and emergency preparedness also play a vital role in addressing emerging threats and global challenges, such as climate change, infectious disease outbreaks, and technological hazards. Climate change is increasing the frequency and intensity of natural disasters, including hurricanes, floods, wildfires, and heatwaves, posing significant risks to human health, infrastructure, and ecosystems. By integrating climate adaptation and mitigation measures into disaster management plans, communities can build resilience to climate-related hazards and reduce vulnerability to their impacts.

Similarly, infectious disease outbreaks, such as pandemics, require robust preparedness and response capabilities to control the spread of disease, protect healthcare workers, and mitigate the impact on public health systems and economies. This includes surveillance and early warning systems, capacity-building for healthcare facilities and laboratories, development and distribution of vaccines and therapeutics, and public health education and communication campaigns.

Technological hazards, such as chemical spills, nuclear accidents, and cyber-attacks, also pose unique challenges for disaster management and emergency preparedness. By investing in technological infrastructure, training personnel, and implementing risk reduction measures, authorities can enhance their ability to prevent, detect, and respond to technological emergencies effectively. Disaster management and emergency preparedness are essential for protecting lives, property, and the environment in the face of natural and human-made disasters. By adopting a comprehensive and proactive approach to risk reduction, planning, preparedness, response, and recovery, communities can build resilience and adaptability to withstand and recover from emergencies, ensuring the safety and well-being of individuals and societies now and in the future.

7.2.3. Healthcare Systems and Policies

Healthcare systems and policies are critical components of public health infrastructure that govern the delivery, financing, and regulation of healthcare services to ensure equitable access, quality care, and improved health outcomes for individuals and populations. Healthcare systems vary widely across countries and regions, reflecting differences in political, social, economic, and cultural contexts, as well as historical developments and healthcare priorities.

One of the key functions of healthcare systems is to provide access to essential healthcare services to all individuals, regardless of their ability to pay. Universal health coverage (UHC) is a guiding principle that aims to ensure that everyone has access to needed healthcare services without suffering financial hardship. Achieving UHC requires comprehensive health financing mechanisms, including taxation, social health insurance, private health insurance, and out-of-pocket payments, as well as strategies to expand coverage to underserved populations, such as rural communities, marginalized groups, and low-income individuals.

Healthcare systems also play a crucial role in promoting preventive care and population health initiatives to reduce the burden of disease and improve overall health outcomes. This includes vaccination programs, screening and early detection of diseases, health education and promotion campaigns, and environmental and occupational health regulations aimed at preventing illness and injury. By investing in preventive measures and addressing social determinants of health, such as education, income, housing, and access to nutritious food, healthcare systems can promote health equity and reduce health disparities within populations.

Quality of care is another essential aspect of healthcare systems, encompassing the effectiveness, safety, timeliness, efficiency, equity, and patient-centeredness of healthcare services. Quality improvement initiatives, clinical guidelines, accreditation standards, and performance measures are used to monitor and assess the quality of care provided by healthcare facilities and professionals, identify areas for improvement, and promote evidence-based practices and patient safety.

Healthcare policies play a central role in shaping the structure, organization, and delivery of healthcare services, as well as influencing health outcomes and population health. Policy decisions related to healthcare financing, workforce planning, service delivery models, technology adoption, pharmaceutical regulation, and health information systems have profound implications for access to care, health system performance, and healthcare expenditures. Effective healthcare policies require collaboration and coordination among government agencies, policymakers, healthcare providers, insurers, employers, and other stakeholders to address complex challenges and achieve desired health outcomes.

Healthcare systems and policies also face numerous challenges and opportunities in response to evolving health needs, demographic trends, technological advancements, and global health threats. Aging populations, rising prevalence of chronic diseases, increasing healthcare costs, healthcare workforce shortages, and health inequities pose significant challenges for healthcare systems worldwide. At the same time, advances in medical research, digital health technologies, telemedicine, precision medicine, and data analytics offer opportunities to transform healthcare delivery, improve patient outcomes, and enhance the efficiency and effectiveness of healthcare systems.

Moreover, global health challenges, such as pandemics, infectious disease outbreaks, antimicrobial resistance, climate change, and health security threats, highlight the interconnectedness of healthcare systems and the importance of international cooperation and collaboration in addressing shared health concerns. By strengthening health systems, promoting evidence-based policies, fostering innovation, and advancing health diplomacy, countries can build resilient healthcare systems capable of responding to current and future health challenges while advancing health equity and improving the well-being of individuals and communities worldwide.

7.3. Relationship Between Diet and Health in Children and Adolescents

Adolescence and childhood are times of ongoing development and growth. An infant's weight doubles at five months of age and triples at one year of age due to rapid growth. In the second year, the child grows four times its birth weight in addition to an additional 7–8 cm of height. The pre-adolescent stage is characterized by an average annual growth in height of 6–7 cm and weight gain of 1.5–3 kg, along with the development and maturation of various tissues and organs.

Older kids and teenagers should drink a lot of milk to meet their high calcium needs. Ghee and cooking oils (25–50 g) ought to be eaten. Excessive consumption of fats can be prevented. Consuming too much salt is not recommended, especially for kids whose families have a history of high blood pressure. Adolescence is a time when unhealthy eating habits and unhealthy behaviors like chewing tobacco, smoking, and alcohol consumption are most likely to develop. Children and adolescents should be encouraged to engage in appropriate lifestyle practices, physical activity, such as games and sports, and the consumption of a nutritious, well-balanced diet.

7.3.1. Primary Changes Occurring in Children and Adolescents as They Grow

Growth is an ongoing process that starts at conception and concludes when sexual maturity is reached. Neuro-psychic growth is accompanied by somatic growth. This long journey can be succinctly divided into three stages: childhood, adolescence, and young adulthood, each distinguished by the unique physical, physiological, and mental changes that are taking place in the child. A child, adolescent, or young adult's growth and development are greatly influenced by the actions of their parents. Different parenting strategies are needed for each of these time periods. For the greatest outcome, interactions in general as well as dietary restrictions, discipline, hygienic standards, and growth-phase-specific pedagogy are crucial.

The first phase, childhood, may be divided, in turn, into:

- Infancy: this extends from birth through the first two years of age and includes the periods identified as newborn (first month of life), unweaned and weaned (first teeth);
- Early childhood or pre-school: from ages 3 to 5;
- Middle childhood, or "school-age" which covers the period from ages 6 to 11.

Adolescence, also known as puberty, is the second stage, which spans the years 11 to 16 for girls and 11 to 18 for boys. And lastly, young adulthood, which spans the ages of 16 to 20 for girls and 18 to 25 for boys.

These three stages describe the child's development from birth, taking into account their anatomical, physiological, and behavioral changes. In reality, though, growth starts 30 days after conception, at which point the head is the size of a pin and the body is four millimeters long. The arms and legs are not yet present, but the heart beats 65 times per minute. The hands and arms don't start to form at the sides of the body until day 35, or a mere five days later. After that, the arms and shoulders start to take shape. By day 40, the first finger indentations appear, and by day 45, they are clearly visible.

The fetus measures about nine centimeters in length at three months. The body's lower regions are still poorly developed. By the time the child is seven months old, his weight has increased to 2.5 kg. The various organs' growth and functioning are essentially complete and sufficient at this age to ensure survival, even outside the mother's womb; however, this will only reach its peak at the conclusion of the entire nine-month gestation period.

Large volumes of water, oxygen, and nutritional materials are needed for this rapid growth. The fetus is a self-sufficient entity during this phase, with its own circulatory system and organs that progressively start operating independently. The placenta and the child have no other means of communication than the umbilical cord. The placenta's function and the mother's nutrition are the only sources of nutrition for the fetus.

7.3.1.1. Early Childhood (From Birth to Age 5)

From the moment of birth, the primary changes involve weight, length of the body, the cranium, dentition, stomach and cardiovascular system:

- The normal average weight of an Italian newborn is approx. 3,250 grams for males and approx. 3,110 grams for females. During the first six months, weight increases by approx. 20–30 grams per day, and 10–15 grams per day during the second six-month period. The weight of a newborn doubles by the fourth month, triples at one year and quadruples at two years;
- The length of a full-term newborn's body is ca. 50 cm. This increases 8 centimeters every three months for the first two three-month periods, while from the age of 6 to 12 months, it will increase by only 8 cm. Generally, a baby is approx. 50 centimeters long at birth, 70 centimeters long at its first birthday and 80 centimeters long at age two;
- In newborns, the cranium is large compared with the body. It is equal to one-fourth the length of the entire body (in an adult it is seven-eighths), and this is because the lower limbs, which are short at birth, subsequently grow much more in comparison with the head and trunk. The cranial bones of an infant are not fused, but rather divided with membranous spaces known as "fontanels" which close between months 14 and 16;
- *Dentition begins in the sixth to eighth* month and lasts until adulthood. It is divided into two major phases: first dentition (from approx. 6–8 mos. to 25–30 mos.) with the appearance of 20 teeth and the second dentition (from approx. 5–6 years to 20–30 years), to reach the full set of 32 teeth;
- The stomach has a capacity of 30–40 cc at birth, which increases gradually to 250 cc by the age of one year. At birth, the cardias (the area that joins the esophagus and stomach) is not able to fully perform its function of preventing the reflux of gastric juices back into the esophagus, a function children acquire later, normally at around 18 months. The slow maturation of the valvular function of the cardias helps to explain both the regurgitation and the ease of vomiting typical in unweaned infants. In proportion, the liver of unweaned infants is much larger than that in adults;
- The cardiovascular system is characterized by a spherical heart and a major axis that is virtually horizontal. During the subsequent development phase, the heart rotates and the major axis takes its more vertical position. At birth, pulse rate is very high (130–180 pulsations per minute), but gradually decreases and by the second year it is 120 pulsations per minute, around the age of 4–5 years, it drops to 100, then to 90 around the age of ten, and, finally, around the age of 15, the heart rate becomes that of an adult. Respiration is superficial, abdominal in type. Inspiration is shorter and expiration longer. Frequency of respiration in newborns is very high (40–50 respiratory acts per minute) and gradually diminishes to 25 respiratory acts per minute at the age of one.

Generally, a healthy child's weight and height are primarily influenced by genetics inherited from parents, as well as factors such as diet, hygiene, physical environment, and emotional connections. A child's genetic potential can only be fully realized with proper nurturing and a healthy lifestyle, including love and attention. Negative external circumstances, like poor nutrition or neglect, can hinder a child's growth and development, preventing them from reaching their full height potential determined by genetics.

7.3.1.2. School-Age (6 to 11 Years of Age)

The child's official entrance into society occurs on the first day of school. Following the fast physical and psychomotor growth that defines infancy and the early years of childhood, school-age growth is slower but still constant (approx. each year, gaining 2 kg in weight and 6 cm in height). During this stage, the child's personality and character continue to develop and mature, and he or she starts to assume greater social roles and take on his first obligations. Playmates and classmates have an increasingly significant role in one's life. A child's heightened sensitivity to his surroundings and increase in intelligence signal the start of a process of both personal and group socialization. The child starts to participate in more and more activities, such as sports and school. Since the child's activities start to be assessed by both his parents and others outside the family, the activities progressively lead to personal responsibility.

7.3.1.3. Adolescence (11 to 16 Years of Age)

The transitional period from childhood to adulthood is known as adolescence. To complete this passage, the person must become independent and forge an identity apart from the family. Young people are then motivated to rebel against their families and the authority of their parents. They do this by acting in a way that is intolerant and defiant and by experiencing extreme emotional ups and downs. Adolescence is defined by the major biological changes associated with puberty, as well as the intense emotional experiences that accompany these changes. These experiences stem from the adolescent's search for new equilibriums in his relationship with the world and with himself, which are driven by bodily changes and impulses. Additionally, the adolescent may experience these changes earlier or later than others their own age, which can cause anxiety and uncertainty.

However, because of these physical changes, the adolescent is treated differently than he was when he was a child by both strangers and the people he normally interacts with. He is expected to behave like an adult, despite the fact that he is still not seen as autonomous or capable of making some decisions regarding his future on his own. The demands placed on him have changed. The adolescent is particularly conscious of this shift in relationships, and he bases his own behavior toward himself and the outside world on this realization. The adolescent no longer accepts being completely dependent on his own family and the various forms of social-emotional support the family has up until that point. This is the first, and frequently a conflictual, indication of this shift. The increase in the amount of stimuli the adolescent pays attention to, based on an increase in his own interests related to his emotions and feelings, as well as the outside world, causes other changes regarding the world around him. Even a small degree of independence gives him the freedom to try new things and develop new ways of acting that go along with new ways of relating to other people. The alterations that take place question the modes of presentation and schema that have up until now controlled the person's relationship with his or her own body, with other people and groups, as well as with activities, things, and social institutions.

7.3.2. Relationship Between Diet and Chronic Diseases in Children

Adults with excess body weight have a well-established link between increased risk of developing chronic diseases and their weight. However, the general public still finds it difficult to acknowledge that this relationship exists with children. Indeed, research to date has demonstrated the significance of risk factors and childhood behavior that contribute to the development of chronic illnesses (diabetes, cardiovascular disease, and cancer) as adults. In instance, it has been shown that there is a connection between the quantity and dietary makeup of eating habits that are adopted during childhood and adolescence and chronic illnesses that are acquired during adulthood.

One of the earliest studies, carried out in the 1930s by Boyd Orr and revisited in 1998 by Frankel, Gunnel and Peters, confirmed a positive correlation between calorie intake during growth and the risk of cancer-related death in adulthood. A recent review by the International Agency for Research on Cancer (IARC) came to the same conclusion, emphasizing a link between obesity in childhood and adolescence and the likelihood of developing chronic illnesses. Must and Limpman found that an excessive consumption of proteins, particularly those from animal sources, can lead to weight gain and obesity, increasing the risk of breast, uterine, and colon cancer. The health status in adulthood is also influenced by the family, social, and economic environment in which a child grows up. Social deprivation and malnutrition in childhood have been associated with a higher risk of cardiovascular diseases and diabetes later in life. Additionally, having overweight family members increases the likelihood of adopting an unhealthy diet, sedentary lifestyle, and obesity.

Three critical factors, if not avoided during adolescence, can have a significant impact on the risk of contracting chronic pathologies during adulthood:

- Exposure to risk factors, such as adopting an unhealthy diet, drinking or smoking, or manifesting excessive weight gain;
- Following a sedentary lifestyle, for example, replacing hours of physical activity with watching TV, playing video games or sitting in front of a computer;
- Ignoring prevention and controlling risk factors.

7.3.3. Relationship between Diet and Health in Pre-School and School-Age Children: Relationships and Principles

Given that young children grow quickly during this time, it would seem that giving them enough energy is essential. The macronutrients fats, carbs, and proteins are found in food items that can give kids energy. The amount of protein consumed by a child in their first years of life is almost the same as that of an adult, but they consume almost twice as many carbohydrates and almost four times as much fat (for every gram of macronutrients consumed per unit of body weight). This illustrates how important energy is, especially in the early years of life. Energy is needed for the digestion, metabolism, and storage of nutrients (thermogenesis), the laying down of new tissue (growth), the maintenance of vital activity (respiration, cardio-circulatory activity, renal and cerebral functions) during rest (basal metabolism), and physical activity. A child's recommended daily energy intake is equal to their energy expenditures (basal metabolism, thermogenesis, and physical activity) plus their energy requirements for growth (i.e., employed to produce new tissue).

The amount of energy needed for growth is substantial in relation to the total during the first year of life, but it drops quickly—it actually drops from 35% in the first month of life to just 5% after a year. A child uses 50–60% of their daily energy for basal metabolism, 30–40% for physical activity, 5–8% for thermogenesis, and only 2% for growth after the first year, up until the age of 9–10.

7.3.3.1. Principles and Relationships

The relationship between diet and health in preschool and school-age children is fundamental to their growth, development, and overall well-being. Establishing healthy eating habits early in life can have long-lasting effects on children's health outcomes, including their physical growth, cognitive development, immune function, and risk of chronic diseases later in life.

Several key principles guide the relationship between diet and health in children:

1. **Nutrient Adequacy:** Preschool and school-age children have specific nutrient requirements to support their growth and development. A balanced diet that includes a variety of nutrient-dense foods such as fruits, vegetables, whole grains, lean proteins, and dairy products is essential to ensure that children receive adequate nutrients, including vitamins, minerals, protein, carbohydrates, and fats.
2. **Energy Balance:** Maintaining a healthy energy balance is crucial for preventing childhood obesity and related health problems. Children should consume an appropriate number of calories to support their growth and activity levels while avoiding excessive calorie intake from high-calorie, low-nutrient foods and beverages such as sugary snacks, fast food, and sweetened beverages.
3. **Variety and Moderation:** Encouraging children to eat a variety of foods from all food groups helps ensure that they receive a wide range of nutrients essential for their health. Teaching moderation in food choices, including portion control and balanced meals, promotes healthy eating habits and reduces the risk of nutrient deficiencies and overconsumption of unhealthy foods.
4. **Role Modeling and Environment:** Parents, caregivers, teachers, and other adults play a critical role in shaping children's eating behaviors and food preferences through their own dietary choices and behaviors. Creating a supportive environment that promotes healthy eating, such as providing nutritious meals and snacks, limiting access to unhealthy foods, and modeling positive eating habits, can help foster lifelong healthy eating patterns in children.
5. **Education and Skill Building:** Teaching children about nutrition, food preparation, and the importance of making healthy food choices empowers them to make informed decisions about their diet and health. Nutrition education programs in schools, hands-on cooking classes, and opportunities for children to grow and harvest their fruits and vegetables can enhance their knowledge and skills related to healthy eating.
6. **Social and Cultural Influences:** Cultural beliefs, traditions, and social norms can influence children's food choices, eating behaviors, and dietary

patterns. Recognizing and respecting cultural diversity in food preferences and meal practices while promoting healthy eating principles can help support children's dietary health within the context of their cultural backgrounds.

7. **Prevention of Food Allergies and Sensitivities:** Early introduction of a variety of foods, including potential allergens, during infancy and early childhood may help reduce the risk of developing food allergies and sensitivities. However, for children with known food allergies or sensitivities, it is essential to provide appropriate dietary modifications and avoid exposure to allergenic foods to prevent adverse reactions and promote optimal health.
8. **Safe Food Handling and Hygiene:** Practicing proper food safety measures, including safe food handling, storage, preparation, and hygiene practices, is critical for preventing foodborne illnesses and promoting children's health. Educating children and caregivers about food safety principles and reinforcing good hygiene habits, such as hand-washing before eating and cooking foods to the appropriate temperature, helps minimize the risk of foodborne infections.

By applying these principles and fostering a supportive environment that promotes healthy eating habits, caregivers, educators, and healthcare professionals can help ensure that preschool and school-age children develop positive relationships with food and maintain optimal health and well-being throughout childhood and beyond.

7.4. Healthy Diet for Child

Providing a nutritious, well-balanced diet for your child is one of the most significant things you can do for their wellbeing. You may be aware of the challenges in getting kids to eat even a spoonful of spinach, let alone the recommended five portions of fruits and vegetables per day. Perhaps it was one of those weeks when your child's only green intake consisted of a green toy. Thankfully, there are lots of simple ways to get your kids to eat their five a day and beyond by serving them fruits and vegetables.

7.4.1. Setting a Good Example

1. Lead by example. As a result, it is critical for parents to set a positive example for their children by making healthy eating choices. Parental self-discipline is necessary to set a good example for their children to follow when it comes to eating healthy foods. If parents are regularly consuming unhealthy foods as snacks, how can kids be expected to behave any differently?

Parents need to provide loving and firm guidance in making healthy and wise choices regarding food and snacks.

It is most important to eat plenty of vegetables and fruits yourself. If you model positive behaviors, chances are your kids will copy you. Watch your body and facial expression as well when you try something new.

2. Give your kids a wide variety of foods to choose from, and let them watch you eat and enjoy different foods—especially fruits and vegetables. When babies first start eating at tables, they are frequently given fruit and vegetable baby food. As a result, your eating habits will have a significant

impact on what your children enjoy to eat. If you don't usually eat fruit or serve veggies with your meals, don't be shocked if your children pick up those habits [https://www.wikihow.life/images/thumb/1/1a/Get-Your-Children-to-Eat-their-Vegetables-and-Fruits-Step-2-Version-2.jpg/aid389518-v4-728px-Get-Your-Children-to-Eat-their-Vegetables-and-Fruits-Step-2-Version-2.jpg.webp].

3. Anticipate some opposition and be prepared to handle it. Since kids dislike having their routines changed, it's normal for them to voice their disapproval of any recent changes made to the family meal plan. Explain to the kids, in a calm manner, "this is what we're having for dinner." If they refuse to eat the meal as scheduled, just cover it and save it for when they express their hunger. Recall that your house is not a cafeteria-style restaurant where kids get to pick what they eat and what they don't. Say, "Well that's good because I saved your dinner for you," when the child later expresses hunger. Reheat as necessary.
4. Explain to children what each vegetable contains by way of providing healthy benefits. For example, carrots have vitamin A which is good for skin and eyes. Make the connections between food and what it does for our bodies.
5. Get the children involved with kitchen preparation. For example, have them help when making salads or main meals together. They will be able to recognize what they are eating if they get to see it and feel it. It's also a great chance to discuss the food and get to understand its value better.

7.4.2. Using Vegetables and Fruit as Snacks

1. Select nutritious kid-friendly snacks like crisp produce paired with delectable dips. Make sure your home is well-stocked with nutritious snacks that are convenient for kids to grab. Cookies and other sugar-coated confections are best enjoyed on special occasions or as an occasional sweet treat. Giving kids cookies or other sugary treats when the family dinner is being prepared or almost ready to be served is never a good idea. To help them wait, think about providing a few nibbles of the salad or veggies that are already prepared for the meal.
2. Take advantage of after school hunger. When your children come home, have a plate ready with crunchy celery, carrots, and cucumbers on it. Serve it with dip if it makes it more enticing for them.
3. Have fresh, already cut vegetables for car trips or walks. Kids eat a lot when they are hungry or even bored, and if it's already prepared, they'll easily snack on the healthy foods.

7.4.3. Making Vegetables and Fruits More Appealin

1. Try a different vegetable every day and prepare it in different ways. Vegetables can be served, raw, baked, steamed, grilled, in a salad, in juice form, stir-fried and broiled. Try a wide variety and in different ways until you find the vegetables that your child will like and in the style, they will like to eat them in.
2. Mix the vegetables into your child's favorite meal. If your child likes macaroni and cheese, make it with steamed broccoli or peas mixed in.

If your child likes spaghetti, mix in tomatoes, mushrooms, or peas and carrots into the sauce. Sometimes mixing right into their favorite foods makes them eat it without even noticing.

3. Try juicing vegetables and mixing with fruit. Make your child part of the juicing experience and they may be more inclined to drink them. Combinations such as carrot, apple, and celery juice are usually sweet to the taste and a big hit. Don't juice too often. It's far healthier to eat the food than to drink it.
4. Offer vegetables and fruit with dip. Most children love to dip items (i.e. French fries in ketchup) so provide them dipping choices such as a salad dressing they might like and let them dip away. Always make vegetables ready to eat and available with lunch, dinner, and snack. By having them readily available your child will eat when they are ready.
5. Find foods that your kids already like to eat, like smoothies, muffins, or yogurt. Find recipes that allow you to add fruit or vegetables to them, like banana or zucchini muffins.
6. Present visually appealing fruits and vegetables. Try creating edible faces by using pieces of broccoli for the mouth, carrot circles for the eyes, pepper strips for the eyebrows, and baby sweet corn for the nose. Children will take great pleasure in assisting with the composition, particularly if you purposefully omit a few anatomical details. Add wild hairstyles using ribbons of courgette, watercress, or cabbage.
7. Introduce color into your children's diet with stir-frying. It is quick, so they get to see instant results. Try stir-frying peas, pepper strips, bean sprouts, and Chinese cabbage, or a mixture of sweet corn, small chunks of carrot and peas.

7.4.4. How to Feed Your Child a Balanced Diet?

It's critical to feed your child a nutritious diet at every meal. It keeps them nourished, provides them with the energy they need to develop, play, and learn, and helps prevent certain diseases like diabetes that can arise from inadequate nutrition. Healthy meal preparation and serving for kids can present a number of difficulties, from time constraints to finicky palates, but they can be addressed with some direction and preparation.

Instead of planning meals based on the nutrients needed, where each meal is planned based on percentages of daily values of macro and micronutrients, the Institute of Medicine advises planning meals based on food choices from the food groups, where each meal is planned based on what type of food is consumed. When meal plans are created using the food-based approach, kids usually get all the nutrients they require. This is how the majority of schools in America choose which foods to serve (Figure 7.2).

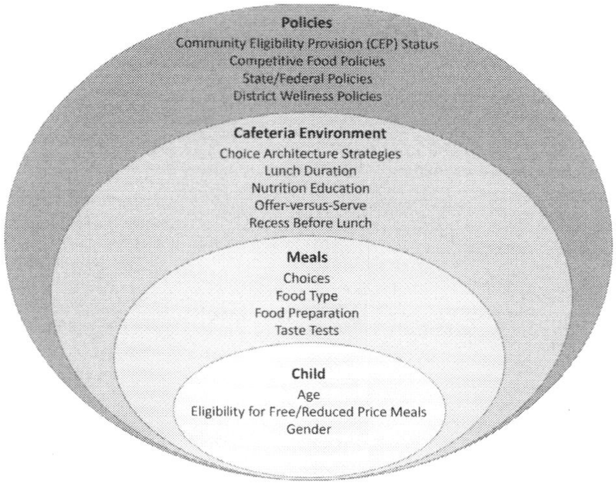

Figure 7.2. *School meal planning-points.*

Source: Cohen, J. F. W., Hecht, A. A., Hager, E. R., Turner, L., Burkholder, K., & Schwartz, M. B., (2021). Strategies to improve school meal consumption: A systematic review. Nutrients, 13(10),3520. https://doi.org/10.3390/nu13103520.

7.4.4.1. Meal Planning

1. Recognize what to serve for each meal. The nutritional requirements of a child vary throughout the day. Your child will receive the best possible combination of foods at each meal and snack for that time of day. Particularly for younger children and toddlers, every meal should be high in nutrients to meet their bodies' needs as they grow quickly. Here are a few minimum serving sizes. Since each child is unique, some might require more. Additionally, some kids might need extra calories on some days because of growth spurts or increased activity. Since your child is learning how to control their calories and listen to their body, it's crucial to follow their lead when it comes to eating habits.
2. Start each day with a balanced breakfast. Eating breakfast does more than break the fast. It sets the stage for the day. When breakfast is eaten, children are better able to focus and learn. Breakfast also tells the body to start burning calories and keep burning calories throughout the day. Each age group has different needs.

Children aged 1 to 2 years old should have 1/2 cup of milk or 1/4 cup of fruits or vegetables or 100% juice, and 1/4 cup or 1/2 slice of enriched or whole grains (bread, bagels, oatmeal, grits, etc.) for breakfast.

- Children aged 3 to 5 years old should have, 3/4 cup of milk or 1/2 cup of fruits or vegetables or 100% juice, and 1/4 cup or 1/2 slice of enriched or whole grains (bread, bagels, oatmeal, grits, etc.) or 1/3 cup cold cereal for breakfast.
- Children aged 6 to 12 years old should have 1 cup of milk or 1/2 cup of fruits or vegetables or 100% juice, and 1/4 cup or 1 slice of enriched or whole grains (bread, bagels, oatmeal, grits, etc.) or 3/4 cup cold cereal for breakfast.

3. Make sure your child has a healthy lunch and dinner to sustain their energy levels throughout the day. Because they grow while they sleep, children need to eat a healthy lunch and dinner that are low in refined sugar to maintain their energy levels throughout the day and night. Since the body takes longer to digest and use complex carbohydrates than simple carbohydrates, like those found in candy or white bread, children who eat whole grain bread or brown rice have better sleep at night.

- Children aged 1 to 2 years old should have 1/2 cup of milk, 2 servings consisting of 1/4 cup each of fruits or vegetables or 100% juice, 1/4 cup or 1/2 slice of enriched or whole grains, and 1 oz. (28 g) of protein for lunch and dinner. Protein should be a lean meat or meat alternative (cheese, beans, etc.).
- Children aged 3 to 5 years old should have 3/4 cup of milk, 2 servings consisting of 1/2 cup each of fruits or vegetables or 100% juice, 1/4 cup or 1/2 slice of enriched or whole grains or 1/3 cup cold cereal, and 1.5 oz. (43 g) of protein for both lunch and dinner. Protein should be a lean meat or meat alternative (cheese, beans, etc.).
- Children aged 6 to 12 years old should have 1 cup of milk, 2 servings consisting of 3/4 cup each of fruits or vegetables or 100% juice, 1/2 cup or 1 slice of enriched or whole grains or 3/4 cup cold cereal, and 2 oz. (56 g) of protein for lunch and dinner. Protein should be a lean meat or meat alternative (cheese, beans, etc.).

4. Prepare balanced snacks because they help with energy needs and keep children from becoming too hungry by the next meal. Maintaining a consistent fuel supply in the body helps children avoid urges to overeat after prolonged hunger periods, and it also helps avoid stomach aches and acid reflux.

- Children aged 1 to 2 years old should have any combination of two from the following as a snack throughout the day, except for milk and juice (will not provide enough calories): choose from 1/2 cup of milk, 1/2 cup of fruits or vegetables or 100% juice, 1/4 cup or 1/2 slice of enriched or whole grains, and 1/2 oz. (14 g) of protein. Protein should be a lean meat or meat alternative.
- Children aged 3 to 5 years old should have any combination of two from the following, as a snack throughout the day except milk and juice (will not provide enough calories): choose from 1/2 cup of milk, 1/2 cup of fruits or vegetables or 100% juice, 1/4 cup or 1/2 slice of enriched or whole grains or 1/3 cup cold cereal, and 1/2 oz. (14 g) of protein. Protein should be a lean meat or meat alternative.
- Children aged 6 to 12 years old should have any combination of two from the following as a snack throughout the day, with the exception of milk and juice (will not provide enough calories): choose from 1 cup of milk, 3/4 cup of fruits or vegetables or 100% juice, 1/2 cup or 1 slice of enriched or whole grains or 3/4 cup cold cereal, and 1 oz. (28 g) of protein. Protein should be a lean meat or meat alternative.

7.4.4.2. Planning Ahead

1. Make a meal plan for the upcoming week in advance. To offer your child variety and introduce them to new foods, it's crucial to have a variety of options for meals and snacks. By exposing kids to a wider variety of foods, you can help them develop an increased tolerance for a wider range of tastes and textures.

- As most kids like to have some control over their lives, and eating is one area where they frequently do so, it might be beneficial to include them in the planning process. You could ask them if they'd like to try any of the foods after showing them pictures of them. Additionally, you could figure out how to incorporate new ingredients into their favorite dishes. For example, you could add cauliflower to macaroni and cheese because it blends in well and adds flavor and texture to their diet.

2. Give yourself plenty of time to grocery shop. Feeding your child a balanced diet does not mean everything has to be homemade, but you will want to pay attention to the labels on packaged food.

- For instance, your child enjoys chicken nuggets so you buy frozen chicken nuggets to meet the protein requirement. When you read the label, you realize the chicken nuggets have more than just chicken in them; they have soy protein, gluten, and sodium phosphate added to them. Although these items are not bad for your child, they are not that good for your child either. These ingredients help fill your child up without giving them the proper protein and nutrition they need.
- Reading nutrition labels will help you identify all the other frozen options available. Giving yourself time to familiarize yourself with food labels will make it easier to identify which packaged food to serve your child and shopping will start to become easier.

7.4.4.3. Preparing Ahead

1. Prepare as much food in advance as possible. It can be helpful to have options readily available to curb the impulse to buy ready-made snacks and dinners.

- Many ready-made snacks are high in calories and sodium and very low in nutrients. Buying fast food for lunch or dinner has the same issue—it fills the child up without supplementing their diet with the nutrients they need. It is ok to have fast food or junk food every once in a while, but plan for it and you will be less likely to splurge too often.

2. Look for the healthier options. For example, instead of fried with a sandwich, prepare apple slices for your child's lunch, and choose milk instead of soda.
3. Pre-portion as much as possible. Cutting vegetables and fruits and pre-portioning them is a great way to help save time.
4. Prepare pantry staples in advance. Rice and pasta hold well in the refrigerator when made in advance but whole wheat pasta tends to dry out, so store it with a little extra water to keep it from drying out too much.
5. Cut meat into portions while still raw and then freeze. A small food scale can be purchased for under $10 at most stores and will make it easier to portion meat.
6. Get your child involved with making the meals. By getting your child involved, they get to feel like they accomplished something. It also helps get them familiar with any new foods in advance so that when it is time to eat, they won't be surprised. This can make mealtime a fun time to look forward to.

7.4.5. How to Keep Your Child Healthy?

It should go without saying that you adore your child. Maintaining your child's happiness and health is a part of being a caregiver. To ensure your child's health, watch out for potential injury hazards and shield them from illness. Make sure your kids play outside and maintain an active lifestyle. Additionally, keep an eye on their mental health by having regular, honest communication with them.

7.4.5.1. *Establishing Healthy Habits*

1. Establish a sleeping schedule. It is important for your child to get around 10 hours of sleep every night, depending on age. Going to sleep at the same time each evening will help this happen. Stick carefully to this routine and only push back the bed time if it is absolutely necessary. When possible, allow your child to sleep in if they went to bed late.

- Sleep is important to health in many ways. It allows your body to recover quickly from illness or fight off potential infections. It also boosts your metabolism. Good sleep can calm your emotions and result in a healthier mindset as well.
- It is recommended that preschoolers get between 10 to 13 hours, elementary and middle-schoolers between 10 to 13 hours, and teenagers between 8 to 10 hours. This is dependent on personal preference as well. Some children simply prefer to sleep more or slightly less than average.

2. Encourage a healthy diet. Purchase a variety of fruits and vegetables, whole-grain products, and lean meats for your household. Go for fresh, organic produce whenever you can. Carefully read labels to determine portion sizes and make meals that conform to those guidelines. Offer healthy snacks, such as hummus and carrot sticks, throughout the day.

- Invite your child to help you with meal prep. Let them choose a healthy recipe for dinner. Take them with you to the grocery store and turn reading labels into a game. Make food more interesting for finicky eaters by crafting healthy personal pizzas (with their own selected toppings) or by positioning fruit into a smiley face on their plate.
- If your child refuses to eat their veggies, keep offering them. Try out other vegetable options and preparations as well. A child who dislikes straight steamed broccoli may love it when it is topped with a bit of shredded cheddar cheese.

3. Offer lots of drinking water. A child should drink the number of 8 oz. water glasses that correspond to their age (up to a limit of 64 oz. total at 8 years of age). So, a 4 year old child should drink 4 glasses containing 8 oz. of water per day. This total does not include milk, juice, or other liquids, just water.

- Your child should only start drinking water after they reach 6 months of age. Prior to this, they should drink formula and/or breast milk.
- To add some variety, a child can also drink milk after their first birthday. A 2 year old should drink up to two 8 oz. glasses of milk per day. You can also offer juice, in moderation.
- A child's brain is composed of 80% water, so staying hydrated is particularly important for optimal cognitive development. Teach your

child to look at their urine to make sure it is more clear than yellow. If they spot yellow, then they should grab a glass of water.

4. Keep junk foods to a minimum. Avoid purchasing sugary, fatty, or heavily processed foods. If you don't buy them, then your child will turn to a healthy alternative that is available in your fridge or pantry. Watch out for 'sneaky' foods that appear healthy but are actually the opposite. This can include items labeled "low-fat" or even low-juice fruit drinks.

- Other 'sneaky' junk foods can include various crackers labeled as kid friendly that actually contain high amounts of sugars or syrups. Watch out for fruit gummies as well. They often contain high amounts of sugar as well. It is better to simply offer your child a piece of fruit (Figure 7.3).

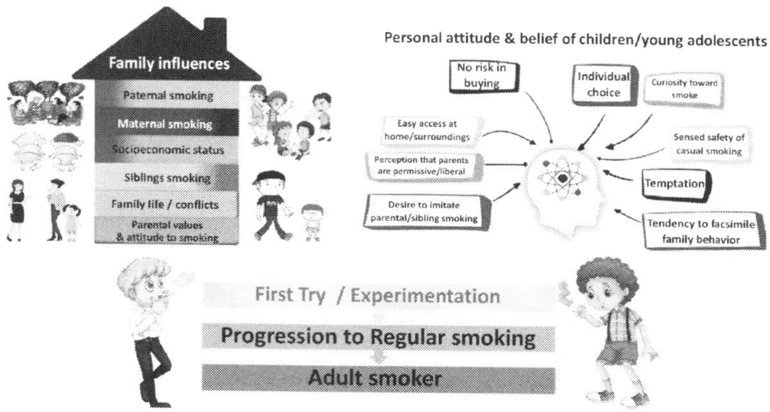

Figure 7.3. *Tobacco addiction in children.*

Source: Sharma, R., Martins, N., Tripathi, A., Caponnetto, P., Garg, N., Nepovimova, E., Kuča, K., & Prajapati, P. K., (2020). Influence of family environment and tobacco addiction: A short report from a post-graduate teaching hospital, India. International Journal of Environmental Research and Public Health, 17(8), 2868. https://doi.org/10.3390/ijerph17082868.

7.4.5.2. Preventing Illness and Injury

- Avoid exposing your child to smoke. Smoke can linger after you put out a cigarette, so it is important to keep your children away from areas where you are smoking or where you have been smoking. If you are a smoker, enroll in a program to quit and ask smoker relatives to do so as well. Secondhand smoke is harmful to children as they develop.
  - Children exposed to secondhand smoke are more likely to contract a variety of breathing problems and illnesses including (but not limited to) bronchitis and **pneumonia**. Smoke can also make existing medical problems worse, such as asthma. Babies are also at an increased risk for sudden infant death syndrome (SIDS).
- Avoid exposing your child to sick persons. When it is possible, keep your child away

from people who are currently sick. Your child encounters plenty of germs during the day but direct exposure to an infection is just not worth it.

- Stay in touch with your relatives, your child's friends, and your child's school to watch out for exposure to various infections. For example, if your child is invited to a sleepover but one of the other children present is sick with strep, it is probably best to decline the invitation. Keep in mind that viral infections are impossible to avoid completely, so don't go overboard if your relatives or friends have a mild cold.

- Promote germ avoidance. Teach your child to frequently wash their hands. They should do so after using the restroom and before they eat or touch their mouth or face. Give them a small bottle of hand sanitizer to carry around and use if a sink is not available. Instruct them to not share water bottles or drinks with others and to keep their hands out of their mouths (much easier said than done with toddlers).
  - Show your child how to sing the "Happy Birthday" song twice when washing their hands with warm, soapy water. This is the amount of time it takes to remove most germs.
  - Show your child how to sneeze into their elbow and how to cover their cough with a hand as well. This way they can help prevent the spread of their germs as well.
- Develop a plan for sick days. If your child is at home with you, then keep them there until they feel better. If your child goes to school or daycare, find out that location's policy on sickness. Some schools require that a child is fever-free for 24 hours before they return. Make no mistake, your child will get sick at some point. Knowing how you will provide for their care will result in less stress for you and your child.
  - Part of planning ahead is also knowing the proper doses of medication for your child. Stock up on common anti-fever medications such as acetaminophen (Tylenol) or ibuprofen. It is best to avoid a run to the pharmacy for basic medications whenever possible.
- Schedule well child visits. Your child should have a well-child check-up every two to three months up until 2 years of age. After 2 years of age, your child will begin to visit their doctor each year for a basic check-up. Find a pediatrician who you trust and make sure to stick to this schedule. Your child's doctor will take a variety of preventative measures each visit, including tracking your child's growth and development.
  - Use child visits as an opportunity to ask any questions that you have regarding your child's physical, mental, or emotional development. It may help to write down questions before you arrive. For example, you

might ask, "Should my toddler be using a spoon and fork yet?"

- Your child will also generally receive vaccinations at well check visits. These vaccinations offer protection against an assortment of more serious illnesses such as polio. A yearly flu shot can also help prevent a lot of misery from the flu.
- Don't forget the importance of taking your child to the dentist as well. At least once every year, your child's teeth need to be cleaned and checked out.

• Minimize in-home hazards. Place all toxic chemicals and cleaners in an inaccessible area. Hide all cords and wires. Secure furniture that could topple over. Remove any sharp or dangerous objects. Even after your child is beyond the baby stage, keep an eye out for potentially dangerous items in your home.

- You may want to ask that your relatives or family friends safely proof their homes as well, especially when your child visits. Medications, for example, need to be stored in a location that is inaccessible for a child.

7.4.5.3. Encouraging Physical Activity

1. Sign them up for sports. Start experimenting with sports at an early age by enrolling your child through your local rec center or school. Or, you could sign your child up for lessons at a local sports facility. Swimming, dancing, and soccer are just a few examples of worthwhile sporting options. Being involved in sports will help your child to get at least 60 minutes of physical activity per day, the minimum suggested amount.

• Be prepared to go through a number of sports before you find the ones that your child will enjoy. This is a normal part of the process. Avoid pressuring your child to pursue a sport that they strongly dislike. Instead, look for alternative options.

• Sports are also great for mental health. The pressure to focus employed by sports like martial arts is great for children struggling with control issues, like ADD.

2. Get your kids outside. Head outside with your child and a jump rope or a bike for a few hours. Go on a nice long walk or hike with your kid. Play an extended game of tag followed by a park picnic. Soaking in the sunshine gets your child their daily dose of Vitamin D. This vitamin can then boost immunity and help prevent a variety of infections. Remember to apply sunscreen to your child before heading outdoors!

• Fresh air is also just healthy. It is good to take a break from the air inside your home as it could actually possess a variety of unhealthy pollutants.

• Always make sure to apply sunscreen before heading outside.

3. Limit technology time. Try to limit TV time to a maximum of two hours per day. You should also try to regulate the use of the computer, video games, and even their cell phone (if they have one) as well. Placing time and use limits on these devices will encourage your child to get out of doors and explore the world around them (Figure 7.4).

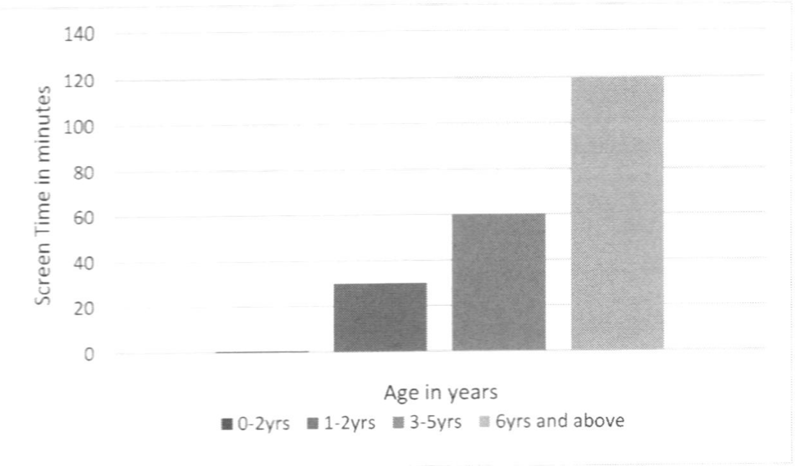

Figure 7.4. *Recommended screen time for children of different age groups in minutes.*

Source: *Panjeti-Madan, V. N., & Ranganathan, P., (2023). Impact of screen time on children's development: Cognitive, language, physical, and social and emotional domains. Multimodal Technologies and Interaction, 7(5), 52. https://doi.org/10.3390/mti7050052.*

- Do not put a TV in your child's bedroom. The use of technology can have a negative impact on sleep patterns. Instead, read a book to your child before bedtime or follow another relaxing routine.

4. Teach them that food is fuel. Spend time with your child researching healthy food options online. Look to see how particular foods translate into calories in and out of your body. Give your child the challenge of identifying the best possible food to eat before their sporting event. All children want to be strong and having them understand the impact of food is one way to get there.

- For example, before your child's soccer game, ask them if a fast-food burger or a homemade sandwich would help them perform the best. Discuss the pros and cons of both options

A Closer Look

Screening

To ascertain whether pediatric physical, occupational, and/or speech therapy is required, a screening is performed. A therapist watches your child doing tasks and in different positions to assess whether a thorough evaluation is required. In many pediatric therapy clinics, screenings are provided for free and last 15 to 20 minutes.

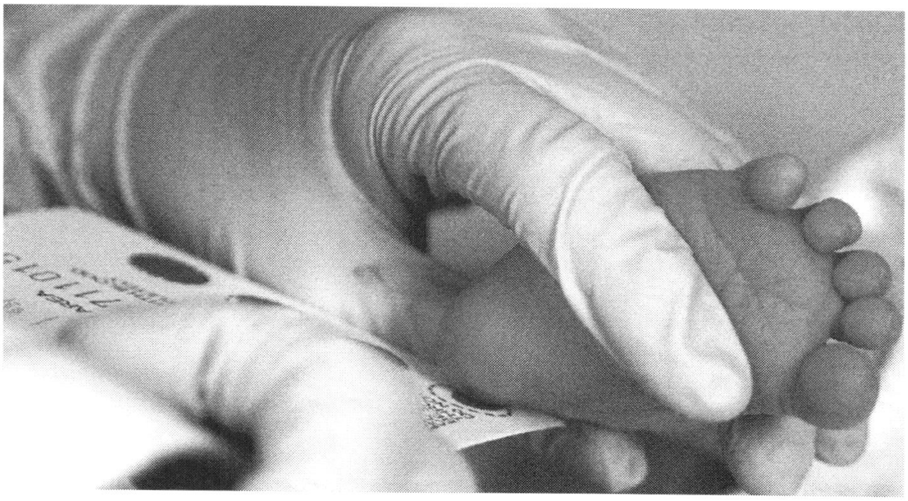

Source: By U.S. Air Force photo/Staff Sgt Eric T. Sheler – USAF Photographic Archives (image permalink), Public Domain, https://commons.wikimedia.org/w/index.php?curid=3268429.

Your child will be able to realize their greatest potential if delays are identified early and any necessary therapy services are obtained. Children can overcome obstacles and improve their quality of life with intervention. Every child should be screened to determine whether extra support is needed for their motor, sensory, or communication development, just as many states now mandate hearing and vision screenings. This does not imply that screenings should wait until kids are old enough to attend school. As early as two months of age, early motor delays can be identified.

Particularly if you and your healthcare provider are concerned, screenings are crucial. Still, there are some challenges that are difficult to identify. This is why we think screening is necessary to make sure all children are developing appropriately. It is preferable to screen as soon as possible. Children under the age of three who are experiencing delays in their physical, cognitive, or social-emotional development can receive federally funded services through Early Intervention.

Summary

- Promoting children's health is paramount for ensuring their overall well-being and future success. It involves a comprehensive approach that addresses physical, mental, emotional, and social aspects of health, laying the foundation for healthy development and lifelong wellness.
- In order to understand health promotion and health maintenance, it is important to understand the definition of health first.
- Physical activity provides many physical and psychological health benefits. However, there is growing disparity between recommendations and reality among most of our children.
- Mental and spiritual health is important concepts to address in health promotion and health maintenance visits. Parents can be encouraged to keep a record of mental health issues to bring to health supervision visits.
- Proper nutrition is crucial for everybody, but it is especially important for kids because it is directly linked to their overall growth and development.
- In adolescence, somatic growth is accompanied by rapid psychological and behavioral development which leads the adolescent to feel a progressively more intense need for independence and freedom; this also has a significant impact on eating habits.
- Childhood obesity is a significant health, social and economic problem of increasing importance for Western countries.
- Growth is a continuous process which begins at conception and ends with the attainment of sexual maturity. Somatic growth accompanies neuro-psychic growth.
- Feeding your child a healthy diet at each meal is important. It keeps them nourished and gives them the energy to grow, play and learn, while helping them to avoid developing certain disorders, such as diabetes, as a result of poor nutrition.

References

1. Datta, P. (2007). *Pediatric Nursing*. Jaypee Brothers, Medical Publishers. p. 506.
2. Fraser, J. (2014). *Pediatric Nursing in Australia*. Cambridge. ISBN 978-1-107-68500-0.
3. Sterling, Y. M. (2013, May 1). "Pediatric clinicians as advocates." *Journal of Pediatric Nursing, 28*(3), 309–310.

Chapter

8

COMMUNITY HEALTH

Contents

Unit Introduction 241
8.1. Overview of Community Health 244
8.2. Epidemiology and Disease Control 251
8.3. Disaster Management and Emergency Preparedness 260
8.4. Healthcare Systems and Policies 268
Summary 280
References 280

Unit Introduction

The general well-being of communities is impacted by numerous issues. In many urban settings, infectious diseases like tuberculosis can become uncontrollably widespread. Violence, accidents, injuries, environmental pollutants, and preventable diseases continue to pose a threat to children's health and wellbeing. Pregnant women, young children, and other vulnerable groups have seen a marked rise in morbidity and mortality due to unequal access to healthcare and insurance coverage. Despite these obstacles, all clinicians have the ability to enhance patient outcomes and develop the infrastructure necessary for disease monitoring and management.

Community health clinicians strive to guarantee that expectant and new mothers have the means to properly care for both themselves and their children in traditional public health settings. They can be found in lead abatement programs that oversee the care of children with lead poisoning, as well as in the WIC Program (the Special Supplemental Nutrition Program for Women, Infants, and Children), which provides well-baby assessments, vaccinations, and newborn screenings.

The ability to adapt and willingness to provide care in a variety of settings, such as schools, churches, homeless shelters, and community health clinics, makes community health clinicians highly valued. These clinicians offer patients comprehensive care in the comfort of their own homes, at planned gatherings like health fairs, and in facilities and agencies that cater to the specific medical needs of their clients. In nurse-managed clinics on college campuses and in elementary and secondary schools, advanced practice clinicians in the community increase access to care and reduce costs.

They create and carry out corporate wellness initiatives, promoting the well-being and productivity of workers within their companies. To address complex community challenges, community health clinicians collaborate with a variety of partners and providers. This can be seen most clearly in the current initiatives to detect, reach, and treat HIV/AIDS positive individuals as well as in the work to assist older adults in effectively managing their long-term health issues and continuing to live in their homes.

In 2002, the Public Health Security and Bioterrorism Response Act expanded the responsibilities of public health professionals. This legislation elevated the role of community health nursing in emergency response, emphasizing the importance of providing mass prophylaxis and effectively managing biochemical threats. Community health nurses, particularly those working in public health settings, are now recognized as essential first responders, a duty that was previously reserved for law enforcement and emergency response personnel. In times of public health crises, these clinicians will take charge of organizing and administering immediate care.

Specializations in clinical, school, or corporate nursing, pharmaceutical sales, home care, case management, and public health nursing are available to community or public health nurses. Advanced degree holders in community health nursing may also be able to pursue careers in clinical research and higher education. Although the qualifications required for these varied fields can differ, clinicians should at the very least have a bachelor's degree and solid clinical experience. In response to the nursing shortage, certain public health settings have loosened their minimum requirements. When it comes to health issues, clinicians who opt for home care or traditional public health should be well-versed in them and have no trouble with change, autonomy, and uncertainty. When applying to this specialty, clinicians should emphasize not only their clinical expertise but also their advocacy, analytical, and critical thinking skills. Because communities are ever-changing, clinicians must be flexible to give patients the care they require. While many community health jobs require little to no weekend or holiday work, their pay may be less than that of comparable positions at large healthcare facilities.

Orientation and Directional Terms

Term	Definition	Illustration
Public Health Security	Public health security is the effort to protect people's health from acute public health events that can endanger people across international boundaries and geographical regions.	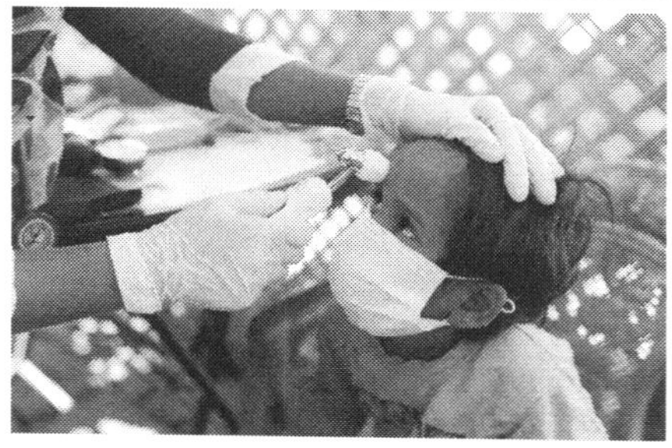
Obstetric care	Obstetric care is a medical specialty that involves the management of pregnancy, childbirth, and the postpartum period.	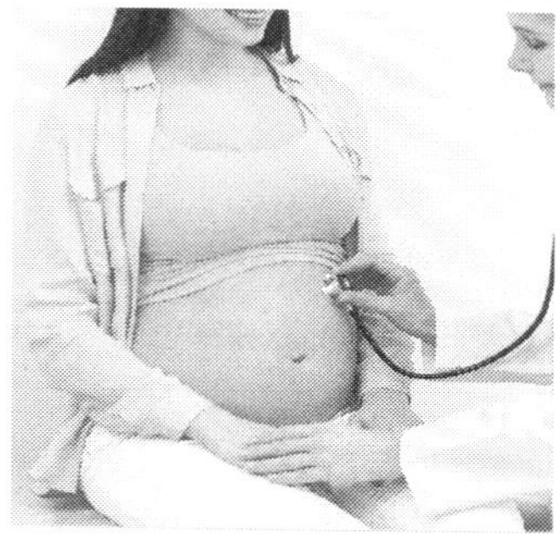
Epidemiology	Epidemiology is a medical science that studies the distribution and determinants of health and disease in a population.	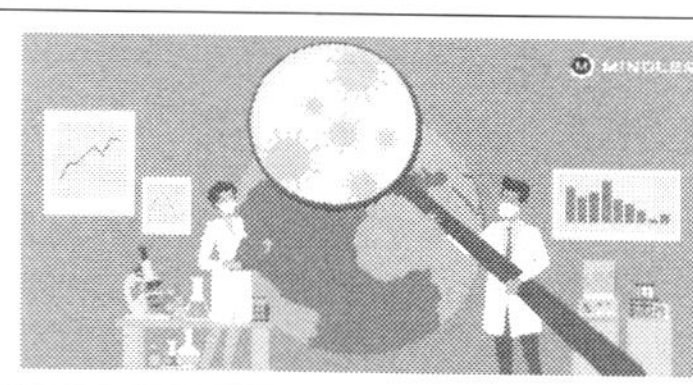
Morbidity	Morbidity is a state of being unhealthy or symptomatic of a disease or condition.	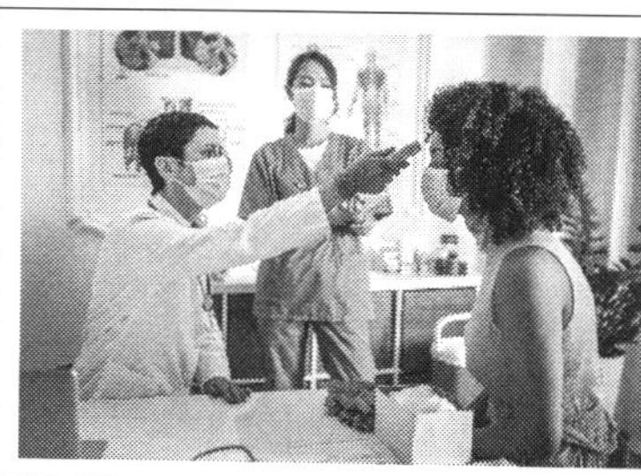
Microorganism	A microorganism, also known as a microbe, is a living thing that is too small to be seen without a microscope.	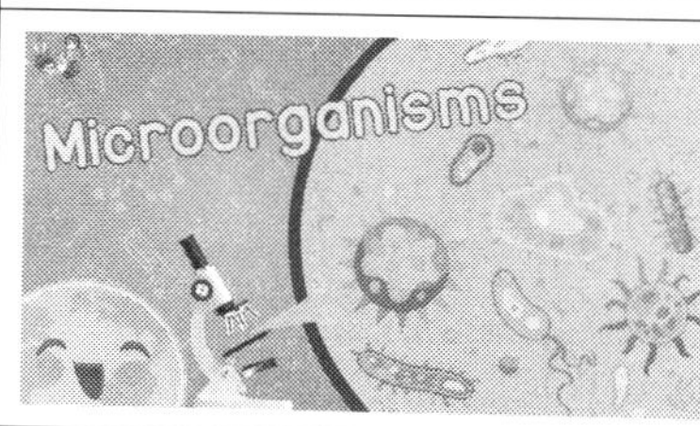

8.1. Overview of Community Health

For hundreds of years, communities have depended on nurses. Clinicians play a critical role in providing medical expertise and compassionate patient care during major illness, injury, or childbirth. Because clinicians have such a profound effect on people's lives, our perception of them can become almost legendary. For example, Clara Barton, the American Red Cross founder and a nurse during the Civil War, was referred to as "the angel of the battlefield."

However, since the position of a nurse became commonplace in all hospital settings, our knowledge of how to deliver healthcare has changed. Healthcare professionals are starting to focus on how a community's general health and safety can contribute to fewer illnesses, longer life expectancies, and fewer injuries rather than just treating an individual's medical needs.

Numerous clinicians have taken on important roles in this endeavor. Improved population health and a decrease in illness and disability are the goals of community health nurses, also referred to as public health nurses. The social sciences, public health, and nursing are all incorporated into this all-encompassing approach to healthcare. Let's examine this significant role in the healthcare system in more detail, as well as the educational requirements community health clinicians must meet to have an influence. The treatment of disease has always been the main focus of medical practice in the US. The healthcare system steps in to help people recover their health when they get sick or hurt. Our brains are hardwired to believe that you visit the doctor when you're sick.

This healthcare paradigm is essentially reactive. In recent times, there has been a growing interest among social scientists and healthcare providers to consider developing a proactive healthcare system. What are the underlying causes of illness and disability within a population and how do we weed them out? In the early 2000s, a number of books and journal articles were written about the social determinants of health and infectious disease. What if the medical crises that physicians and clinicians respond to could be prevented in the first place? Less access to care or inherited susceptibilities to disease were found to be less significant risk factors for poor health outcomes than low levels of education, membership in marginalized communities, and signs of poverty. Even though solving these frequently related problems is undoubtedly difficult, advancements in healthcare obviously require a comprehensive strategy.

The community health nurse is a professional who strives to decrease the social and environmental factors that contribute to illness in a community to enhance the health of numerous people. Community health clinicians are involved in planning, developing policies, and advocating. They specifically promote social justice ideals to enhance everyone's health outcomes.

Ø **Where Do Community Health clinicians Work?**

Community health clinicians provide care to a wide range of populations in a variety of settings. Community health clinicians may or may not have direct interaction with specific community members depending on where they work. Here are 5 examples of organizations and facilities that rely on community health nurses:

1. **Community Health Centers:** In this context, a community health nurse might provide direct medical care to community members. Community health clinicians also create educational

materials and campaigns on pertinent subjects like contraception, sexual health, and other preventive care. To gain more exposure to a broader range of community members, community health clinicians may choose to work in settings other than the community health center.

2. **Correctional Facilities:** A correctional facility is a place where a large number of people are kept in close quarters. Here, preventing the spread of infectious diseases is a common goal of community health nurses. They manage staff and prisoner education programs, put in place measures to control infectious diseases, and collaborate closely with local and state health departments.
3. **Schools:** Community health clinicians can educate students in schools about healthy habits and illness prevention. Youngsters who have this knowledge at their disposal can live longer, healthier lives. In addition to helping kids manage current health issues, community health clinicians in schools can step in if kids are being abused or neglected.
4. **Aid Organizations:** A large number of community health clinicians are employed by groups like Doctors without Borders or the Red Cross. Similar to the work at any community health center, these clinicians frequently assist with disaster relief, access to clean drinking water, and the prevention of infectious diseases in addition to other local needs.
5. **Government Agencies:** Government-affiliated community health clinicians frequently provide little direct medical care to local residents. Rather, they focus on developing and implementing policies to bring about widespread change for a variety of demographics.

8.1.1. Common Responsibilities of a Community Health

A community health nurse's areas of expertise include population health policy reform, health promotion, and community building. Owing to their wide range of duties, community health nurses' responsibilities change based on their workplace and the needs of the community they serve. In addition to providing routine medical care like vaccinations, screenings, and medication, community health clinicians may also work on advocacy, program development and implementation, and research on the social and environmental factors that influence health outcomes.

8.1.1.1. How to Become a Community Health?

Becoming a community health nurse usually involves a little bit more education and training than other registered nursing roles. In addition to having a solid nursing background, a community health nurse must be knowledgeable about social science and public policy.

8.1.1.2. Education Requirements

Aspiring community health clinicians must, at the very least, complete an Associate's Degree in Nursing (ADN) program and pass the NCLEX-RN exam. However, it should be noted that a Bachelor of Science in Nursing may be preferred by many employers. Around 61% of the 2,173 community health nurse job postings that we analyzed required a minimum BSN. Community health clinicians might also want to think about pursuing a master's degree in public health or a similar discipline.

8.1.2. Public Health Issues Related to Maternal and Child Health

Mothers' and kids' health are linked and influenced by a variety of factors. Each year, millions of expectant mothers, new moms, and children suffer from severe illness or pass away, usually from treatable or preventable causes. Around 99% of maternal and child fatalities take place in developing nations, with Africa being the most severely affected. Maternal and child health (MCH) has received increasing attention in the last 10 years; since 1990, both maternal and under-five mortality have significantly decreased, and MCH improvements are thought to be essential to promoting economic growth.

Effective interventions are available, but progress has been impeded, especially in the area of maternal health, by a lack of funding and restricted access to services. There is mounting evidence that the COVID-19 pandemic has negatively impacted nutrition and maternal and child health, slowing or even reversing some of the gains made in the last 10 years. This is because the pandemic has disrupted vital services, such as regular immunization campaigns, and has exacerbated malnutrition.

8.1.3. Impact

An estimated 5 million children under the age of five, mostly infants, pass away each year from conditions that are mainly treatable or preventable. Furthermore, millions more women suffer grave consequences from pregnancy and childbirth, and about 295,000 women lose their lives to these conditions annually. These difficulties are particularly common in underdeveloped nations. In addition, sub-Saharan Africa is the world's most affected region, with Southern and South-Eastern Asia following; these three regions combined are responsible for almost 90% of maternal and under-five fatalities.

8.1.3.1. Maternal Mortality

Severe bleeding, usually following childbirth (postpartum hemorrhage), accounts for over a quarter (27%) of all maternal deaths. Other significant causes include hypertension (14%), unsafe abortions (8%), and sepsis (11%). Anemia, HIV, and malaria are among the illnesses that make pregnancy more difficult and cause approximately 28% of maternal deaths. The lifetime risk of maternal death is increased by high fertility rates and inadequate prenatal care, which are frequently brought on by limited access to family planning and reproductive health (FP/RH) services. Though it has been increasing, only 66% of pregnant women worldwide and even less in sub-Saharan Africa and Southern Asia are receiving the minimum recommended four antenatal care visits.

8.1.3.2. Newborn and Under-Five Mortality

Over one-third (35%) of newborn deaths are caused by complications resulting from premature births. These are followed by complications related to delivery (24%) sepsis (15%) congenital abnormalities (11%), pneumonia (6%), tetanus (1%), diarrhea (1%), and other causes of death (7%). One of the main risk factors and an indirect cause of neonatal death is low birth weight. In terms of causes of death, pneumonia (12%), diarrhea (8%) injuries (6%) malaria (5%) measles (2%) HIV/AIDS (1%) and other causes of death (21%) are the leading causes of child deaths (47%). Children who are malnourished are much more susceptible to these illnesses, as are those who do not have access to sanitary facilities and clean water.

8.1.3.3. Intervention

Emergency obstetric care and skilled birth care are important interventions that lower the risk of maternal mortality. Increasing the use of easy, low-cost interventions like breastfeeding, keeping babies warm and dry, and treating serious newborn infections can significantly lower the number of newborn deaths. Over the past 20 years, there have been notable decreases in child morbidity and mortality due to the implementation of interventions like immunizations, oral rehydration therapy (ORT), and insecticide-treated mosquito nets (ITNs) when they have been scaled up. Other successful child health initiatives include treating neglected tropical diseases (NTDs), enhancing nutrition, and facilitating better access to and use of clean water, sanitation, and hygiene practices like handwashing. It is also crucial to improve access to services and strengthen health systems. This can be achieved, for example, by establishing community-based clinics. Research has shown that interventions work best when they are part of an all-encompassing continuum of care.

8.1.4. Global Goals

There are several key global goals for expanding access to and improving MCH services, including:

Ø **SDGs 2 & 3: Save Mothers and Children's Lives and End All Forms of Malnutrition:** Global MCH targets were adopted in 2015 as part of Sustainable Development Goals (SDGs) 2 and 3 and are to, by 2030:

- Reduce the global MMR and end preventable deaths of newborns and under-five children (as targets under SDG 3, which is "ensure healthy lives and promote well-being for all at all ages"); and
- End all forms of malnutrition (as a target under SDG 2, which is "end hunger, achieve food security and improved nutrition, and promote sustainable agriculture").

The 2010 launches of the Scaling Up Nutrition (SUN) and Every Woman, Every Child (EWEC) movements are two examples of international initiatives aimed at assisting nations in their efforts to achieve these targets. The U.S.N. By combining the efforts of partners who commit to advancing MCH and related efforts, the -led EWEC movement seeks to operationalize the 2015 Global Strategy for Women's, Children's, and Adolescents' Health (2016–2030), with the aim of, among other things, ending preventable maternal, newborn, child, and adolescent deaths and stillbirths by 2030. The SUN movement is an initiative that acknowledges the close relationship between nutrition, maternal health, and child survival and seeks to unify partner efforts to support households and women in particular.

Ø **Global Nutrition for Growth Compact:** The Global Nutrition for Growth Compact includes a goal of reducing stunting in children and nutrient deficiencies in women and children. Endorsed in 2013 by more than 40 developing countries and donor governments, including the U.S., as well as other stakeholders, it committed them to, by 2020:

- Ensuring that at least 500 million pregnant women and children under two are reached with effective nutrition interventions;
- Reducing the number of children under five stunted by at least 20 million; and
  - Saving at least 1.7 million under-fives by preventing stunting and increasing breastfeeding and treatment of severe acute malnutrition (Figure 8.1).

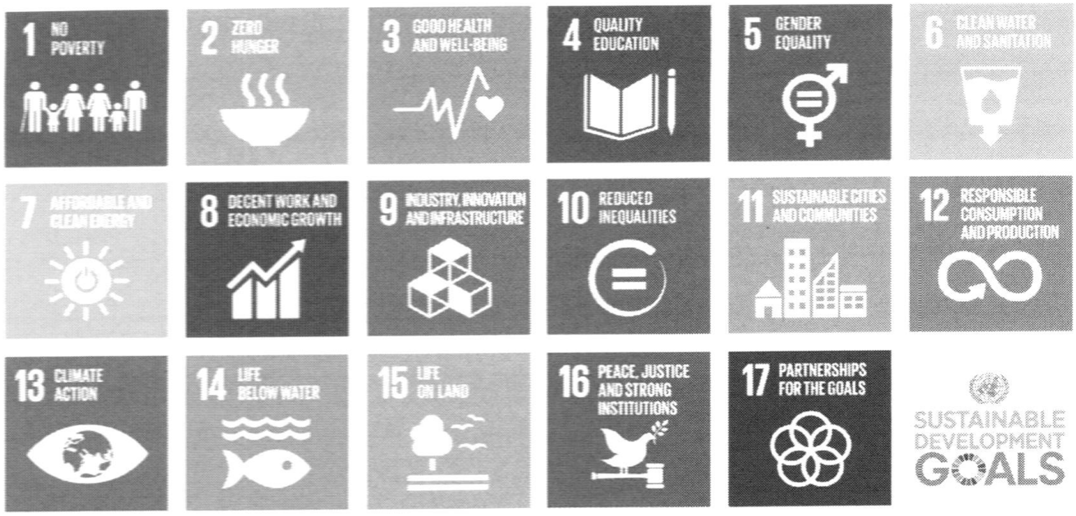
1 NO POVERTY
2 ZERO HUNGER
3 GOOD HEALTH AND WELL-BEING
4 QUALITY EDUCATION
5 GENDER EQUALITY
6 CLEAN WATER AND SANITATION
7 AFFORDABLE AND CLEAN ENERGY
8 DECENT WORK AND ECONOMIC GROWTH
9 INDUSTRY, INNOVATION AND INFRASTRUCTURE
10 REDUCED INEQUALITIES
11 SUSTAINABLE CITIES AND COMMUNITIES
12 RESPONSIBLE CONSUMPTION AND PRODUCTION
13 CLIMATE ACTION
14 LIFE BELOW WATER
15 LIFE ON LAND
16 PEACE, JUSTICE AND STRONG INSTITUTIONS
17 PARTNERSHIPS FOR THE GOALS
SUSTAINABLE DEVELOPMENT GOALS

Figure 8.1. *The sustainable development goals.*

Source: *Sætra HS. A Framework for Evaluating and Disclosing the ESG Related Impacts of AI with the SDGs. Sustainability. 2021; 13(15):8503. https://doi.org/10.3390/su13158503.*

The Tokyo Nutrition for Growth Summit held in December 2021 provided an opportunity for governments to review the status of progress, including the impact of the COVID-19 pandemic on efforts, and to make new commitments in support of reaching SDG 2 by 2030; the next Summit will be hosted by France in 2024.

8.1.5. U.S. Government Efforts

The U.S. has spent more than 50 years contributing to MCH initiatives worldwide. The initial US. Beginning in the 1960s, international MCH efforts concentrated on child survival research, including groundbreaking ORT research carried out by the U.S. military, the U.S. The National Institutes of Health (NIH) and the Agency for International Development (USAID). Early initiatives included efforts to combat malaria as well as fortifying international food aid with vitamin A, a deficiency of which can impair immune system function, cause blindness, and slow down growth in young children. The U.S. enhanced funding for its child health initiatives in FY 1985 by almost doubling the amount allotted for child survival activities to $85 million. Then, in 1989, USAID created its first project focused on maternal health, and in 2001, it unveiled a plan for the survival of newborns. Over time, funding has grown, and in FY 2022 it reached $10.435 billion, the highest level to date. By 2035, the U.S. government hopes to have eliminated avoidable maternal and child deaths.

8.1.6. Organization

USAID serves as the lead U.S. implementing agency for MCH activities, and its efforts are complemented by those of the Centres for Disease Control and Prevention (CDC), NIH, and the Peace Corps. Collectively, U.S. activities reach over 40 countries.

8.1.6.1. USAID

A variety of MCH interventions are funded by USAID (*see* Table 8.1), with a focus on 25 "priority countries," the majority of which are in Africa and Southern Asia. Reaching the most vulnerable groups and enhancing mothers' and kids' access to high-quality care and services nationwide are priorities. S. In terms of global health initiatives, the agency's short-term goal was to save the lives of 600,000 women and 15 million children in priority countries between 2012 and 2020; these nations account for roughly 70% of all maternal and child deaths worldwide. Although the goal was not met, USAID notes that its work over the previous 10 years has helped save the lives of more than 9 point 3 million children and 340,000 women. In addition, USAID unveiled a multisectoral nutrition strategy in 2014 for the first time, with the goal of strengthening the connections between its development, global health, and humanitarian initiatives to better address the root causes and immediate consequences of malnutrition as well as to strengthen food security and resilience in communities that are already at risk.

Table 8.1. *The SDGs, Assessed Variables, and Sources of Data*

SDG	Assessed Variables—Associated SDG Target	References
1. No poverty	Poverty rate (%)—1.1	[58]
2. Zero hunger	Prevalence of undernourishment rate (% of population)—2.1.1.	[59]
3. Good health and well-being	Maternal mortality rate per 100,000 live births—3.1.1.	[60]
4. Quality education	Out-of-school children rate—4.1.	[61]
5. Gender quality	Female education (%) higher level—5.1	[62]
6. Clean water and sanitation	Drinking water safely managed service (%)—6.1.	[63]
7. Affordable and clean energy	Share of modern renewables in total final energy consumption (%)—7.2.1.	[64]
8. Decent work and economic growth	GDP annual growth per capita (USD)—8.1.1.	[58]
9. Industry, innovation, and infrastructure	Research and development expenditure as a percentage of GDP—9.5.1.	[65]
10. Reduced inequalities	Gini index—10.3	[58]
11. Sustainable cities and communities	Population living in slums (% of urban population)—11.1.1.	[66]
12. Responsible consumption and production	Fossil fuels consumption (tons)—12.2.2.	[67]
13. Climate action	CO_2 emissions (metric tons per capita)—13.2.	[68]
14. Life below water	Mean percentage of each marine key biodiversity area covered by protected area—14.5.	[69]
15. Life on land	Tree cover loss (ha)—15.2.	[70]
16. Peace, justice, and strong institutions	Rule of law index—16.3	[71]

Source: *Ordonez-Ponce E. Exploring the Impact of the Sustainable Development Goals on Sustainability Trends. Sustainability. 2023; 15(24):16647. https://doi.org/10.3390/su152416647.*

8.1.6.2. Other U.S. MCH Efforts

In addition to running immunization programs and offering technical and scientific support, DC also aims to increase capacity across a wide range of MCH (and related RH) fields. It additionally functions as a Collaborating Center for Reproductive, Maternal, Perinatal, and Child Health for the World Health Organization. To address MCH, NIH conducts implementation research and basic science projects, occasionally in collaboration with foreign nations. Around the world, the Peace Corps conducts volunteer work related to MCH. Furthermore, the internationally accepted definition of reproductive health includes both FP and MCH, so global FP/RH efforts are also essential to improving MCH, even though Congress allocates funds to and USAID manages these programs independently.

Other U.S. Global health and related initiatives, such as Feed the Future, USAID's NTD Program, the President's Malaria Initiative (PMI), the President's Emergency Plan for AIDS Relief (PEPFAR), and clean water projects funded by the Water for the Poor and Water for the World Acts, address issues that endanger the health of many expectant mothers, new mothers, and children.

8.1.6.3. Multilateral Efforts

The U.S. government partners with several international institutions and supports global MCH funding mechanisms.

Key among them are:

- Gavi, the Vaccine Alliance (a multilateral financing mechanism aiming to increase access to immunization in poor countries to which the U.S. is one of the largest donors;
- The Global Financing Facility (GFF, a partnership to improve the health of women, children, and adolescents through innovative financing in which the U.S. is an investor);
- The Global Polio Eradication Initiative (GPEI, a public-private partnership aiming to advance efforts to eradicate polio to which the U.S. is the second largest donor; and
- The United Nations Children's Fund (UNICEF, a U.N. agency aiming to improve the lives of children, particularly the most disadvantaged children and adolescents, to which the U.S. is the largest donor; UNICEF is one of the largest purchasers of vaccines worldwide).

8.1.6.4. Funding

Total U.S. funding for MCH and nutrition, which includes the U.S. contributions to Gavi and UNICEF as well as support for polio activities, has increased over time. It rose from $728 million in FY 2006 to $1.435 billion in FY 2022, its highest level to date. MCH funding totaled $1.28 billion in FY 2022 and includes $848 million for bilateral efforts (of which $253 million was for polio activities) and $429 million for multilateral efforts ($290 million for Gavi and $139 million for UNICEF). Nutrition funding, all of which was for bilateral efforts, totaled $158 million in FY 2022. The current administration has proposed a similar level of MCH and nutrition funding for FY 2023.

Most U.S. funding for MCH and nutrition is provided through the Global Health Programs account at USAID, with additional funding provided through the Economic Support Fund account. MCH funding is also provided through the International Organizations & Programs account at the State Department for the U.S. contribution to UNICEF and through CDC's global immunization programs.

Although not included as part of core MCH funding, in FY 2021 the U.S. also appropriated $4 billion in emergency COVID-19 funding to Gavi to support COVID-19 vaccine procurement and delivery through COVAX.

8.1.7. Key Issues for the U.S.

In the previous 10 years, both foreign and U.S. S. Activities have refocused funding and attention on MCH initiatives. The COVID-19 pandemic poses a threat to past gains and ongoing progress as the international community works to support and fund efforts to meet the MCH and nutrition targets of SDGs 2 and 3. Concerns have been raised about the pandemic's negative effects on MCH and MCH programming, including disruptions in basic MCH services like routine immunization. Reversing and minimizing its effects continue to be U's main priorities. S. and additional initiatives.

Other key issues and challenges for U.S. efforts include:

- Continuing to expand access to and ensure the quality of MCH services, while building local capacity;
- Reaching the most vulnerable, particularly adolescent girls and young women;
- Supporting advances in research and uptake of new technologies and vaccines;
- Further integration of MCH efforts with other U.S. global health programs (such as family planning and reproductive health as well as global HIV under PEPFAR) and broader U.S. development efforts (including education and food security);
- Coordinating efforts with the activities of other donors and partner countries to maximize the impact of available resources; and
- Addressing the immediate and long-term effects of the COVID-19 pandemic on maternal and child health.

8.2. Epidemiology and Disease Control

The term epidemiology refers to "applying this study to control health problems and the distribution and determinants of health-related states in specified populations." The term epidemiology refers to "applying this study to control health problems and the distribution and determinants of health-related states in specified populations."

The mother's death jeopardizes the development of the newborn baby who might have survived and that of the other young children in the family. Pregnant women are often in their prime and are the primary caregivers for their families, so their health and well-being are important to them. Many women work outside the home to support their families and also take full responsibility for childcare and household chores. This puts a double burden on them. Nevertheless, the high rate of maternal mortality in many developing nations provides compelling evidence that women's health needs are neglected, even in spite of the crucial role that women play in society.

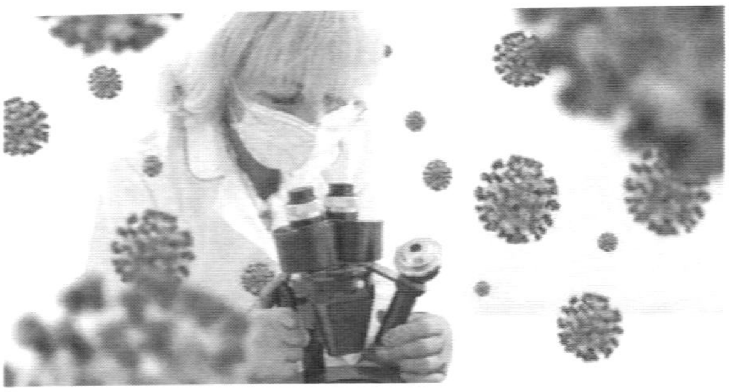

Source: https://www.healthcare-management-degree.net/wp-content/uploads/2021/01/What-is-Epidemiology-and-What-Does-an-Epidemiologist-Do.jpg.

It is unknown how many women lose their lives to pregnancy-related causes each year. Misclassification and underreporting of maternal fatalities are widespread. Most people who pass away are impoverished and reside in isolated, rural areas; as a result, few people know about their deaths. Deaths and their causes are rarely reported in the parts of the world with the highest rates of maternal mortality. Despite the fact that hospital data show high mortality rates, the majority of the information is inaccurate and incomplete. Furthermore, deaths that happen at home or during transport are not included in data that is based only on hospital or other healthcare facility data. The cause of death and the timing of the death in relation to the woman's pregnancy status are important factors to consider when determining whether a woman's death qualifies as a maternal death. This information is frequently not easily accessible. Maternal deaths are misclassified when the death certificate's cause of death misrepresents the actual connection between the woman's pregnancy and her demise. The confluence of these variables results in reported rates of maternal mortality that are prone to understate the actual severity of this significant public health concern, thereby diminishing the significance of drawing international comparisons based on these data.

The true severity of the issue is up to 70% greater than what is indicated by reported rates of maternal mortality. Maternal mortality can be greatly underestimated, even in nations where the majority of deaths are medically certified. For example, the Centers for Disease Control and Prevention (CDC) in the United States estimated, based only on vital statistics data, that the number of deaths attributable to pregnancy and its complications from 1982 to 1996 was actually 1.3 to 3 times the rate. To get accurate data on maternal mortality, extra effort must be made. In the past, epidemiologic surveys tended to focus on the biological processes of mortality and morbidity, while demographic studies typically focused on the socioeconomic determinants of maternal health. The necessity for both scientific disciplines to integrate their work has come to light more recently. By working together, they may be able to provide the better health information required to assess the effectiveness of health interventions in a population as well as to characterize the scope and identify the determinants of maternal mortality and morbidity.

Up until now, only a few locations throughout the world have seen the regular collection of data on maternal mortality and morbidity using a standardized methodology. To improve trends in morbidity and mortality, baseline data must be gathered to more precisely evaluate the effects of interventions. These evaluations highlight the extent of pregnancy-related deaths among women, which aids in concentrating policymakers' attention and resources. This module covers the following topics: 1) the scope and causes of maternal morbidity and mortality; 2) definitions of the measures of morbidity and mortality; 3) methods of measuring morbidity; 4) epidemiologic studies of morbidity and mortality; and 5) implications of research and data collected on these topics. We can start to understand what needs to be done to improve prevention strategies for lowering maternal morbidity and mortality at the community level, within the formal healthcare system, and in other social sectors by looking into maternal deaths.

Maternal health metrics shouldn't be limited to mortality. Interventions aimed at reducing maternal mortality will also reduce maternal morbidity because there is a clear overlap between the factors that cause maternal deaths and those that cause maternal morbidity.

8.2.1. Chain of Infection

The chain of infection includes the three factors that lead to infection: the etiologic agent, the method of transmission, and the host. These links should be characterized before control and prevention measures are proposed. Environmental factors that may influence disease occurrence must be evaluated (Figure 8.2).

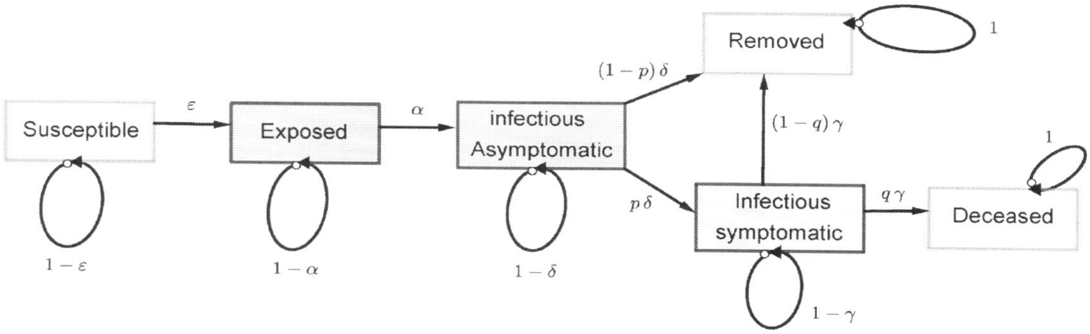

Figure 8.2. *Summary of important aspects involved in the chain of any infection.*

Source: *Ripoll, J., & Font, J., (2023). A discrete model for the evolution of infection prior to symptom onset. Mathematics, 11(5), 1092. https://doi.org/10.3390/math11051092.*

8.2.1.1. Etiologic Agent

Any microorganism with the ability to cause infection could be the etiologic agent. An agent's capacity to cause disease is referred to as its pathogenicity; the virulence and invasiveness of the organism are additional characteristics that define pathogenicity. The term "virulence" describes the degree of infection, which can be described by stating the infection's morbidity (disease incidence) and mortality (death rate). The plague agent *Yersinia pestis* is an example of a highly virulent organism; it nearly always causes severe disease in the susceptible host.

An organism's capacity to infiltrate tissue is referred to as its invasiveness. The noninvasive Vibrio cholerae bacteria cause symptoms by releasing an exotoxin into the intestinal canal that affects the tissues. Shigella bacteria in the intestinal canal, on the other hand, are invasive and migrate into the tissue. Without a doubt, no microbe is avirulent. Even though an organism has very low virulence, infection with it can still result in disease if the host is highly susceptible, such as when immunosuppressed therapeutically. For instance, the oral polio vaccine contains a highly attenuated form of the poliomyelitis virus, which has low virulence overall but can cause paralysis in certain highly susceptible individuals. The agent's description should take other aspects into account.

The number of organisms required to cause disease, known as the infecting dose, varies depending on the type of organism, the host's defenses, the mode of transmission, the site of the organism's entrance into the host, and the host species. Specificity is another aspect of an agent; certain agents, like Salmonella typhimurium, can infect a wide variety of hosts, while others can only infect a limited number of hosts. For example, only humans can contract styphi. Additional agent factors include the production of enzymes, antibiotic sensitivity, resistance transfer plasmids, and antigenic composition, which can differ within a species (e.g., streptococcus or influenza viruses).

An organism's reservoir is where it lives, metabolizes, and reproduces. The location where an organism is transferred, either directly or indirectly through an intermediary object, to a host that is susceptible is known as its source. The source and reservoir of S typhi can differ; for instance, the gallbladder of an infected person may serve as the reservoir, but food contaminated by the carrier may serve as the source of transmission. The source and reservoir may also be the same person, as in the case of a persistent nasal carrier of S aureus that spreads the organisms from this location. When deciding where to implement control measures, the distinction may be crucial.

8.2.1.2. Method of Transmission

The agent travels from the source to the host via the transmission method. The four main ways that something can spread are through contact, a shared vehicle, the air, or a vector.

The agent can propagate through direct, indirect, or airborne droplet transmission in contact transmission. Also known as person-to-person transmission, direct contact transmission occurs when organisms are transferred directly from the source to the susceptible host without the need for an intermediary object. One instance is the spread of the hepatitis A virus through hand-to-hand contact. When organisms are transferred from an inanimate source to a host through an inanimate object, this is known as indirect transmission. One instance is the spread of pseudomonas bacteria from one person to another via a shaving brush.

The term "droplet spread" describes organisms that move less than three feet—that is, very short distances—through the atmosphere from a source to a host. As a result, the organisms are not actually airborne. The measles is one illness that can spread through droplets.

Agents transmitted by a common inanimate vehicle are referred to as common-vehicle transmission, and exposure to such agents can result in multiple cases. This group comprises illnesses where the agents of infection are not only drugs and parenteral fluids but also food or water. Salmonellosis transmitted through food, shigellosis transmitted through water, and bacteremia brought on by intravenous fluid use contaminated with a gram-negative organism are a few examples. Airborne transmission, the third mode of transmission, describes the spread of infection through dust or droplet nuclei. The particles must travel more than three feet through the air from the source to the host to be considered truly airborne.

Droplet nuclei are the leftover material left over after fluid from droplets evaporates. They are sufficiently light to travel more than three feet from their source and can float in the air for extended periods of time. The main way that tuberculosis spreads is through the air; a coughing patient may produce aerosols of droplet nuclei containing tubercle bacilli. Dust particles have the potential to contain infectious agents, which could resuscitate and spread to hosts. An instance of this happened during a salmonellosis outbreak in a neonatal nursery. The infants contracted the disease after dust contaminated with salmonella from a vacuum cleaner bag resuspended after the equipment was used frequently.

Arthropods serve as the vectors in the fourth mode of transmission, known as vector-borne transmission. Transmission of vectors can occur internally or externally. When organisms are carried mechanically on the vector—such as Salmonella bacteria that contaminate flies' legs—this is known as external, or mechanical, transmission. When the organisms are carried inside the vector, internal transmission takes place. The term "harborage" refers to a situation in which a flea ingests plague bacilli from an infected person or animal and contaminates a susceptible host when it feeds again; the organism is not altered while in the flea. This occurs when the pathogen is not altered by its carriage within the vector. Biologic transmission is the other type of internal transmission. In this form, the organism undergoes biological changes as it passes through the vector (malaria parasites in the mosquito vector, for instance). Multiple pathways can be utilized to spread an infectious agent. For instance, salmonella can spread through contact with a human carrier or a common medium like food. All four routes are potential means of transmission for Francisella tularensis.

8.2.1.3. Host

The host is the third component in the infection chain. In addition to entering fetuses through the placenta, the organism can enter hosts through the skin, mucous membranes, lungs, gastrointestinal tract, or genitourinary tract. Though this is not always the case, meningococci that enter the host through the mucous membranes can still cause meningitis. The ensuing illness frequently corresponds with the site of entry. Disease development in a host is influenced by both non-specific and specific host defense mechanisms, as well as agent characteristics (see above).

The skin, mucous membranes, secretions, excretions, enzymes, the inflammatory response, genetics, hormones, nutrition, behavioral patterns, and the existence of other illnesses are examples of nonspecific defense mechanisms. Certain defense mechanisms, or immunity, can be produced artificially through active or passive immunization, or naturally through exposure to the infectious agent. Any link in the infection chain is susceptible to environmental influences.

Low humidity can harm mucous membranes, temperature can promote or prevent the growth of organisms at their reservoir, air velocity can help droplet nuclei travel through the air, and UV radiation can kill the microorganisms.

It is critical to assess the impact of environmental factors in any disease investigation. Environmental control measures are sometimes implemented based less on epidemiologic evidence and more on sentiment. It should be clear that a variety of factors interact to cause disease to occur (Table 8.2). Here is an outline of a few of these factors.

Table 8.2. *Emerging and Re-Emerging Zoonotic Viruses*

Virus	Year of first human case* Year of major outbreak** (per country)	Country	Reference
SARS-CoV	2003	Vietnam Singapore Thailand The Philippines Indonesia Malaysia	[illegible]
Influenza A(H5N1)	2003	Vietnam	[illegible]
Influenza A(H5N1)	2004	Thailand	[illegible]
Influenza A(H5N1)	2005	Indonesia Cambodia	[illegible]
Dengue virus	2007	Cambodia	[illegible]
Influenza A(H5N1)	2007	Lao PDR Myanmar	[illegible]
Chikungunya virus	2008	Malaysia	[illegible]
Chikungunya virus	2009	Thailand	[illegible]
Ebola	2009	The Philippines	[illegible]
Influenza A(H1N1)	2009	All SEA countries	[illegible]
Chikungunya virus	2009	Myanmar	[illegible]
		Indonesia	[illegible]
Dengue virus	2013	Thailand	[illegible]
		Lao PDR	[illegible]
Chikungunya virus	2013	Singapore	[illegible]
		Lao PDR	[illegible]
Dengue virus	2014	Brunei	[illegible]
MERS-CoV	2014	Malaysia	[illegible]
MERS-CoV	2015	Thailand The Philippines	[illegible]
Dengue virus	2015	Myanmar	[illegible]
Dengue virus	2016	Indonesia	[illegible]
Zika virus	2016	Singapore	[illegible]
		Thailand	[illegible]
		Vietnam	[illegible]
Chikungunya virus	2017	The Philippines	[illegible]
Dengue virus	2019	Malaysia	[illegible]
		The Philippines	[illegible]
Monkeypox	2019	Singapore	[illegible]
SARS-CoV-2	2020	All SEA countries	[illegible]
Chikungunya virus	2020	Cambodia	[illegible]
Dengue virus	2020	Singapore	[illegible]
Monkeypox	2022	Vietnam Thailand The Philippines Indonesia	[illegible]
Dengue virus	2022	Vietnam Timor-Leste	[illegible]

SARS-CoV, Severe Acute Respiratory Syndrome; MERS-CoV, Middle East Respiratory Syndrome; SARS-CoV-2, Severe Acute Respiratory Syndrome Coronavirus 2; PDR, People's Democratic Republic; SEA, Southeast Asia.

*Year of first human case: SARS-CoV, Influenza A(H5N1), Ebola, Influenza A(H1N1), MERS-CoV, Monkeypox, SARS-CoV-2.

**Year of major outbreak: Zika virus, dengue virus and Chikungunya virus.

Source: Saba, V. P. M., Gumpangseth, N., Songhong, T., Yainoy, S., Monteil, A., Leaungwutiwong, P., Missé, D., & Wichit, S., (2023). Emerging and re-emerging zoonotic viral diseases in Southeast Asia: One health challenge. Front. Public Health, 11, 1141483. doi: 10.3389/fpubh.2023.1141483.

8.2.2. Epidemiologic Methods

The three main methods used in epidemiology are experimental, analytical, and descriptive. While any of the three can be employed to look into the occurrence of disease, descriptive epidemiology is the approach that is most frequently used. Following the description of a disease's basic epidemiology, specialized analytical techniques can be applied to further investigate the illness, and a particular experimental strategy can be created to evaluate a theory.

8.2.2.1. Descriptive Epidemiology

In descriptive epidemiology, information about the disease's occurrence is gathered from all pertinent sources using a variety of techniques. Next, the information is compiled by person, place, and time. When characterizing the epidemiologic data, four time trends are taken into account. The term "secular trend" refers to the occurrence of disease over an extended period of time, typically years; it is influenced by the population's level of immunity as well as potentially nonspecific factors like improved socioeconomic and nutritional conditions. For instance, the United States' secular trend for tetanus cases since 1920 indicates a slow but steady decrease.

The periodic trend is the second time trend. The periodic trend, which is a brief alteration in the general secular trend, might point to a shift in the antigenic properties of the pathogen. For instance, the antigenic structure of the common influenza A virus changes every two to three years, which causes a cyclical rise in the incidence of clinical influenza brought on by a lack of innate immunity in the populace. Furthermore, an increase in the incidence of the disease can arise from a reduction in the general immunity of a population or a subset of it (a phenomenon referred to as herd immunity).

This is evident in certain vaccine-preventable diseases when there are recurring drops in the immunization rate within a specific population. As a result, there might be more cases overall, which would raise the herd immunity level overall. After then, there are fewer new cases until the herd's immunity is low enough to permit transmission to happen once more, at which point new cases start to emerge.

The seasonal trend is the third time trend. This pattern shows how seasonal variations in environmental factors that improve the agent's capacity for replication or transmission lead to variations in the incidence of disease. For instance, outbreaks of food-borne illness are more common in the summer because of the bacterial growth-promoting conditions. When the monthly incidence of salmonellosis is analyzed, this trend is clearly visible (Figure 8.3).

The epidemic occurrence of disease is the fourth temporal trend. An epidemic is characterized by a sharp rise in incidence brought on by common elements that facilitate spread. Three distinct sites must be taken into account when describing epidemiologic data by place: the individual's location at the time the disease manifested, the source of the infection where the source contracted the infection, and the source itself where the etiologic agent was introduced. As a result, a person who has eaten food at a restaurant may develop a serious illness at home during a food poisoning outbreak. It's possible that the undercooked chicken in the car was contaminated on a chicken farm. It is crucial to take these distinctions into account when trying to stop more cases.

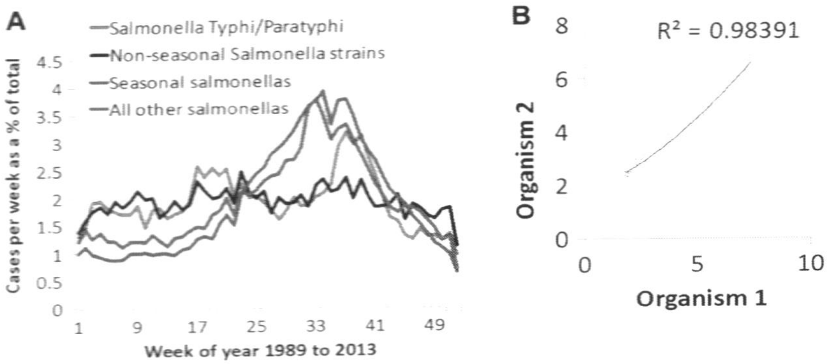

Figure 8.3. *An example of a disease showing a seasonal trend. The seasonality of several human infectious disease pathogens in England and Wales.*

Source: Cherrie, M. P. C., Nichols, G., Iacono, G. L., et al., (2018). Pathogen seasonality and links with weather in England and Wales: A big data time series analysis. BMC Public Health, 18, 1067. https://doi.org/10.1186/s12889-018-5931-6.

The afflicted individual is the third focus of descriptive epidemiology. Age, sex, occupation, personal habits, socioeconomic status, immunization history, presence of underlying disease, and other relevant characteristics should all be recorded.

8.2.2.2. Analytic Epidemiology

Analytic epidemiology, which examines disease determinants for potential causal relationships, is the second epidemiologic technique. The case-control (or case-comparison) method and the cohort method are the two primary analytical techniques. The case-control approach looks into the cause of the effect (disease) after starting with the effect. Individuals who have the disease comprise the case group, while those who do not have the disease make up the comparison group. The differences between these two groups are then compared to see if they could account for the disease's occurrence. To determine what factors may have influenced the occurrence in the group that developed disease, a case-control study might involve choosing participants with meningococcal meningitis and a comparison group that is matched for age, sex, socioeconomic status, and place of residence but does not have the disease.

The cohort method is the second analytical technique. It studies two populations prospectively: a group that has been in contact with the suspected causal factor under investigation and a similar group that has not. Upon observing both groups, the factor's effect ought to become evident. Observing two comparable groups of people—one made up of people who received blood transfusions and the other of people who did not—is an example of a cohort approach. One can establish a correlation between blood transfusions and hepatitis by looking at the prospective incidence of hepatitis in both groups. In other words, if the transfused blood contained hepatitis B virus, the recipient cohort should have a higher incidence of hepatitis than the non-transfused cohort.

The case-control approach has the advantage of being more affordable, reproducible, and easier to conduct than the cohort approach. On the other hand, bias could be introduced during the selection of the two groups, it might be challenging to omit subclinical cases from the comparison group, and patients' memories of past events might be inaccurate. Cohort studies have the advantage of being more accurate in data collection and providing a direct estimate of the disease risk resulting from factor contact; however, they are more costly and take longer to conduct. An additional analytical technique is the cross-sectional study, which involves surveying a population for a set amount of time to ascertain the association between a disease and concurrent variables that could affect its occurrence.

8.2.2.3. Experimental Epidemiology

The experimental approach is the third epidemiologic method. An experimental model with one or more chosen factors manipulated is built based on a hypothesis. The manipulation's outcome will either support or refute the hypothesis. The assessment of a novel drug's impact on a disease is one instance. A subset of the diseased population is identified, and a random selection process is used to determine who gets the medication. If the drug's use is the only distinction between the two, then the drug's efficacy should be reflected in the clinical variations between the groups.

8.2.3. Epidemic Investigation

An epidemic investigation outlines the elements that contribute to a disease outbreak; after the conditions surrounding the disease's occurrence are established, suitable controls and preventative measures can be found. When conducting an epidemic investigation, information is gathered, sorted by person, place, and time, examined, and conclusions are made.

The first step in the investigation should be to establish the epidemic's existence by counting suspected cases from historical surveillance data and comparing it to the number of cases that were first reported. When the investigator has examined patients and reviewed laboratory and hospital records, they should also talk about the disease's prevalence with doctors or other medical professionals who have observed or reported cases. Then, these diagnoses ought to be confirmed. To distinguish between patients who represent real cases, those who represent suspected or presumed cases, and those who ought to be excluded from additional research, a case definition needs to be created. It may be necessary to look for more cases or gather more patient data before estimating the number of cases.

The main task of this first stage is gathering data, which needs to be arranged by person, place, and time. A hypothesis regarding the disease's occurrence should be developed, along with the identification of the population that is at risk. Specimens ought to be gathered and brought to the lab if necessary. Further specialized research might be necessary. Further information from these investigations needs to be examined to verify or modify the hypothesis. Following analysis, control and prevention strategies ought to be created and, to the greatest extent feasible, put into action. This data should be put into a report that is created and given to people looking into the outbreak and putting control and/or preventative measures in place. It might be appropriate to carry out ongoing surveillance to assess how well the control and preventative measures are working.

In the US, the CDC supports state health departments by offering laboratory and epidemiologic support services upon request. Its assistance includes different training programs run by the CDC and the states, as well as disease investigations and diagnostic laboratory activities. The state health departments and the CDC collaborate closely on projects. In addition, doctors regularly attend public health training programs and consult with CDC staff on a range of health-related issues. The early research on acquired immune deficiency syndrome serves as an example of how epidemiology can be used to characterize a disease before its etiology is known (AIDS). When a rise in requests for pentamidine to treat *Pneumocystis carinii* pneumonia was noticed in late 1981, the CDC became aware of the first cases. This sparked particular epidemiological research and surveillance initiatives that yielded crucial data regarding this recently discovered illness.

Fever, appetite loss, weight loss, extreme fatigue, and lymph node enlargement are some of the initial symptoms. The subsequent development of a severe immune deficiency appears to be linked to opportunistic infections. 52% of cases were diagnosed with *P. carinii* pneumoniae; 26% with Kaposi sarcoma; and 7% with both *P. carinii* pneumoniae and Kaposi sarcoma. Other bacterial, fungal, viral, or parasitic infections linked to immunodeficiencies affect 15% of AIDS patients. There were 1,092 deaths among the first 2,640 cases that the CDC received, translating to a case-fatality rate of 41%. Around 70% of the cases at the time of diagnosis were in the 20–49 age range, with approximately 95% of the cases being male. Of the cases reported, about 40% came from New York City, 12% from San Francisco, 8% from Los Angeles, and the remaining cases came from 32 other states. At least 16 other countries reported cases. Around 90% of the patients were classified based on potential risk factors, and the groups most at risk included homosexuals or bisexuals (70%), injectable drug users (17%), Haitian immigrants to the US (92.5%), and hemophiliacs (1%).

Examining these preliminary data—gathered prior to the identification of the AIDS etiologic agent—confirmed the theory that the main routes of transmission were through intercourse, intravenous needle contact, and receiving tainted blood or blood products. It didn't seem likely that casual contact would spread. According to epidemiologic data, AIDS was classified as an infectious disease. It is now known that infection with a retrovirus belonging to the human T cell leukemia/lymphoma virus family causes AIDS; this virus is known as human immunodeficiency virus type I (HIV-l). An examination of the data that was later gathered indicates that the original theories were correct.

8.3. Disaster Management and Emergency Preparedness

Natural disasters, man-made calamities, or a mix of the two that pose serious risks to a community's health, safety, security, or well-being are referred to as humanitarian emergencies. More than three-quarters of those impacted by disasters are thought to be women and children, and one in five women who are of childbearing age may be pregnant.

Basic health systems, which include services for maternity, newborn, and child health, frequently collapse as a result of disasters. Furthermore, disasters tend to happen more frequently in nations with high rates of maternal, newborn, and infant mortality. To provide sexual and reproductive health as well as newborn, child, and adolescent care, national health systems should have emergency preparedness plans backed by skilled professionals, particularly midwives. This will ensure that high-quality medical care is provided even in the most difficult humanitarian situations.

"Any occurrence that causes damage, ecological disruption, loss of human life, or deterioration of health and health services on a scale sufficient to warrant an extraordinary response from outside the affected community area" is what the World Health Organization (WHO) defines as a disaster. More than 2 billion people were impacted by natural or technological disasters between 1990 and 1999, which resulted in 600,000 fatalities. There are many different kinds of disasters, such as hurricanes, tsunamis, floods, famine, drought, and disasters linked to epidemics (Figure 8.4).

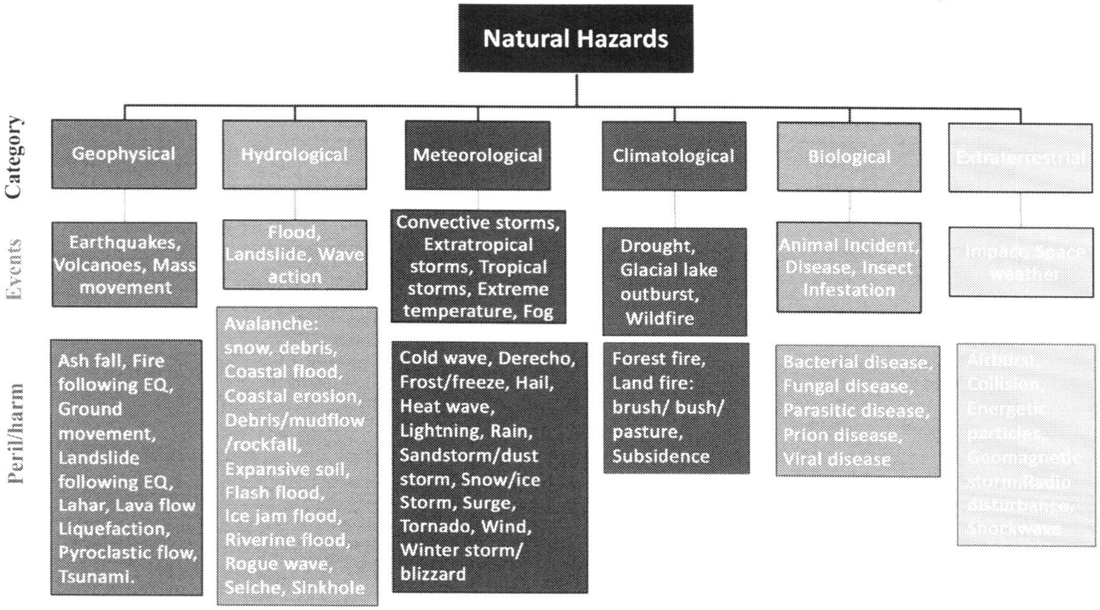

Figure 8.4. *Natural disasters (1971–2001).*

Source: *Chaudhary, M. T., & Piracha, A., (2021). Natural disasters – Origins, impacts, management. Encyclopedia, 1(4), 1101–1131. https://doi.org/10.3390/encyclopedia1040084.*

The average number of natural disasters between 2000 and 2008 was 392. In 2009, there were 350 natural disasters and in 2010 there were 373. The location of a catastrophic event is directly related to the number of people affected. Disasters that have had the highest impact are the drought in India in 2002 (300 million victims), the Indian Ocean tsunami in 2004 (226,408 deaths), cyclone Nargis in Myanmar in 2008 (138,366 deaths), and the Haitian earthquake in 2010 (296,800 deaths). Although Hurricane Katrina was the third deadliest hurricane in the United States, killing approximately 1500 people (and costing $81 billion), the availability of US resources minimized further human deaths.

The areas most severely affected by natural disasters are undoubtedly those in low-resource countries where infrastructure, transportation, and healthcare are already in jeopardy. The 2010 earthquake in Haiti severely damaged the country's healthcare system. Doctors compared their experience to practicing medicine in the 1930s, when saws were used to amputate limbs and vodka was used to sterilize instruments. The discrepancy between the resources that were actually available and the supplies that physicians needed to care for their patients caused them difficulty. While the number of fatalities from disasters is declining, the number of impacted individuals is rising. Natural disasters will still happen, despite the fact that it is impossible to forecast their trends.

8.3.1. Gender Differences in the Aftermath

Research has shown that disasters impact men and women differently due to biological, social, cultural, and reproductive health variations. For example, during the Seveso technological disaster in Italy in 1976, exposure to dioxin led to different outcomes for men and women. Studies revealed that more men died from rectal and lung cancer, while more women succumbed to diabetes 15 years later. The Indian Ocean tsunami in 2004 also showcased gender disparities in mortality rates, with a ratio of 3:1 for women to men. This was attributed to factors such as men's physical strength, women's lack of swimming skills, and the risk of entanglement due to women's long hair.

Men and women are impacted by social determinants in different ways. For instance, when the 1993 Maharashtra, India, earthquake struck, women and children perished at a higher rate than men because the women were at home and the men were working in the fields. On the other hand, because of societal norms, men were impacted by the Chernobyl disaster in 1985 more than women. Greater radiation exposure resulted from the soldiers and male civilians cleaning up the site. Cultural norms have made it difficult for women to ask for assistance after a disaster, particularly in places where it is strictly forbidden for women to interact with men. Social norms have shown that women are more likely to be responsible for taking care of the elderly, children, and injured or ill. Women are obviously impacted by reproductive factors, though. Research has indicated that women experience higher rates of miscarriages, early births, intrauterine growth restriction (IUGR), low birth weight babies, sexual assault, and unwanted pregnancies following disasters.

8.3.2. Effect of Disasters on Women

8.3.2.1. Violence Against Women

Women and girls are more vulnerable to sexual assault and domestic abuse when they are uprooted. Women and girls are subjected to increased exploitation and abuse, including domestic violence, as a result of their increased helplessness and vulnerability. In exchange for food, shelter, or even security, women may be forced or coerced into having sex. Girls are more likely to become victims of human trafficking and may be coerced into child marriages. Because of supply and demand, the sex industry prospers in these hard times. The United Nations Refugee Agency has determined the causes of sexual assault. Male dominance, psychological stress in refugee camps, inadequate protection and assistance for women, drug and alcohol addiction, and general lawlessness are a few of these causes.

Long after the tragedy has passed, the psychological effects of sexual abuse, manipulation, or both may make it more difficult for women to reintegrate into society. In times of crisis, medical professionals may lack the necessary training to care for victims of sexual assault. Sexual violence is seldom discussed when the main focus is on methods for saving lives or limbs. Inquiring about a victim's sexual history in detail, attending to any physical wounds, offering emergency contraception and preventative treatment for STIs, reporting the offender or offenders, and establishing security and order in shelters and camps are all effective ways to care for victims of rape. Health professionals who specialize in assisting victims of sexual assault can also assist in identifying children who may be in danger (such as orphans and children who have been taken from their families). It is also important to direct women to resources that will guarantee their safety from future sexual assaults.

8.3.2.2. Access to Contraceptive Care and Prevention of STIs

During emergencies, regular behaviors undergo significant changes. It's possible that women who use contraception won't have access to the medications or devices, or they might forget to take or use them. Furthermore, when people crave intimacy and closeness, stress and despair can lead to, at best, comfort-seeking behaviors and, at worst, violent sexual behaviors. Therefore, unprotected coitus puts women at risk for STIs and pregnancy. Prioritizing the prevention of unwanted and unplanned pregnancies should be the top priority for emergency response protocols. Injectable contraceptives, if available, are the best option because they spare women from having to remember to use contraception in an emergency (Table 8.3).

Table 8.3. *Examples of Contraception-based Studies*

First Author, Year of Publication	Methods, Country	Participants	Interventions	Outcomes	Total Patients in Parenteral	Total Patients in COC	Mean (SD) Age in Parenteral	Mean (SD) Age in COC
Ahrendt, 2006 [38]	Randomized trial in 10 European countries from May 2002 to Apr 2004.	1017 women, at least 18 years old.	Vaginal ring (etonogestrel 120 µg + EE 15 µg) versus COC (drospirenone 3 mg + EE 30 µg).	Contraceptive efficacy, compliance, acceptability, adverse events, continuation.	499	484	26.6 (6.1)	26.6 (6.2)
Audet, 2001 [37]	39 centers in the United States and 6 centers in Canada.	Healthy women aged 18 to 45 years.	Patch (norelgestromin 150 µg + EE 20 µg) versus oral contraceptive (levonorgestrel 50/75/125 µg + EE 30/40/30 µg).	Pearl index, cycle control, compliance, adverse events.	811	605	28.0 (6.6)	27.8 (6.4)
Creinin, 2008 [36]	–	581 women.	Vaginal ring (etonogestrel 120 µg + EE 15 µg) versus transdermal patch (norelgestromin 150 µg + EE 20 µg).	Adverse events.	241	238	26.2 (5.6)	25.1 (5.5)

Fan, 2016 [35]	Phase-III, open-label, randomized multicenter trial in China.	1137 healthy women.	NuvaRing or COC.	Contraceptive efficacy, cycle control, dysmenorrhea, compliance.	714	232	31.8 (4.0)	31.2 (3.9)
Gilliam, 2010 [34]	–	273 women, 18–45 years.	Vaginal ring (etonogestrel 120 μg + EE 15 μg) versus COC.	Compliance.	135	137	22.3 (N/A)	22 (N/A)
Kaunitz, 2014 [32]	Open-label, randomized, parallel-group, multicenter study.	Women, 17–40 years of age.	Transdermal patch (120 μg levonorgestrel + 30 μg EE) versus 100 μg LNG and 20 μg EE.	Contraceptive efficacy, compliance, tolerability.	1043	344	26.4 (5.7)	26.4 (5.7)
Kaunitz, 2015 [25]	Open-label, randomized, multicenter, parallel-group clinical trial.	Women, 17–40 years of age.	Transdermal patch (120 μg levonorgestrel + 30 μg EE) versus 100 μg LNG and 20 μg EE.	Adverse events.	998	330	26.4 (N/A)	26.4 (N/A)
Kaunitz, 2015 [33]	Multicenter crossover study, presumably conducted in USA, dates not specified.	Women, 17–40 years.	Transdermal patch, (levonorgestrel 120 μg + EE 30 μg) versus COC (levonorgestrel 150 μg + EE 30 μg).	Pregnancy (Pearl Index), breakthrough bleeding and spotting, noncompliance, patch wearability, and adverse events.	1450	188	26.4 (5.6)	26.7 (5.7)

Merz, 2015 [31]	Double-blind, double-dummy, randomized, controlled, parallel-group, multicenter trial conducted at 28 centers in the United States.	Healthy women, 18–45 years of age.	Transdermal patch (0.55 mg EE and 2.1 mg GSD) versus COC (0.02 mg EE and 0.1 mg levonorgestrel).	Bleeding pattern, cycle control, safety.	199	198	29.1 (7.3)	27.2 (6.8)
Mohamed, 2011 [39]	Randomized trial conducted in Cairo, Egypt between 1 May 2008 and 31 July 2010.	600 women between 17 and 42 years.	Vaginal ring (etonogestrel 120 µg + EE 15 µg) versus COC (drospirenone 3 mg + EE 30 µg).	Cycle control (via diary cards), withdrawal bleeding, breakthrough bleeding or spotting, adverse events.	300	300	29.7 (4.1)	30.9 (4.2)
Oddsson, 2004 [30]	Open-label, randomized, comparative, multi-center trial in Belgium, Brazil, Chile, Denmark, Finland, France, Germany, Italy, Norway, Spain, and Sweden	1090 healthy women.	–	Contraceptive efficacy, cycle control, dysmenorrhea, compliance.	512	518	27.0 (6.2)	27.2 (6.3)

Rad, 2005 [29]	48 healthy premenopausal women between 18 and 34 years old.	–	Vaginal ring (nestorone 150 μg + EE 15 μg) versus COC (levonorgestrel 150 μg + EE 30 μg).	Pregnancy and continuation. Study focused on hemostasis variables.	23	24	24 (N/A)	N/A (N/A)
Urdl, 2005 [28]	Open-label, randomized trial in 65 centers in Europe and South Africa.	1517 healthy women aged 18 to 45 years.	Transdermal patch (norelgestromin 150 μg + EE 20 μg) versus COC (desogestrel 150 μg + EE 20 μg)	Pregnancy, continuation, compliance, cycle control, satisfaction, adverse events.	846	643	28.8 (6.5)	28.3 (6.5)

Source: *Vleskó, G., Meznerics, F. A., Hegyi, P., Teutsch, B., Unicsovics, M., Sipos, Z., Fehérvári, P., Ács, N., Várbíró, S., & Keszthelyi, M., (2024). Comparison of combined parenteral and oral hormonal contraceptives: A systematic review and meta-analysis of randomized trials. Journal of Clinical Medicine, 13(2), 575. https://doi.org/10.3390/jcm13020575.*

During disasters, attention to preventive measures for sexually transmitted infections (STIs) and HIV/AIDS may be overlooked. People living with HIV may face challenges accessing their medications, increasing their risk of spreading the disease. Therefore, it is crucial to prioritize STI prevention as part of emergency response efforts (Table 8.4).

Table 8.4. *STI Pathogens*

Spectrum of Pathogens	
Parasites	*Trichomonas vaginalis, Sarcoptes scabiei, Phthirus pubis*
Fungi	Trichophyton mentagrophytes subspecies Note: *Candida albicans* is only facultatively pathogenic and does not cause STIs.
Bacteria	*Chlamydia trachomatis (serotypes D-K, serotypes L_1–L_3), Klebsiella granulomatosis, Neisseria gonorrhoeae, Treponema pallidum, Haemophilus ducreyi; Mycoplasma genitalium.*
Viruses	Human papillomaviruses, Herpes simplex virus, HIV, Hepatitis B virus, Hepatitis C virus, Molluscum contagiosum virus, monkeypox virus.

Source: Wihlfahrt, K., Günther, V., Mendling, W., Westermann, A., Willer, D., Gitas, G., Ruchay, Z., Maass, N., Allahqoli, L., & Alkatout, I., (2023). Sexually transmitted diseases – An update and overview of current research. Diagnostics, 13(9), 1656. https://doi.org/10.3390/diagnostics13091656.

8.3.2.3. Prenatal Care and Delivery in Emergencies

Prenatal care and delivery can be difficult in countries with limited resources because of the subpar facilities and lack of emergency equipment. Even in the best of circumstances, pregnancy complications like placenta previa and placenta accreta, retained placenta, obstructed labor, and fetal distress can be difficult to deal with. Healthcare providers and facilities are overworked during a natural disaster. Maternal and neonatal morbidity and mortality are increased by pregnancy complications and unsafe childbirth practices.

Following a disaster, there is a notable decrease in the provision of prenatal care. Initially, pregnant women are looking for food, water, and shelter in an attempt to survive the calamity. If a woman is able to track her fetal movement, she might not believe that she needs to see a doctor until after giving birth. Poor maternal and fetal outcomes can arise from the failure to diagnose high-risk pregnancies involving preeclampsia, placenta previa, IUGR, or gestational diabetes.

During one disaster, even in areas where prenatal care was available, the rate of inadequate prenatal care increased from 1.3% to 3.9%. Among women living within 2 miles of the World Trade Center, there was a higher rate of infants with IUGR, infants who were small for gestational age, and infants who had a small head circumference.

Many doctors who work in disaster relief are skilled surgeons or emergency room doctors who have rarely or never delivered a baby via cesarean section. When they notice fetal heart rate decelerations, their inexperience with reading fetal monitors can sometimes lead them to make snap decisions to perform cesarean deliveries. Expert obstetricians and midwives may be better able to spot the decelerations and improve the likelihood of a vaginal birth. This strategy would also prevent the mother from developing sepsis and a possible wound infection. It is imperative to emphasize the importance of breastfeeding during disasters. Obtaining clean water to sterilize bottles or purchase formula is difficult. It is essential to teach and assist new mothers in starting and continuing breastfeeding. According to data, lactation can be started or restarted by nonlactating mothers who are less than six months pregnant.

In low-resource countries, it is rare to find the level of care that professionals are used to during catastrophic disasters. Critical choices are made quickly, and patients are treated in order of medical priority, starting with those who have the best chance of surviving. Emergency medicine, orthopedics, pediatric, and trauma surgery volunteers are the first to be called in during these crises. Gynecologists and obstetricians are typically not taken into account. The needs of mothers and children during the acute or recovery phases of the crisis must be considered in the response to disasters. Perhaps more obstetricians and gynecologists should get involved in disaster relief work given their experience with obstetric emergencies, such as postpartum hemorrhage, placenta accreta, and cesarean hysterectomies, as well as their capacity to observe a nonreassuring fetal heart tracing and assess whether it indicates a danger to the fetus. STIs and the treatment of sexual assault victims can be handled by obstetricians and gynecologists, while surgeons handle crush injuries and infectious disease control. In general, victims of disasters need to receive complete care. To enhance the long-term health outcomes for women and families, relief teams need to include a specialist in maternal and women's health.

8.4. Healthcare Systems and Policies

Congress was debating legislation to overhaul the U.S. healthcare system, but decided to wait until the following year to take any action. The way healthcare is financed and provided may alter if the Congress passes healthcare reform legislation next year. How a reformed system will strike a balance between concerns about cost containment and quality of care—particularly for women and children—is a major worry for many. Everyone is at risk from the possibility that cost-cutting initiatives will incentivize underservice, but individuals who are already at a disadvantage due to their financial situation or unique healthcare needs may be particularly concerned.

Owing to a long-standing concern for women's and children's health and wellbeing, on July 7–8, 1994, the IOM and the NRC hosted an invitational workshop to discuss the special healthcare needs of women and children in the context of healthcare reform. The main topics brought up in the presentations and discussions on the first day of the workshop are summarized in this brief report, which was written with the workshop steering committee's guidance. The workshop's second day covered a wide range of topics related to evaluating the standard of care for children.

The results of healthcare reform will greatly affect women and children. The report "Including Children and Pregnant Women in Healthcare Reform" is still a useful resource for efforts to ensure that women and children receive adequate healthcare, according to workshop participants. However, they expressed concern that important public health and community services have received little funding and attention, that federal legislation may not guarantee universal coverage, and that its benefits package might not meet the needs of women and children, especially those with disabilities. The public health system, which is made up of the federal, state, and local health departments, offers crucial population-based public health services like environmental monitoring, epidemic control, and vital statistics and surveillance. Furthermore, personal health services like well-child care and prenatal care are frequently offered by state and local public health departments, along with enabling services like case management, transportation, and home visits.

Because women and children are disproportionately represented among the uninsured, it is important to expand health insurance coverage. In 1992, 15% of American children, or almost 10 million, lacked health insurance of any kind, despite recent federally mandated expansions in Medicaid coverage that have partially countered declines in private coverage. At the moment, 40% of kids aren't covered by the job-based health insurance of their parents. 62 million working women between the ages of 18 and 44 who were fertile did not have health insurance in 1991.

Access to essential medical services is hampered by not having health insurance. However, it became clear from the workshop discussions that women's and children's healthcare needs cannot be fully met by better benefit packages or by having full health insurance coverage. The community services and public health that many maternity and child health programs support also require adequate support. For instance, to access available prenatal care and reproductive healthcare services, women may require child care or transportation. Services including nutrition programs, protection from intentional and unintentional injuries, mental health programs, health education, and family planning programs may promote the best possible physical and psychosocial development in children and adolescents. Legislators must be well-informed about a wide range of advantageous health promotion initiatives in addition to the medical care that women and children require as they draft legislation for healthcare reform.

8.4.1. Healthcare Needs of Women, Children, and Adolescents

A reformed healthcare system should provide for the healthcare needs of all Americans. The current national focus on healthcare reform offers a unique chance to address the specific healthcare needs of children, adolescents, and women in their reproductive years.

8.4.1.1. Healthcare Needs of Women

A growing interest in safeguarding and advancing women's health is evident in initiatives like the National Institutes of Health's new women's health research agenda and the emergence of multiple advocacy groups supporting women's health, broadly understood to include social, psychological, and medical aspects. In addition to regular medical care and mental health services, workshop discussions brought attention to the need that women in their childbearing years, and especially those who are pregnant, have for a wide range of reproductive healthcare services. The participants suggested that these reproductive health services should, at the very least, consist of regular breast and pelvic exams (including Pap tests), diagnosis and treatment of STDs, prenatal, intrapartum, and postpartum care, and contraceptive services and supplies. in compliance with established frequency schedules; risk evaluation; and sufficient counseling and education to back up each of these interventions.

The idea that access to abortion and sterilization should be provided as part of reproductive health services without undue delay was endorsed by a large number of workshop attendees. Delaying an abortion into the second trimester significantly raises the possibility of health issues. Workshop presentations pointed out that most existing commercial indemnity plans already cover both abortion and sterilization as surgical services, despite the ongoing political controversy surrounding their inclusion in a required national benefits package.

Participants in the workshop argued that a variety of obstacles contribute to the explanation of comparatively poor patterns of contraceptive use in the United States when compared to a number of other developed nations. Some drew attention to the fact that a large number of private insurance providers do not fully cover family planning services. For some women, cost-sharing requirements, such as deductibles and co-payments that divide the cost of services and contraceptives between the patient and the insurance plan, maybe a significant obstacle to using contraception. It is particularly crucial to comprehend and remove obstacles to the use of contraceptives because over half of pregnancies in the US are unplanned at the time of conception. This leads to excessively high rates of abortion, delayed access to prenatal care, and a variety of unfavorable pregnancy outcomes. As a result, workshop attendees stated that large co-payments for contraceptive services and supplies should be avoided in insurance policies, whether they are private or public.

Obstacles to women's access to healthcare, particularly for those at high risk, extend beyond the domains of reproductive health and contraception. Participants in the workshop pointed out that a range of societal, economic, and other obstacles could prevent women from generally accessing healthcare. For example, women are more likely than men to be uninsured or underinsured due to the fact that many of them work at jobs that do not offer health insurance benefits, which makes it difficult for them to get the care they need. This is especially true for young women who are in their prime childbearing years. Furthermore, it appears from certain recent studies on cardiovascular disease that women may not always receive the same level of care that men receiving the same diagnosis receive.

8.4.1.2. Healthcare Needs of Children

Even though the majority of children are generally healthy, they still need healthcare that places a strong emphasis on immunizations and other preventive measures as well as monitoring their physical and psychosocial development. Sensitive times when proper care is crucial for healthy development and progress should also be given special consideration. Just 6% of children under the age of 18 (3.8 million) had chronic health conditions that made it difficult for them to engage in daily activities like playing or going to school in 1991.

Participants in the workshop pointed out that minor deviations from a child's typical developmental trajectory could have long-term effects. For instance, it has been suggested that toddler speech and language difficulties may be linked to recurrent otitis media with fluctuating hearing loss. In the short- and long-term, delays in diagnosing an issue or getting the right treatment may have irreversible effects that raise morbidity, mortality, and costs. Children rely on their parents, other adults, and community institutions, such as schools, to identify and address any new health issues to safeguard their health and well-being. While children's dependence on adults diminishes with time, they still largely depend on them for care that supports healthy development as well as for the ability to identify problems and seek treatment.

Participants in the workshop observed that to prevent issues and mitigate the effects of conditions that negatively affect children, many children require both medical care and other health and social services to achieve optimal health and development. Socioeconomic and environmental variables, such as poverty and neighborhood violence, pose significant health risks to children but are not typically the focus of clinical preventive services. The medical system frequently has to provide acute or long-term care for illnesses brought on by trauma, exposure to poisonous substances (e.g., lead), or emotional disorders; social and environmental variables have a significant impact on all of these conditions. In addition to more conventional medical techniques, the design of successful health promotion or primary prevention programs frequently calls for extensive environmental and social interventions. For example, a variety of social services might be required to support a safe home environment, offer comprehensive care for children with chronic illnesses, or address specific behavioral issues that might not normally be associated with health issues.

8.4.1.3. Healthcare Needs of Adolescents

Adolescence is a special developmental stage that includes behavioral, psychological, and cognitive changes in addition to the physiological changes associated with puberty. Adolescents need to have access to family planning services, drug rehab centers, mental health services, medical care for illnesses and injuries, as well as a variety of educational and informational programs focused on forming healthy habits. Risky health behaviors contribute to a number of their health issues, including increased rates of substance abuse, unintended pregnancy, and STDs. violence as well as injuries. Participants in the workshop mentioned that a lot of teenagers get medical care at community clinics or through programs offered in schools, which aim to support healthy behavior and guarantee that all teenagers have access to healthcare. By getting involved in adolescence, one can introduce and establish healthy, new behavior patterns that may last a lifetime, as well as stop the onset of behavior that harms one's health.

Adolescents are the age group least likely to seek care in office settings and use healthcare services less frequently overall. Teens may encounter several obstacles to receiving healthcare: they may no longer feel comfortable seeking care next to infants or young children; they may not want to involve their parents in their care; or their parents' insurance may not cover their needs. Participants in the workshop mentioned that teens face many obstacles when it comes to accessing healthcare; therefore, they need ways to get care on their own, with a guarantee of privacy so that their parents are only informed when necessary. Patients should not be refused care due to their incapacity to pay cost-sharing, particularly in areas like mental health, substance abuse, and reproductive health (including diagnosis and treatment of STDs and contraception), where family support may be particularly hard to come by.

8.4.2. Healthcare Benefits for Women and Children

Participants in the workshop made the point that, in the context of universal health insurance, more work needs to be done to create a comprehensive benefits package for women and children. The need for greater focus on family planning services, mental health and substance abuse treatment, health education and counseling, and services for children with special healthcare needs, such as care coordination, long-term care, or home- and community-based therapeutic services, was highlighted during the discussion of healthcare benefits for women and children. Participants in the workshop looked at a variety of benefit design strategies, including benefit packages from several ongoing congressional healthcare reform proposals.

"Amount payable for a loss under specific insurance coverage (indemnity benefits) or as the guarantee that certain services will be paid for (service benefits)" are the two definitions of benefits. The United States is dependent on both government-funded insurance programs and an optional system of employment-based health benefits (private insurance, e.g., Medicaid and Medicare). Certain vulnerable populations, such as families whose income exceeds Medicaid limits but who cannot afford private insurance, are currently not covered by either government- or employment-based programs.

Furthermore, for some services like mental health, family planning, and preventive care, coverage under private insurance may be less extensive than that provided by government-funded insurance. Participants in the workshop concluded that for women and children to receive the best medical care possible, a comprehensive national benefits package would be required. It was stressed, nevertheless, that expanding health insurance coverage or enhancing benefits won't be sufficient to address all of the medical requirements of women and children. Participants stressed in particular that children with chronic health issues require adequate benefits for long-term care and ancillary services like care coordination. The significance of providing benefits for mental health and drug abuse services was also mentioned by several people.

The coverage of particular medical services is addressed in legislative proposals for healthcare reform. (or advantages) in two regards. One method involves defining particular services in healthcare reform laws, along with their quantity, extent, and duration of coverage. An organization or agency, like a national health benefits board, is identified in a different method that establishes a general set of covered services or categories in legislation and specifies the amount, scope, and duration of coverage along with the co-payments for specific services. Certain legislative proposals, for instance, list the services they would cover under broad headings like prescription drugs, family planning and prenatal care, preventive medicine, hospice and home healthcare, mental health and substance abuse services, physician and hospital services, and vision, hearing, and dental care. At the workshop, a different approach to creating a benefits package was presented.

In this approach, benefits are given to match each individual's needs on a case-by-case basis, leading to a benefit that is clinically determined as opposed to the conventional benefit-driven treatment. For instance, some major corporations have used this strategy to negotiate the provision of mental health and drug abuse services with health maintenance organizations (HMOs). To ensure that patients receive the right kind of care at the right level for their individual needs, all treatment is managed in accordance with clinical protocols and criteria, negating the need for arbitrary limits on these services.

8.4.2.1. Defining Medical Necessity

According to workshop attendees, whether or not a particular health service is considered medically necessary determines whether or not it is covered by health insurance plans. Some contended that there are ambiguities in this term and that it can have multiple meanings. Medical necessity, which is sometimes used interchangeably with medical appropriateness, is defined by the IOM (1993a) as the need for a particular medical service based on clinical expectations that the health benefits will outweigh the health risks. However, as was mentioned during the workshop, the legal definition of "medical necessity" frequently works to restrict a health plan's contractual duty to a beneficiary. The decision-making standards that health plans employ to ascertain medical necessity are not specified in standard clauses in health insurance contracts. A limited interpretation of medical necessity by certain insurers and health plans may result in the limitation or exclusion of certain services that could have more extensive health benefits.

Narrow interpretations of medical necessity may place special restrictions on care for everyone, not just women and children. The creation of a pediatric standard of care may help to alleviate this issue for kids. A distinct pediatric standard is justified by three key distinctions between adults and children: (1) developmental vulnerability. (2) Dependency; and (3) Illness and Injury Patterns. A pediatric coverage standard should enable a fair assessment of the cost of a service in relation to what is medically necessary, as was discussed at the workshop. A list of healthcare services that plans should offer to children would be part of the standard of care, along with a requirement that the extent and duration of those services be in line with the development and growth of the children, their status as dependents, their level of risk, and best clinical practices.

8.4.3. Coordinated Healthcare Services for Women and Children

The workshop participants reached the consensus that a coordinated and collaborative approach is necessary for healthcare reform, particularly for programs that support maternal and child health, as many of the outdated models for delivering healthcare are no longer suitable. The entire spectrum of health services required by women and children cannot be efficiently provided by either the public health system or the current system for delivering traditional personal health services. For example, public health services have not traditionally focused on personal health services, which include the diagnosis and treatment of the majority of medical illnesses. Personal health services are also limited in their ability to manage socioeconomic threats to health, violence, or homelessness. To prevent and monitor health problems, workshop participants suggested that effective systems of care ensure collaboration between medical services and programs related to education, nutrition, welfare, and public health. A combination of community-based education and nutrition programs before and early in pregnancy, medical and monitoring services during pregnancy, sufficient social support during and after pregnancy, and access to specialized, technologically advanced services for high-risk pregnancies and community-based services for normal and high-risk pregnancies, for instance, is necessary to ensure optimal pregnancy outcomes. As a result, a lot of people believe that to guarantee comprehensive healthcare, cooperation between the public health system and providers of personal health services will be required. For instance, adding school health services, counseling, and enabling services like case management and recurring home visits may increase the efficacy of standard pediatric care provided in a doctor's office.

8.4.3.1. Access to Healthcare

Although having insurance coverage is often seen as a way to access healthcare, it does not guarantee that individuals in need will actually receive the services they require, access refers to the ability of individuals and groups to obtain necessary medical services. Despite an increase in the number of physicians in recent years, few are located in rural or inner city areas and many are hesitant to accept Medicaid patients. This lack of accessibility has created obstacles for low-income and uninsured women and children, leading them to rely more heavily on community healthcare providers like hospital clinics, public health clinics, and community and migrant health centers.

8.4.3.2. Managed-Care Organizations

The primary driving force behind healthcare reform in the United States was the need to control costs for medical services. In this regard, managed care has been proposed as a means of enhancing access and preserving the standard of care while reducing the rate of increase in medical expenses. Over the past few years, there has been a significant increase in both public and private sector participation in managed care plans. In fact, many states have made it mandatory for Medicaid recipients to enroll in managed care plans. Regardless of how healthcare reform advances, managed care is here to stay, according to workshop participants, and its existence affects vulnerable populations' access to necessary healthcare services. Public or private managed care programs are unlikely to expand to include comprehensive treatment services for high-risk populations outside of those covered by the health plan, nor to create community-based preventive services like social work. The significance of the public health sector's role in guaranteeing women's and children's access to a wide array of programs that support their proper growth, development, and health was emphasized by the participants. Significant questions were raised regarding how managed care would affect Medicaid recipients. A few attendees of the workshop pointed out that Medicaid patients may have less access to healthcare services due to managed care, especially since referrals are restricted. Participants in the workshop recommended that the federal government take these factors into account when deciding whether to waive Medicaid.

8.4.3.3. Public Programs for Maternal and Child Health

Medicaid, the maternal and child health programs of Title V of the Social Security Act (which provides services to low-income women and children, including children with special healthcare needs), the Supplemental Food Program for Women, Infants, and Children, and the federal family planning program of Title X of the Public Health Service Act are just a few examples of federal and state public health programs that support women and children. Community-based preventive care programs, as well as migrant and community health centers, are other pertinent public health initiatives (i.e., vaccination campaigns, and initiatives to prevent lead poisoning) supported by the Centers for Disease Control. Participants in the workshop voiced grave concerns, saying that the services currently offered by programs for maternal and child health should not be compromised by healthcare reform.

The current proposals to reshape the healthcare system will result in significant changes to many long-standing public health initiatives. The long-term implications of the suggested modifications on these programs and the populations they serve, however, are not at all evident. Specifically, it is unclear how the managed care organizations that many reform plans propose will interact with the public health programs. It is obvious that some work needs to go into figuring out how these numerous disparate parts will work together under a redesigned system and whether or not this new set of programs will be sufficiently sensitive to the needs of women and children. The participants in the workshop expressed the significance of maternal and child health programs within the framework of all-encompassing healthcare reform. The participants endeavored to delineate the requisite components and frameworks for maternal and child health initiatives that supplement the services offered by managed care schemes or alternative avenues for direct medical attention.

Participants in the workshop suggested that in addition to more conventional medical techniques, the design of successful health promotion or primary prevention programs will frequently call for extensive environmental and social interventions. Medical care can lessen some of the negative health effects and make it easier to access a range of other services that can support children's development and health, even though it cannot solve social and environmental issues. Healthcare providers might offer certain services, while public health organizations might offer others. Public health organizations frequently receive funding from the federal government in the form of Maternal and Child Health Block Grants. Education and services provided in schools also have a significant impact on a child's development and well-being. Programs for preventing injuries, family violence, and the harmful effects of the environment are examples of community-wide prevention initiatives that go beyond the confines of the clinical setting. (i.e., lead). Family-centered care may make it more likely that kids will have sufficient access to preventive medical care.

Participants proposed that home visiting programs, which offer family-centered care, could be one means of guaranteeing children's sufficient access to preventive care. Typically, a home visiting program starts when a woman is pregnant and lasts for the first two years of her child's life. Home visiting programs have demonstrated efficacy in providing infant health and development programs, mental health services, and other preventive health services to children and their families. Children with developmental delays and ongoing medical needs, as well as at-risk parents—such as those who are young, unmarried, poor, and illiterate—have been the main beneficiaries of these programs.

A few states are creating integrated strategies to address women's and children's healthcare needs more effectively. According to workshop attendees, some states have merged financing and care sources to develop better mental health initiatives for kids and teenagers. For example, Minnesota recently enacted an integrated funding law that permits local agencies to combine public funds from the local level and match those funds with Medicaid funds to create mental health programs for children. Ohio is redesigning its Medicaid program to provide health benefits to underserved populations under a new initiative called Ohio Care.

Participants in the workshop reached the following consensus: cooperation between public health and providers of personal health services will be required to guarantee the availability of comprehensive healthcare for women and children; the current public health system can facilitate the integration and coordination of maternal and child health programs. In the wake of healthcare reform, the public health system would be able to track providers' adherence to care standards, look into cases of unwarranted morbidity, and gather and evaluate data on population-based outcomes related to maternal and child health. Together with facilitating and supporting community outreach and interactions between healthcare, education, and social support agencies, the public health system could also suggest priorities for services to families.

A viewpoint that was discussed during the workshop is that it should be the duty of the public health system to guarantee that all women and children have access to primary and preventive healthcare. The public health system may still need to provide healthcare to children and families who are not served by the private healthcare system, even though it is not always necessary to do so directly. A few workshop attendees believed that the federal program for mother and child health could be improved by giving it more administrative visibility and support in developing policies by establishing a national advisory board. While the U.S. healthcare system changes, it will be necessary to reorganize the components intended for women and children before the system can function as intended.

Participants in the workshop came to the conclusion that developing a new vision that prioritizes programs for women and children as well as defining a plan to implement this vision to enhance and progress their healthcare should be top priorities for the maternal and child health community. After the national health insurance debate is over, federal leadership can assist in establishing clinical guidelines for the whole field of maternity and child health. To ensure that women and children receive the greatest care possible, federal leadership should also encourage innovative redesign and improvement initiatives that would combine public and private health programs.

A Closer Look

Childbirth

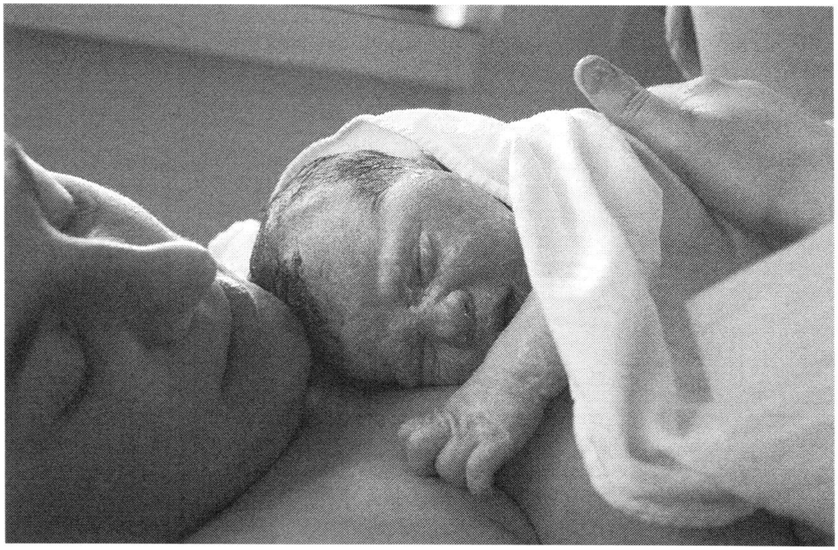

Source: By Tom Adriaenssen – https://www.flickr.com/photos/inferis/110652572/, CC BY-SA 2.0, https://commons.wikimedia.org/w/index.php?curid=639667.

Three phases of labor precede and follow childbirth: the dilation, expulsion, and placental phases. Every woman gives birth in a different amount of time. Each childbirth experience is unique, as are the beginnings of labor and delivery. Since every birth is unique, having a second child might not be the same as the first. The majority of births occur naturally, or spontaneously, between weeks 37 and 42 of pregnancy. Although the uterus, or womb, usually begins to tighten and cause contractions to occur, there may be other indications that labor is about to begin. Painful cramps that last 45 to 60 seconds and occur more frequently than every 10 minutes are called contractions.

As labor advances, contractions become more frequent, intense, and last longer than they did at first—typically occurring several minutes apart. The majority of women experience lower back and/or lower abdomen pain. When your contractions are regular, or about five to six minutes apart, time them and call the hospital or unit. When the contractions begin, call the hospital if you're worried, far from the hospital, have given birth quickly in the past, or have experienced problems with prior pregnancies or deliveries. As soon as labor begins, the pressure from the contractions causes your cervix to start slipping to the sides, giving your baby more room to pass through the birth canal.

The birth canal consists of:

- The pelvis – the bony part of the birth canal;
- The muscles in the pelvis;
- The vagina – the soft part of the birth canal.

Because of its funnel-shaped structure, the pelvis's dimensions vary depending on the level of the pelvis. This implies that for the baby to adjust and pass through the pelvis during labor, it must rotate slightly. The dilation, expulsion, and placental stages are the three phases of labor. The placental stage takes anywhere from a few minutes to as long as 60 minutes, while the dilation (opening) stage is the longest. The expulsion (pushing out) stage lasts between 30 and 60 minutes.

Various factors influence how long it takes to give birth:

- Whether you've given birth before or not. Giving birth to a first baby usually takes the longest.
- The frequency and effectiveness of your contractions influence how long the labor lasts. Regular and effective contractions are all-important for good progress; the contractions push the baby down into the pelvis and the cervix (neck of the womb) opens.
- Active labor in first-time mothers lasts 4 to 16 hours. For women who have given birth before, labor usually lasts 2 to 11 hours. This varies from woman to woman and from birth to birth.

The "dilation stage" is the initial phase of labor. At this point, in order for the baby to descend into the pelvis and be delivered, the cervix, or neck of the womb, must pull to each side and open. The cervix becomes fully dilated, opening up to 10 cm from its closed state. Delivery is not possible until the cervix is fully dilated. The "bloody show," or some blood-tinged vaginal discharge, occurs as the cervix dilates. This indicates that the pressure from the baby's head and the contractions are causing the cervix to dilate. Although it can happen at any point during labor, the active phase of the dilation stage is typically when your waters break.

The latent phase, which precedes the dilation stage, is the longest stage of labor. When your contractions are consistent and occur less than 10 minutes apart, you enter this phase. At first, the contractions are quite far apart, but as time goes on, they become stronger and occur more frequently. The active phase of labor begins when the cervix dilates by approximately 4–5 centimeters. The cervix dilates (opens) more quickly as the contractions become more powerful. The midwife feels your belly to gauge the intensity of your contractions to monitor the progress of labor. The midwife can examine the baby's head position in the birth canal and the cervix's degree of dilation by performing an internal exam. Throughout labor, it is normal to undergo examinations multiple times; you will be made aware of this prior to the procedure. Additionally, the midwife will update you on the status of your labor.

It's important to alternate between activity and rest during the dilation phase. The baby rotates and passes through the pelvis with the assistance of the mother's movement and activity. Additionally, most women report that having an active contraction is less painful than having a stationary contraction while in bed. The midwife will assist you in transitioning between active living and comfortable resting positions. One of the midwife's primary responsibilities during the dilation stage is to assist you in finding positions that facilitate your baby's descent through the pelvis and birth canal. The midwife advises you to continue moving and using gravity's force while also relaxing your body at this point in the labor process. It takes a lot of energy to work. Thus, you must increase your body's energy levels by consuming liquids and small meals. They'll give you some food and beverages.

From this point on, you will use every contraction to force your baby out. You will be pushing your baby down into your vagina and out with each contraction, combined with the force of the contractions. Finding birthing positions that let you rest in between contractions and push when the next one comes will be necessary. During this stage of labor, switching up your birthing positions can often be beneficial. This facilitates your baby's pelvic rotation and descent. The midwife will assist you in finding comfortable birthing positions that will facilitate the progress of labor.

The head and body of the baby are almost ready to be delivered; the midwife will advise you on how to push at that point. To ensure that the birth is as gentle as possible for the baby and to avoid you crying, you and the midwife will now need to collaborate. The tissue (peritoneum) between your vagina and anus will be supported by the midwife while the head and body of the baby are being born.

Summary

- Community health nurses are valued for their adaptability and willingness to provide care in many settings, including community health clinics, churches, homeless shelters, and schools.
- The health of mothers and children is interrelated and affected by multiple factors. Millions of pregnant women, new mothers, and children experience severe illness or death each year, largely from preventable or treatable causes.
- Epidemiology is the "study of the distribution and determinants of health-related states in specified populations, and the application of this study to control health problems".
- An epidemic investigation describes the factors relevant to an outbreak of disease; once the circumstances related to the occurrence of disease are defined, appropriate control and prevention measures can be identified.
- Humanitarian emergencies are natural disasters, man-made events or a combination of both that represent critical threats to the health, safety, security or wellbeing of a community.
- Participants in the workshop agreed that many old models for health care delivery are no longer adequate and that health care reform needs to promote a coordinated and collaborative approach, especially for maternal and child health programs.
- Community health nurses work in many different locations with many different populations. Depending on where they work, community health nurses might have more or less direct contact with individual members of the community.

References

1. Ager, A., Stark, L., Akesson, B., & Boothby, N. (2010). Defining best practice in care and protection of children in crisis-affected settings: A Delphi study. *Child Development, 81*(4), 1271–1286.
2. Al Gasseer, N., Dresden, E., Keeney, G. B., & Warren, N. (2004). Status of women and infants in complex humanitarian emergencies. *Journal of Midwifery & Women's Health, 49*(4 Suppl 1), 7–13.
3. Annas, G. J. (2010). Standard of care-in sickness and in health and in emergencies. *New England Journal of Medicine, 362*, 2126–2131.
4. Carballo, M., Hernandez, M., Schneider, K., & Welle, E. (2005). Impact of the tsunami on reproductive health. *Journal of the Royal Society of Medicine, 98*, 400–403.
5. Committee on Health Care for Underserved Women, authors. (2010). Preparing for Disasters: Perspectives on Women. Washington, DC: American College of Obstetricians and Gynecologists. (Committee Opinion 457).
6. Harville, E., Xiong, X., & Buekens, P. (2010). Disasters and perinatal health: A systematic review. *Obstetric Gynecology Survey, 65*(11), 713–728.
7. Last, J. M. (Ed.). (2001). *Dictionary of Epidemiology* (4th ed.). New York: Oxford University Press.

8. Lederman, S. A., Rauh, V., Weiss, L., et al. (2004). The effects of the World Trade Center event on birth outcomes among term deliveries at three lower Manhattan hospitals. *Environmental Health Perspectives, 112*, 1772–1778.
9. Pyone, Dickinson, Kerr et.al. (2015). Data collection tools for maternal and child health in humanitarian emergencies: A systematic review. Geneva: World Health Organization. http://www.who.int/bulletin/volumes/93/9/14-148429/en/ (accessed on 17 May 2024).
10. Sapir, D. G. (1993). Natural and man-made disasters: The vulnerability of women-headed households and children without families. *World Health Statistics Quarterly*, 46, 227–233.
11. The deadliest U.S. Hurricanes. Tropical Weather.net Website. Retrieved February 25, 2011, from http://www.tropicalweather.net/deadliest_U.S._hurricanes.htm (accessed on 17 May 2024).
12. Thornton, W. E., & Voigt, L. (2007). Disaster rape: Vulnerability of women to sexual assaults during Hurricane Katrina. *Journal of Public Management & Social Policy*, 13, 23–49.
13. United Nations High Commissioner for Refugees (UNHCR), authors. (2001). Prevention and response to sexual and gender-based violence in refugee situations: Inter-agency lessons learned conference proceedings (27–29 March 2001—Geneva). Geneva: UNHCR. Retrieved February 25, 2011, from http://action.web.ca/home/cpcc/attach/prevention%20and%20responses.pdf (accessed on 17 May 2024).
14. Vos, F., Rodriguez, J., Below, R., & Guha-Sapir, D. (2010). Annual Disaster Statistical Review 2009: The numbers and trends. Brussels: Centre for research on the epidemiology of disasters. Retrieved February 25, 2011, from http://cred.be/sites/default/files/ADSR_2009.pdf (accessed on 17 May 2024).
15. World Health Organization (WHO). Department of Gender and Women's Health, authors. (2002). Gender and health in disasters. Geneva: WHO. Retrieved February 25, 2011, from http://www.who.int/gender/other_health/en/genderdisasters.pdf (accessed on 17 May 2024).
16. World Health Organization (WHO). Department of Injuries and Violence Prevention, authors. (2005). Violence and disasters. Geneva: WHO. Retrieved February 25, 2011, from http://www.who.int/violence_injury_prevention/publications/violence/violence_disasters.pdf (accessed on 17 May 2024).

Chapter 9

CHILD MALTREATMENT

Contents

Unit Introduction 284
9.1. Abuse and Neglect: Scope of the Problem 286
9.2. Classification of Child Maltreatment 289
9.3. Symptoms and Signs of Child Maltreatment 292
9.4. Treatment of Child Maltreatment 296
9.5. Prevention of Child Maltreatment 298
Summary 309
References 309

Unit Introduction

Maltreatment of children under the age of 18 is defined as abuse and neglect. In the context of a relationship involving responsibility, trust, or power, it encompasses all forms of physical and/or emotional abuse, sexual abuse, neglect, carelessness, and commercial or other exploitation that actually or potentially endangers the child's health, survival, development, or dignity.

The term "child maltreatment" describes the mistreatment, abuse, or neglect of children and includes a wide range of negative behaviors that can have a severe and enduring impact on a child's mental, emotional, and physical health. This is a serious global issue that crosses cultural, social, and economic boundaries. It can take many different forms, such as neglect, emotional, sexual, or physical abuse. When a child is purposefully subjected to physical abuse, such as hitting, punching, kicking, or burning, this is referred to as physical abuse. Although this type of abuse frequently results in visible wounds, it can also cause internal trauma, fractures, or other health problems. Any kind of sexual exploitation or coercion against a child, such as rape, molestation, or exposure to pornography, is considered sexual abuse. Sexual abuse can leave children with severe and long-lasting psychological wounds that impact their relationships, mental health, and sense of self. Psychological abuse, also known as emotional abuse, includes actions that damage a child's self-esteem, like unrelenting rejection, ridicule, or criticism. A child's emotional development may be seriously harmed by this type of abuse, which may result in anxiety, depression, or behavioral issues. Neglect, which is commonly defined as the inability to meet a child's fundamental needs, such as clothing, food, shelter, and medical attention, can be caused by a number of things, such as parental mental health problems, substance abuse, or poverty. Children who are neglected may experience malnourishment, poor personal hygiene, or untreated medical conditions.

Abuse of children has long-lasting and complex effects that continue into adolescence and adulthood. Maltreatment survivors are more likely to experience difficulties with their physical and mental health, substance abuse, and establishing and maintaining healthy relationships. Moreover, victims of abuse may find it difficult to parent or may revert to the same patterns of behavior that they encountered as children, which can cause the cycle of abuse to continue into subsequent generations. A multifaceted strategy that includes support services, intervention, and prevention is needed to address child abuse. This involves bringing attention to the issue, encouraging good parenting techniques, fortifying child safety protocols, and offering easily accessible resources to low-income families. Communities can work toward ending the cycle of abuse and establishing a nurturing environment where every child can thrive by placing a high priority on the safety and well-being of children.

Orientation and Directional Terms

Term	Definition	Illustration
Sexual abuse	**Sexual abuse** or sex abuse is abusive sexual behavior by one person upon another.	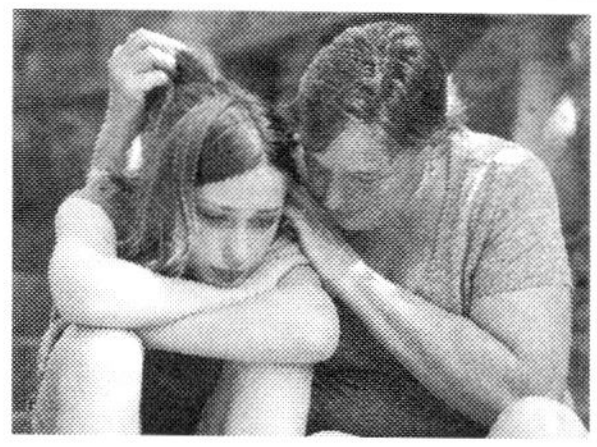
Anxiety	Anxiety is a feeling of fear, dread, or uneasiness that can be a normal reaction to stress.	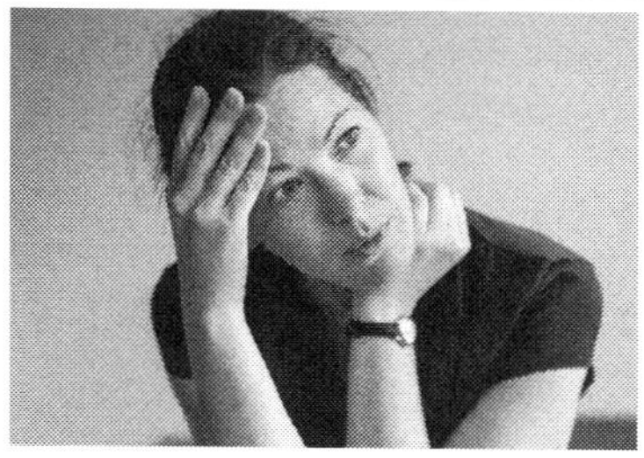
Gynecological disorders	**Gynecologic diseases** in general are diseases that involved the female reproductive track.	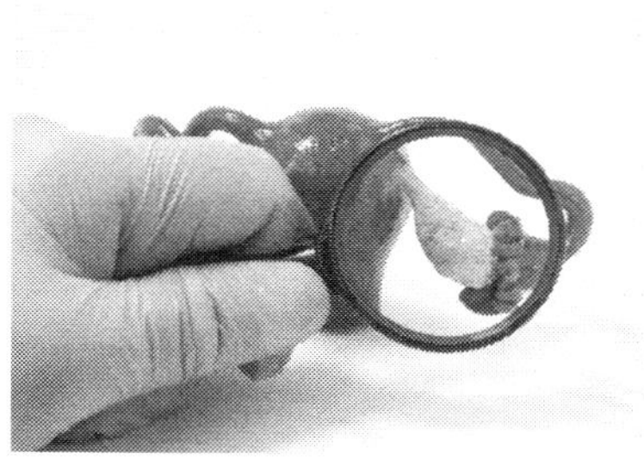
Multifaceted Strategy	A multifaceted strategy is a combination of two or more elements that can be used to address multiple barriers or goals.	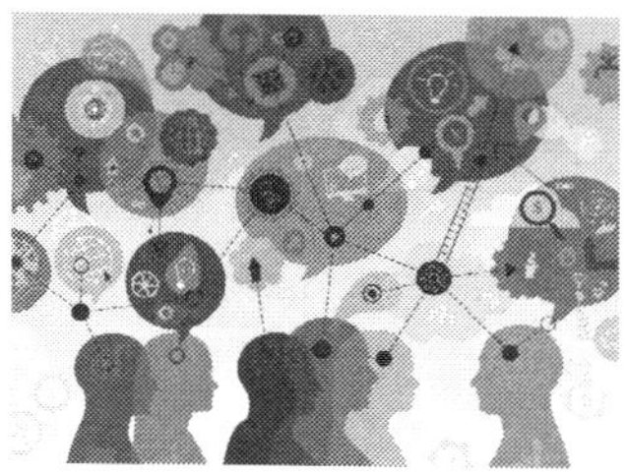
Physical abuse	Physical abuse is any intentional act causing injury or trauma to another person or animal by way of bodily contact.	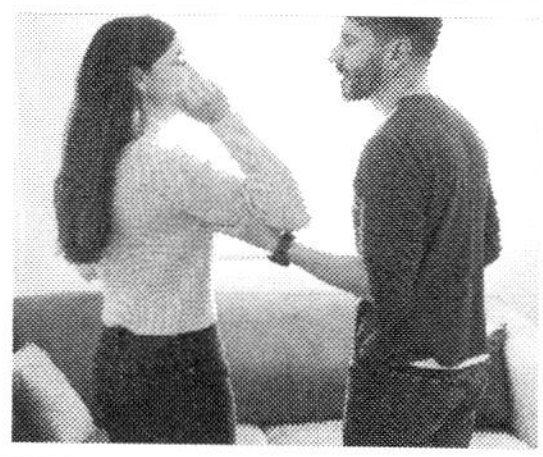

9.1. Abuse and Neglect: Scope of the Problem

Maltreatment of children is a worldwide issue that has detrimental long-term effects. Several low- and middle-income countries have conducted national surveys recently, but data from many other countries are still missing. It is challenging and complex to research child abuse. The current estimates differ significantly based on the nation and the research methodology.

Estimates depend on:

- the definitions of child maltreatment used;
- the type of child maltreatment studied;
- the coverage and quality of official statistics;
- the coverage and quality of surveys that request self-reports from victims, parents or caregivers (Figure 9.1).

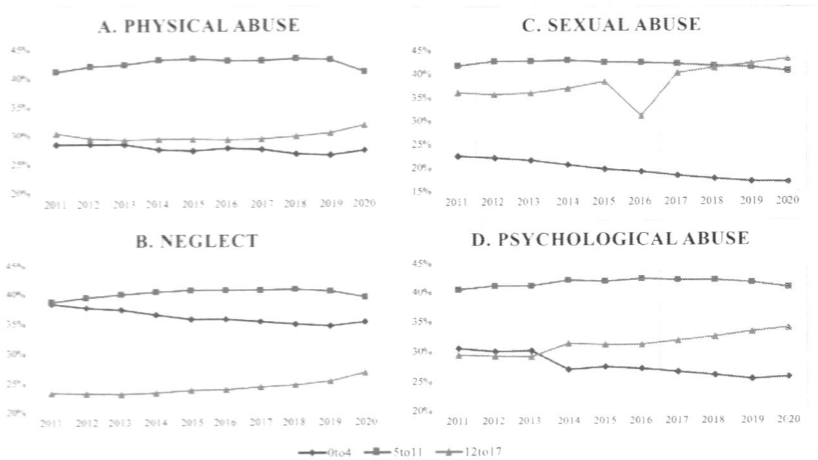

Figure 9.1. *Prevalence of subtypes of maltreatment by age group between 2011 and 2020.*

Source: *Guastaferro, K., & Shipe, S. L., (2024). Child maltreatment types by age: Implications for prevention. International Journal of Environmental Research and Public Health, 21(1), 20. https://doi.org/10.3390/ijerph21010020.*

International studies, however, show that 1 in 5 women and 1 in 13 men report having experienced sexual abuse as children, and nearly 3 out of 4 children between the ages of 2–4 years regularly endure physical punishment and/or psychological violence at the hands of parents and caregivers. An estimated 40,150 children under the age of 18 die from homicide each year, some of which are probably the result of maltreatment of the children. This figure most likely understates the actual scope of the issue because a sizable percentage of child abuse-related deaths are mistakenly linked to falls, burns, drownings, and other incidents. Girls are especially vulnerable to sexual violence, exploitation, and abuse by combatants, security forces, community members, aid workers, and others in armed conflict and refugee settings.

9.1.1. Consequences of Maltreatment

Abuse of children can have serious short- and long-term effects on one's physical, sexual, and mental health. These include physical harm, such as concussions and severe disabilities, especially in young children; psychological distress; anxiety; depression; and STIs, such as HIV. Adolescent girls may experience other health problems, such as unintended pregnancy and gynecological disorders. Child abuse is linked to smoking, alcoholism, and drug addiction, all of which are major risk factors for non-communicable diseases (NCDs) like cancer and cardiovascular disease. It can also have an impact on cognitive and academic performance.

Maltreatment causes stress that is associated with disruption in early brain development. Extreme stress can impair the development of the nervous and immune systems. Consequently, as adults, maltreated children are at increased risk for behavioral, physical and mental health problems such as:

- Perpetrating or being a victim of violence;
- Depression;
- Smoking;
- Obesity;
- High-risk sexual behaviors;
- Unintended pregnancy;
- Alcohol and drug misuse.

Education disparities are also a result of violence against children. Children who were exposed to violence as young children are 13% more likely to drop out of school. Child abuse has an economic impact in addition to negative effects on health, society, and education. This impact includes hospitalization, mental health treatment, child welfare, and long-term health costs.

9.1.2. Risk Factors

There are several known risk factors for child abuse. When trying to understand the causes of child maltreatment, the list below offers a general overview as not all risk factors are present in all social and cultural contexts.

9.1.3. Child

It is important to emphasize that children are the victims and are never to blame for maltreatment. Characteristics of an individual child that may increase the likelihood of being maltreated include:

- being either under four years old or an adolescent;
- being unwanted, or failing to fulfil the expectations of parents;
- having special needs, crying persistently or having abnormal physical features;
- having an intellectual disability or neurological disorder;
- identifying as or being identified as lesbian, gay, bisexual or transgender.

9.1.4. Parent or Caregiver

Characteristics of a parent or caregiver that may increase the risk of child maltreatment include:

- Difficulty bonding with a newborn;
- Not nurturing the child;
- Having been maltreated themselves as a child;
- Lacking awareness of child development or having unrealistic expectations;
- Misusing alcohol or drugs, including during pregnancy;
- Having low self-esteem;
- Suffering from poor impulse control;
- Having a mental or neurological disorder;
- Being involved in criminal activity;
- Experiencing financial difficulties.

9.1.5. Relationship

Characteristics of the relationships within families or among intimate partners, friends and peers that may increase the risk of child maltreatment include:

- Family breakdown or violence between other family members;
- Being isolated in the community or lacking a support network;
- A breakdown of support in child rearing from the extended family.

9.1.6. Community and Societal Factors

Characteristics of communities and societies that may increase the risk of child maltreatment include:

- Gender and social inequality;
- Lack of adequate housing or services to support families and institutions;
- High levels of unemployment or poverty;
- The easy availability of alcohol and drugs;
- Inadequate policies and programmers to prevent child maltreatment, child pornography, child prostitution and child labor;
- Social and cultural norms that promote or glorify violence towards others, support the use of corporal punishment, demand rigid gender roles, or diminish the status of the child in parent–child relationships;
- Social, economic, health and education policies that lead to poor living standards, or to socioeconomic inequality or instability.

9.1.7. Prevention

A multifaceted strategy is needed to both prevent and address child abuse. The advantages to the child of receiving such interventions increase with the earlier they happen in their lives (e.g., cognitive growth, social and behavioral skills, level of education attained) and to society (e.g., decreased crime and delinquency).

Effective and promising interventions include:

- **Parent and Caregiver Support:** Information and skill-building sessions to support the development of nurturing, non-violent parenting delivered by nurses, social workers, or trained lay workers through a series of home visits or in a community setting.
- Education and life skills approaches include the following:
- Increasing enrolment in quality education to allow children acquire knowledge, skills and experiences that build resilience and reduce risk factors for violence

- Programmed to prevent sexual abuse that builds awareness and teach skills to help children and adolescents understand consent, avoid and prevent sexual abuse and exploitation, and to seek help and support
- Interventions to build a positive school climate and violence-free environment, and strengthen relationships between students, teachers, and administrators
  - **Norms and values Approaches:** Programmed to transform restrictive and harmful gender and social norms around child-rearing, child discipline and gender equality and promote the nurturing role of fathers
  - **Implementation and Enforcement of Laws:** Laws to prohibit violent punishment and to protect children from sexual abuse and exploitation.
  - **Response and Support Services:** Early case recognition coupled with ongoing care of child victims and families to help reduce the reoccurrence of maltreatment and lessen its consequences.

To maximize the effects of prevention and care, WHO recommends that interventions are delivered as part of a four-step public health approach:

- Defining the problem;
- Identifying causes and risk factors;
- Designing and testing interventions aimed at minimizing the risk factors;
- Disseminating information about the effectiveness of interventions and increasing the scale of proven effective interventions.

9.1.8. WHO Response

WHO, in collaboration with partners:

- Guides evidence-based child maltreatment prevention; see INSPIRE Seven strategies to end violence against children.
- Provides evidence-based guidance to help frontline healthcare providers recognize children who have suffered from violence and neglect and provide evidence-based first-line support; one can refer to "Child maltreatment: a Clinical Handbook for Health Professionals."
- Advocates for increased international support for and investment in evidence-based child maltreatment prevention.
- Provides technical support for evidence-based child maltreatment prevention programs in several low- and middle-income countries.

9.2. Classification of Child Maltreatment

Different forms of maltreatment often coexist, and overlap is considerable. The 4 main forms include:

- Physical abuse;
- Sexual abuse;
- Emotional abuse;
- Neglect.

Furthermore, it is deemed abuse (child abuse in a medical setting) when a child's medical symptoms are purposefully faked, inflated, or feigned to justify potentially harmful medical interventions.

9.2.1. Physical Abuse

When a caregiver physically abuses a patient or engages in behaviors that put the patient at risk for harm, this is considered physical abuse. Child abuse does not specifically refer to assault by a person who is not the child's caregiver or someone in a position of authority (such as a shooter in a school mass shooting). Shaking, dropping, striking, biting, and burning (e.g., by touching or scalding with cigarettes) are examples of specific forms.

The developmental stages that infants and toddlers may experience—such as colic, irregular sleep patterns, tantrums, and toilet training—may irritate caregivers, making them the most vulnerable. Because they are unable to report their abuse, this age group is also more vulnerable. The most frequent reason why infants sustain significant head injuries is abuse. Abdominal injuries are also common in toddlers. Due to their smaller heads compared to their bodies and their weaker neck muscles, children in these age groups are also more likely to suffer brain and spine injuries.

9.2.2. Sexual Abuse

Sexual abuse occurs when a child is used for the erotic pleasure of an adult or a child who is significantly older (either chronologically or developmentally) (Pedophilic Disorder). State-by-state regulations distinguishing sexual abuse from play differ, but generally speaking, it is deemed inappropriate for people who are > 4-years apart in terms of age (either chronologically or in terms of mental or physical development) to have sex.

Forms of sexual abuse include

- Intercourse, which is oral, anal, or vaginal penetration;
- Molestation, which is genital contact without intercourse;
- Forms that do not involve physical contact by the perpetrator, including exposure of the perpetrator's genitals, showing sexually explicit material to a child, sexting with or posting pictures of a child, and forcing a child to participate in a sex act with another person or to participate in the production of sexual material.

Sexual play, in which young children of similar ages and developmental stages observe or touch each other's genital areas freely, is not considered sexual abuse.

9.2.3. Emotional Abuse

Emotional abuse is inflicting emotional harm through the use of words or actions. Specific forms include:

- Berating a child by yelling or screaming;
- Spurning by belittling the child's abilities and achievements;
- Intimidating and terrorizing with threats;
- Exploiting or corrupting by encouraging deviant or criminal behavior.

In addition, emotional abuse can also take the form of emotional neglect when words or deeds are withheld or ignored (e.g., ignoring or rejecting children or isolating them from interaction with other children or adults).

9.2.4. Neglect

Neglect is the failure to provide for or meet a child's basic physical, emotional, educational, and medical needs. Neglect differs from abuse in that it usually occurs without intent to harm.

Different types of neglect can be defined as:

- Physical neglect includes failure to provide adequate food, clothing, shelter, supervision, and protection from potential harm.
- Emotional neglect is failure to provide affection or love or other kinds of emotional support.
- Educational neglect is failure to enroll a child in school, ensure attendance at school, or provide home schooling.
- Medical neglect is failure to ensure that a child receives appropriate care or needed treatment for injuries or physical or mental disorders.

However, failure to provide preventive care (e.g., vaccinations, routine dental examinations) is not usually considered neglect.

9.2.5. Special Considerations

1. **Child Abuse in a Medical Setting:** In a medical setting, child abuse happens when caregivers purposefully cause or fabricate a child's physical or psychological symptoms or indicators. To mimic illness, caregivers may harm the child with drugs or other substances or contaminate urine samples with bacteria or blood. This kind of child abuse results in needless, harmful, or possibly harmful assessments, tests, and/or treatments, such as operations or surgeries, for the victims.
2. **Cultural Factors:** While severe forms of corporal punishment (such as beatings, burnings, and scaldings) are unquestionably abusive, different cultures have different boundaries between acceptable behavior and abuse when it comes to milder forms of physical and psychological reprimands. Similarly, culturally acceptable practices (like female genital mutilation) are considered abuse in the United States. Nevertheless, some traditional treatments (such as coining, cupping, irritant poultices) can result in lesions (such as bruises, petechiae, or small burns) that raise questions about what constitutes appropriate cultural behavior or misuse.

Sometimes, members of particular religious groups have neglected to get children treated for conditions like meningitis or diabetic ketoacidosis, which can be fatal. It doesn't matter what the parents or other caregivers think; this kind of failure is usually regarded as neglect. Furthermore, some parents in the US refuse to vaccinate their children due to safety concerns (Vaccine Hesitancy). It's unclear if this vaccination refusal represents actual medical neglect. However, when faced with illness, declining to receive medically recommended treatment occasionally necessitates additional research and legal action.

9.2.6. Etiology of Child Maltreatment

1. **Abuse:** Abuse is often a result of a lack of impulse control in a parent or caregiver, influenced by various factors such as parental characteristics, upbringing, and personal experiences. Parents who have not received affection or emotional support in their own

childhood may struggle to provide the same for their own children. This can lead to unrealistic expectations, frustration, and poor impulse control, as they seek to fulfill their own unmet needs through their children. Substance abuse and untreated mental health disorders can further exacerbate these behaviors and increase the risk of maltreatment.

With children who have special needs and/or challenging behaviors, a parent may more easily and frequently reach their breaking point and resort to abusive actions. This lack of bonding is more common in sick or premature babies who are taken from their parents at a young age, as well as in biologically unrelated children (stepchildren, for example), which raises the possibility of abuse. Abuse may arise as a result of situational stress, especially if peers, neighbors, family, or other emotional support is not available. Abuse of any kind, including sexual abuse, affects people from a wide range of socioeconomic backgrounds. Risk is raised by socioeconomic stress (e.g., financial strain, social isolation, young or single parenthood). Abuse on all fronts—physical, emotional, and neglectful—has been linked to poverty and a lower social standing.

2. **Neglect:** A multitude of factors, including parenting challenges, inadequate coping mechanisms, dysfunctional family structures, and stressful life events, frequently culminate in neglect. Families under financial and environmental stress are more likely to experience neglect, especially if one or both parents suffer from an untreated mental illness (usually depression, anxiety, bipolar disorder, or schizophrenia), abuse drugs, or are intellectually disabled. Single-parent households may have fewer resources and a lower income, which puts their children at risk of neglect.

9.3. Symptoms and Signs of Child Maltreatment

Symptoms and signs depend on the nature and duration of the abuse or neglect.

9.3.1. Physical Abuse

Skin lesions are the most common findings. Skin findings are usually subtle (e.g., a small bruise, petechiae on the face and/or neck).

More severe findings may include:

- Handprints or oval fingertip marks caused by slapping or grabbing and shaking.
- Long, bandlike ecchymoses caused by belt whipping.
- Narrow arcuate bruises caused by extension cord whipping.
- Multiple small, round burns caused by cigarettes.
- Symmetric scald burns of upper or lower extremities or buttocks caused by intentional immersion.
- Bite marks.
- Thickened skin or scarring at the corners of the mouth caused by being gagged.
- Patchy alopecia, with varying hair lengths, caused by hair pulling.

Fractures that often indicate physical abuse include metaphyseal lesions, rib fractures, and spinous process fractures. Skull fractures, long bone fractures, and rib fractures are commonly associated with physical abuse. In children < 1 year old, about 75% of fractures are inflicted by others.

Central nervous system injuries can lead to confusion and localized neurologic abnormalities. Traumatic brain injury, especially in infants who have been shaken violently, may not always have visible head injuries. These infants may exhibit symptoms such as comatose or stuporous behavior, retinal hemorrhage, fussiness, and vomiting. Traumatic injuries to organs in the chest or abdominal/pelvic area may also occur without visible signs.

Older kids who experience abuse on a regular basis tend to be fearful, agitated, and have trouble sleeping. They might exhibit signs of anxiety, post-traumatic stress disorder, or depression. Abuse victims can occasionally exhibit symptoms that are mistakenly diagnosed as attention-deficit/hyperactivity disorder (ADHD). Suicidal or violent behavior is possible.

9.3.2. Sexual Abuse

Children rarely come forward on their own to report sexual abuse, and they also don't always show outwardly visible behavioral or physical indicators of it. If a disclosure is made, it is typically done so after a delay of days or even years. Abrupt or drastic behavioral changes may happen occasionally. Phobias or sleep disturbances may emerge, along with aggressiveness or withdrawal. Certain behaviors displayed by children who have experienced sexual abuse are not appropriate for their age.

Physical signs of sexual abuse that involves penetration may include:

- Difficulty walking or sitting;
- Bruises or tears around the genitals, anus, or mouth;
- Vaginal discharge, bleeding, or pruritus.

Pregnancy or a sexually transmitted infection are two more signs. Examining the mouth, anus, and genitalia a few days after the abuse will probably reveal no abnormalities, but the examiner might notice healed lesions or minor alterations.

9.3.2.1. Emotional Abuse

Emotional abuse during the early years of life can stifle emotional expressiveness and reduce curiosity about the surroundings. Emotional abuse frequently leads to underdevelopment and is mistakenly identified as a physical ailment or intellectual disability. Inadequate parental engagement and stimulation may be the cause of a child's delayed social and language development. Children who have experienced emotional abuse may exhibit traits such as insecurity, anxiety, distrust, superficiality in social interactions, passivity, and an excessive concern for appeasing adults. Kids who experience rejection could have extremely low self-esteem. Youngsters who feel intimidated or threatened may exhibit fear and retreat.

The emotional impact on kids usually shows up when they start school and start having trouble forming relationships with their peers and teachers. Emotional effects are frequently overlooked until the child has been moved to a new setting or until their abnormal behaviors have subsided and been replaced by more acceptable ones. Adopted children have a higher risk of becoming criminals or developing drug addictions.

9.3.2.2. Neglect

Undernourishment, exhaustion, unhygienic conditions, inappropriate attire, and inability to flourish are typical indicators of insufficient food, clothing, or shelter provision. Starvation or exposure to extreme weather conditions can lead to stunted growth and death. Inadequate supervision combined with neglect can cause avoidable illness or injury.

9.3.3. Diagnosis of Child Maltreatment

- High index of suspicion (e.g., for history that does not match physical findings or for atypical injury patterns).
- Supportive, open-ended questioning.
- Sometimes imaging and laboratory tests.

Injuries and nutritional deficits are evaluated in other sections of the handbook. It can be challenging to identify maltreatment as the root cause, so suspicion must be kept to a high level. Due to social prejudices, abuse is thought to occur less frequently in children residing in two-parent households with incomes at least at the median level. However, regardless of the makeup of the family or socioeconomic status, child abuse can still happen. Direct questions can occasionally yield answers. Some children, especially those who have experienced sexual abuse, may be sworn to secrecy, threatened, or so traumatized that they are reluctant to speak about the abuse (and may even deny abuse when specifically questioned). However, some children who have experienced maltreatment may describe the events and the perpetrator.

When gathering medical history, it is important to ask children (if developmentally capable) and their non-offending caregivers about the events in a calm setting. In these situations, open-ended inquiries (such as "Can you tell me what happened?" and "Did daddy do this?" or "Did he touch you here?") are especially crucial since they prevent young children from developing false memories of their past. After the initial assessment, it is frequently unclear whether abuse actually took place. When this happens, the mandated reporting of suspected abuse enables relevant authorities and social agencies to look into the matter. If their assessment reveals abuse, then the necessary legal and social actions can be taken.

9.3.3.1. Physical Abuse

Both history and physical examination provide clues suggestive of maltreatment. Features suggestive of abuse in the history are:

- Parental reluctance or inability to give the history of a significant injury.
- History that is inconsistent with the injury (eg, bruises on the backs of the legs attributed to a forward fall) or apparent stage of resolution (eg, old injuries described as recent).
- History that varies depending on the information source or over time (it must be acknowledged that some discrepancies may be attributed to how the information was documented by the clinician).
- History of injury that is incompatible with the child's stage of development (eg, injuries ascribed to rolling off a bed in an infant too young to roll over, or to a fall down stairs in an infant too young to crawl).
- Inappropriate response by the parents to the severity of the injury—either overly concerned or unconcerned.
- Delay in seeking care for the injury.

Major indicators of abuse on examination are:

- Atypical injuries;
- Injuries incompatible with stated history.

Fall-related injuries in children are usually isolated and affect the mouth, chin, forehead, or extensor surfaces of the limbs, especially the shins, knees, elbows, and forearms. It is very uncommon for falls to cause bruises on the backs of the legs or the buttocks. Apart from clavicular fractures, typical falls during play or down stairs are less likely to result in fractures of the tibia (toddler's) and distal radius (Colles). While there is no definitive sign of abuse, certain conditions such as classic metaphyseal lesions, rib fractures (particularly the posterior and first rib), depressed or multiple skull fractures (resulting from supposedly minor trauma), scapular fractures, sternal fractures, and fractures of the spinous processes should raise suspicions of abuse.

When a baby sustains a significant injury and is not walking or at least cruising (i.e., walking with assistance from objects in the environment), physical abuse should be taken into consideration. Young infants who appear to have minor injuries should also receive additional assessment. Even with severe brain damage, the younger infant might seem normal, and every infant that is lethargic should have acute head trauma included in the differential diagnosis. Additional clues include numerous injuries at various phases of healing or development, patterns in cutaneous lesions that point to specific injury sources, and recurrent injuries that point to maltreatment or insufficient supervision.

A dilated eye examination and neuroimaging are recommended for all children < 1 year old with suspected abuse. Retinal hemorrhages occur in 85 to 90% of cases of abusive head trauma vs < 10% of cases of accidental head trauma. However, retinal hemorrhages are not pathognomonic of abuse. They also may result from childbirth and persist for 4 or more weeks. When retinal hemorrhages result from accidental trauma, the mechanism is usually obvious and life-threatening (eg, major motor vehicle crash), and the hemorrhages are typically few in number and confined to the posterior poles.

Children who are < 36 months old (previous recommendation 24 months) with possible physical abuse should undergo a skeletal survey for evidence of previous bony injuries (fractures in various stages of healing or sub-periosteal elevations in long bones). Surveys are rarely done on children > 3 years old. The standard survey includes images of the:

- Appendicular skeleton: Humeri, forearms, hands, femurs, lower legs, and feet.
- Axial skeleton: Thorax (including oblique views), pelvis, lumbosacral spine, cervical spine, and skull.

Physical disorders causing multiple fractures include osteogenesis imperfecta, rickets, and congenital syphilis. In inherited copper deficiency (Menkes syndrome), osteoporosis may lead to bone fractures.

Sexually transmitted infections (2) in a child < 12 years old are nearly always the result of sexual abuse. When a child has been sexually abused, behavioral changes (eg, irritability, fearfulness, insomnia) may be the only clues initially. If sexual abuse is suspected, the perioral and anal areas and the external genitals should be examined for evidence of injury. If the suspected abuse is thought to have occurred recently (≤ 96 hours), forensic evidence should be gathered using an appropriate kit and handled according to required legal standards. An examination involving use of a magnifying light source with a camera, such as with a specially equipped colposcopy, may be helpful to the examiner as well as for documentation for legal purposes.

9.3.3.2. Emotional Abuse and Neglect

To ascertain whether the child is not developing normally, the evaluation focuses on the child's overall appearance and behavior. Social workers and teachers are frequently the first to identify neglect. A pattern of missing appointments and out-of-date vaccinations may be noticed by the doctor. Medical neglect of chronic, life-threatening conditions like diabetes or asthma can result in poor adherence to prescribed treatment plans and an increase in office or emergency department visits.

9.4. Treatment of Child Maltreatment

The child's immediate safety and critical medical needs, including potential STDs, are given priority during treatment. One option should be to refer the patient to a pediatrician who specializes in child abuse. Families should be approached in a supportive rather than a punitive manner in both abuse and neglect situations.

- Treatment of injuries;
- Reporting to the appropriate agency;
- Creation of a safety plan;
- Family counseling and support;
- Sometimes removal from the home.

9.4.1. Immediate Safety

All US states have laws requiring doctors and other professionals who work with children—such as nurses, teachers, daycare providers, and police—to report suspected cases of child abuse or neglect. These professionals are known as mandated reporters (Mandatory Reporters of Child Abuse and Neglect). Each state has its own legal system. Reporting suspected abuse is not required, but it is encouraged for members of the public. Anyone reporting abuse in good faith and with reasonable cause is exempt from both criminal and civil penalties. If a mandated reporter doesn't submit a report, they risk facing both criminal and civil consequences. The reports are sent to the appropriate child protection agency, such as Child Protective Services. Professionals should generally inform caregivers that a report is being made in accordance with the law, and if the report is accepted, they will likely be contacted, interviewed, and visited at their home. In certain situations, the expert may conclude that there is a higher risk of harm to the child and/or the caregiver if they notify them before the police or another agency can help. In those situations, the expert might decide not to tell the parent or caregiver right away.

Social workers and child protective agency representatives assess the events and the child's situation. They can assist a doctor or other professional in determining the likelihood of further harm and, in turn, determine the best course of action for the child in the short term.

Options include:

- Protective hospitalization;
- Placement with relatives or in temporary housing (sometimes a whole family is moved out of an abusive partner's home);

- Temporary foster care;
- Going home with prompt social service and medical follow-up.

Before beginning any additional supportive nutritional care in an age-appropriate manner (eg, gastrostomy tube). A child who flourishes while in the hospital is strong evidence of neglect (or starvation due to poverty). The doctor is crucial in collaborating with neighborhood organizations to promote the child's safest and best course of action. When a child is suspected of being abused, healthcare professionals in the US are frequently asked to write an impact statement, which is a letter usually addressed to a Child Protective Services worker (who can then bring it to the attention of the judicial system). In layman's terms, the letter should include a clear explanation of the history and physical examination results as well as an assessment of the probability that the child was abused.

If a child is malnourished and appears to be the victim of neglect, they should be admitted to the hospital and provided with age-appropriate nutrition before receiving other supportive nutritional care, such as a gastrostomy tube.

9.4.2. Follow-Up

Having access to primary medical care is essential. However, it can be challenging to maintain continuity of care when the families of abused and neglected children move frequently. Scheduled appointments are frequently missed; social workers and/or public health clinicians may be able to assist with outreach and home visits. A nearby child advocacy center can facilitate more efficient, well-coordinated, and kid-friendly multidisciplinary teamwork between community organizations, medical professionals, and the legal system. It is crucial to carefully examine the family environment, previous interactions with different community service organizations, and the needs of the caregivers. In addition to conducting these reviews, social workers can assist with family counseling and interviewing. Social workers also help caregivers in more concrete ways by assisting them in obtaining child care, public assistance, and respite services, all of which can reduce caregiver stress. They may also assist in organizing caregivers' access to mental health services. Regular or continuous social work contact is typically required.

Some communities offer parent-aide programs, which use non-professionals with training to support abusive and neglectful parents and set an example of proper parenting. There has also been success with other parent support groups. Particularly in the case of older children and adolescents, sexual abuse can have a long-lasting impact on a child's development and ability to adapt sexually. Psychotherapy or counseling for the involved adults and the child may mitigate these effects. Abuse by physical means, especially severe trauma to the head, can also have long-term consequences for development. Early Intervention Services is a program designed to assess and treat children with suspected disabilities or developmental delays. If doctors or caregivers have concerns that young children have a disability or delayed development, they can request an evaluation from their state's Early Intervention system (see Early Intervention Services).

9.4.3. Removal From the Home

The main objective of child protective services is to maintain children with their families in a safe and healthy environment, even though emergency temporary removal from the home until evaluation is finished and safety is guaranteed is occasionally carried out. To facilitate the reunification of adopted children with their families, families are frequently offered services aimed at rehabilitating the caregivers. Parental rights may need to be terminated and long-term removal must be considered if the interventions previously outlined are unable to guarantee safety. A court petition must be filed for this important step, and it must be submitted by the relevant welfare department's legal counsel. While the exact process varies from US state to US state, a doctor's testimony in family court is typically required. If the court rules that the child should be taken out of the family, a disposition is set up, usually in foster care or another short-term facility. If at all possible, the child's own doctor or a medical team that specializes in foster children should stay in touch with the parents during the child's temporary placement to make sure that sufficient efforts are being made to assist them. Children placed in foster care occasionally experience recurrent abuse. The doctor needs to be aware of this potential. The child might be allowed to go back to the original caregivers once the dynamics of the family environment improve. On the other hand, mistreatment does not always stop.

9.5. Prevention of Child Maltreatment

Every well-child visit should include prevention of abuse by identifying risk factors and educating parents, caregivers, and children. Families that are at risk ought to be directed to the proper community resources. Parents who experienced abuse are more likely to mistreat their own offspring. These parents are receptive to help and occasionally express their anxiety regarding their history of abuse. Parents who are first-time, adolescent, or have multiple children under the age of five are also more likely to abuse their offspring (Figure 9.2).

Prenatal screening is frequently used to identify maternal risk factors for abuse (e.g., a mother who smokes, has a substance use disorder, has a history of domestic violence). Parent-infant bonding can be weakened by medical issues that arise during pregnancy, delivery, or the early years of infancy and may have an impact on the mother's or the infant's health (see also caring for Sick Neonates). It's critical to find out how the parents are feeling about themselves and the welfare of the child at these times. A healthcare professional who is aware of the signs and able to offer support can have a significant impact on the family and potentially prevent child abuse. How well-adjusted to an infant with numerous needs or health demands can the parents handle? Do the parents support each other both physically and morally? Are there friends or relatives available to help in times of need?

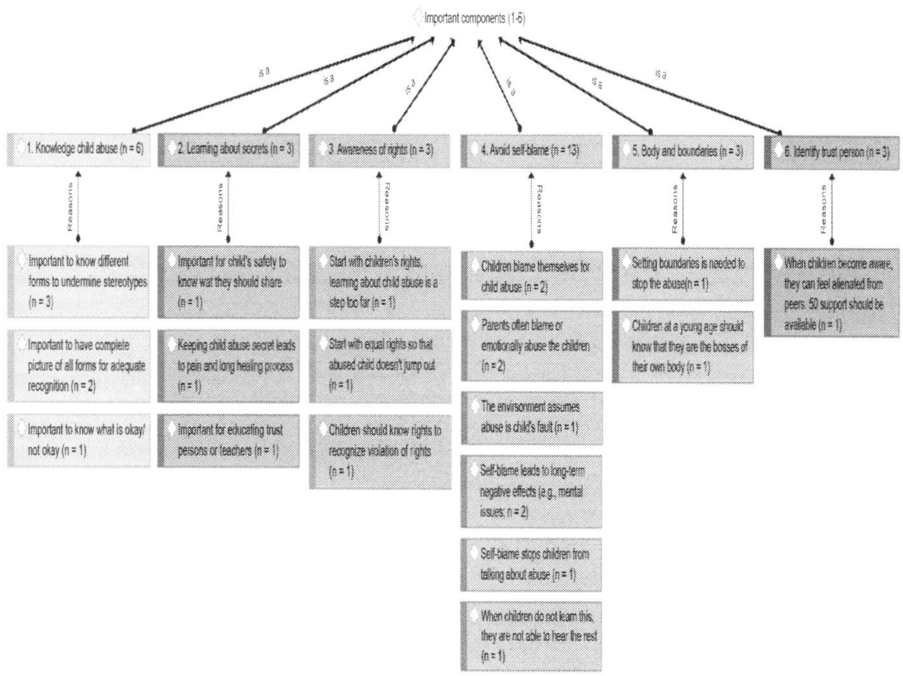

Figure 9.2. *Preventing child abuse.*

Source: *Gubbels, J., Assink, M., Prinzie, P., & van der Put, C. E., (2021). What works in school-based programs for child abuse prevention? The perspectives of young child abuse survivors. Social Sciences, 10(10), 404. https://doi.org/10.3390/socsci10100404.*

9.5.1. Child Maltreatment: A Public Health and Prevention Considerations

Globally, child maltreatment (CM) affects hundreds of millions of children and is a serious public health concern. Numerous short- and long-term health consequences, such as poor mental and physical health, altered biological factors, changes in brain architecture and development, decreased cognitive ability and academic achievement, and impaired psychosocial functioning, have been linked to chronic migraine. Given the scope of the issue and the strain it puts on public health, addressing the CM problem from a public health perspective is obviously necessary. The definitions of child abuse will be reviewed in the section that follows, along with its prevalence, incidence, and effects, which include risks to one's physical health, academic performance and cognitive development, as well as one's emotional and behavioral well-being.

9.5.1.1. Definitions

The term "battered child syndrome" was first used in the early 1960s by Kempe, Silverman, Steele, Droegemueller, and Silver (1962), but researchers and practitioners still struggle to define and operationalize experiences of child abuse and neglect. Not only are CM experiences varied in nature, encompassing a multitude of types and subtypes, but the definition of CM frequently varies based on the context in which it is employed. Specifically, different definitions used by the various sectors addressing CM (e.g., Effective communication across disciplines is frequently restricted by Child Protective Services [CPS], law enforcement and legal communities, medical professionals, public health officials, and other advocates. This variation poses a significant obstacle to the effective surveillance, treatment, and prevention of child maltreatment. The Centers for Disease Control and Prevention (CDC) collaborated with experts in CM research, prevention, and surveillance from a range of settings, including universities, state health departments, hospitals, research firms, and other federal agencies, to develop conceptual definitions of CM and guidelines for use in public health settings. This was done in an effort to facilitate the gathering and use of public health-based CM data. The definitions were created collaboratively, so they complement current definitions, draw from definitions already in use in other sectors, and have been adjusted to meet the needs of public health professionals, whose goal is to stop child abuse and neglect before it starts.

According to the CDC, child maltreatment (CM) is any act or sequence of acts of commission (abuse) or omission (neglect) by a parent or other caregiver that causes harm to a child or raises the possibility of harm. The CDC's brief descriptions of the CM subtypes (includes sexual abuse, psychological abuse, physical abuse, including abusive head trauma), and two types of neglect: neglectful provision and neglectful supervision. These definitions support Article 19 of the United Nations Convention on the Rights of a Child, which expressly shields children from all forms of abuse, exploitation, and violence while in the care of parents and other caregivers. They also correspond with the definitions of the World Health Organization (WHO) (Table 9.1).

Table 9.1. *Allegations of Maltreatment Types Published in a Study*

Year	Neglect	Physical Abuse	Sexual Abuse	Psychological Maltreatment	Total
2011	2,719,392	939,424	307,856	355,594	4,322,266
2012	2,250,666	796,233	263,469	282,174	3,592,542
2013	1,920,956	677,247	222,510	239,026	3,059,739
2014	1,714,509	589,280	189,058	187,901	2,680,748
2015	1,645,641	585,459	178,664	191,510	2,601,274
2016	1,542,898	596,411	174,279	181,084	2,494,672
2017	1,495,698	571,931	166,989	185,915	2,420,533
2018	1,413,308	535,929	167,345	184,952	2,301,534
2019	1,309,072	512,458	157,651	183,623	2,162,804
2020	1,187,440	425,232	139,250	165,856	1,917,778
Total	**17,199,580**	**6,229,604**	**1,967,071**	**2,157,635**	**27,599,672**

Source: *Guastaferro, K., & Shipe, S. L., (2024). Child maltreatment types by age: Implications for prevention. International journal of Environmental Research and Public Health, 21(1), 20. https://doi.org/10.3390/ijerph21010020.*

Child sexual exploitation is one of the hardest childhood adversities to measure and research because it occurs covertly, but it can have some of the worst effects on a person's physical and mental health. Emergency rooms and other medical settings frequently see these kinds of cases at different stages of the victimization process.

9.5.1.2. Incidence and Prevalence

It has become much more difficult to precisely estimate and monitor the extent of CM in relation to other public health issues due to the lack of consistent, trustworthy definitions and related data on the disease. This has resulted in a variety of conclusions regarding the number of children and families affected. Furthermore, because of the experiences with CM, particularly with specific kinds (e.g., sexual abuse), are frequently only known to the victim and the offender, official estimates are usually greatly understated. Despite these restrictions, 34.4 million reports of children as victims of child maltreatment (CM) were received by state and local CPS agencies in the United States (US) in 2012. Of these reports, 78.3% were related to neglect, followed by 18.3% to physical abuse, 9.3% to sexual abuse, and 10.6% to "other" forms of maltreatment.

While self-report data from a national survey of violence against children show that rates of CM are highest among 14 to 17-year-olds, CPS data suggest that young children are at the highest risk for CM (USDHHS, 2013). As a result, the type or nature of CM cases that are brought to the notice of official agencies may differ from those that are not. Because official data frequently contradicts self-reports, it can also skew descriptions of the problem's characteristics and the types of people who are at risk (Pinto & Maia, 2012). As a result, research based on official data sources is likely to significantly underestimate the actual scope of the issue and may not appropriately identify the populations most at risk. In general, collecting data on a variety of indicators from a variety of sources during the assessment and monitoring of CM can help determine the true scope of the issue and enable more precise surveillance and monitoring.

9.5.1.3. Consequences

Research over the past few decades has shown that CM can have serious effects that last long after the maltreatment takes place. The impacts may affect several facets of a person's development and may manifest in childhood, adolescence, or adulthood (e.g., behavioral, psychological, cognitive, and physical). The consequences of these effects range from diminished functioning to death, long-term illness, and brain damage. The consequences that fall into the three overlapping categories of physical health, academic achievement and cognitive development, and emotional and behavioral health will be discussed in detail in the following sections.

9.5.1.4. Physical Health

A person's physical health may be impacted by CM in a variety of direct and indirect ways. Bumps, burns, fractured bones, and STDs are a few examples of the direct medical consequences of physical abuse, sexual abuse, and/or neglect. Young children and infants may be especially susceptible to the immediate physical effects of physical abuse. Youngsters under five are most likely to suffer from abusive head trauma, which can result in fatalities or serious nonfatal effects like vision impairment (e.g., seizures, convulsions, etc.). The risk is highest when the child is between the ages of two and three months for physical disability (e.g., cerebral palsy) and/or deficits in cognition.

In addition to causing acute injuries, CM also foretells a host of physical health issues that are maybe not immediately linked to abuse and neglect. For instance, the Adverse Childhood Experiences (ACE) Study has consistently shown a substantial correlation between exposure to abuse and dysfunctional households in childhood, as well as between abuse exposure and a number of the primary risk factors for the leading causes of death in adulthood (e.g., skeletal fractures, cancer, chronic lung disease, ischemic heart disease, and liver disease). The results of this extensive study also showed that these negative childhood experiences have a cumulative effect on an adult's health status, meaning that the more negative events (e.g., repeated abuse), the higher the risk of unfavorable health consequences.

New findings in brain research suggest that many of the maltreatment-related developmental consequences have partially neurological explanations. Abuse and neglect can lead to abnormal formation and function of important brain regions, which has implications for all areas of development. For instance, chronic abuse-related stress can cause hyperarousal responses in specific brain regions, causing hyperactivity and sleep disturbances. It can also strengthen the connections between neurons involved in the fear response, making the brain more likely to perceive the environment as hostile, which can result in anxious and aggressive behaviors. According to recent research, CM may also result in reduced left hemisphere growth, which raises the possibility of depression and is linked to a higher risk of alcohol and tobacco use.

9.5.1.5. Cognitive Development and Academic Achievement

Adopted children are more likely than their classmates to show signs of learning disabilities and poor academic performance. Even after adjusting for possible individual and familial confounders like maternal drug and alcohol use, prematurity and birth weight, and maternal anxiety and depression, the detrimental effects of both abuse and neglect have been found. According to recent research, kids who witness or experience physical or sexual abuse in their families also exhibit lower executive functioning (e.g., cognitive functions (e.g., working memory, inhibition, auditory attention, and processing speed) in comparison to their classmates, even after accounting for external stressors and internalizing distress.

9.5.1.5.1. Emotional and Behavioral Health

Generally speaking, children who have been maltreated are more likely to show signs of internalizing (e.g., anxiety, depression) and externalizing (e.g., hostility, and drug abuse) actions. Particularly, kids who have experienced abuse in the past are more likely to develop anxiety disorders, depressive disorders, and panic attacks, PTSD, and higher rates of bullying, aggression, and juvenile delinquency than their peers without similar backgrounds. A long-term study found that experiencing maltreatment as a child increased the likelihood of being arrested as a juvenile by 59%.

Adult maltreatment victims exhibit higher rates of alcohol and drug abuse, suicidality, high-risk sexual behavior, and a variety of psychiatric disorders compared to their non-maltreated counterparts. Up to 80% of young adults with histories of maltreatment in one long-term study satisfied the diagnostic criteria for at least one mental illness (e.g.at the age of 21 (major depressive disorder, posttraumatic stress disorder).

The development and maintenance of other close relationships throughout childhood, into adolescence, and into adulthood can be severely harmed by CM due to the influential nature of children's early relationships with their parents. Children who experience abuse are more likely to encounter other forms of violence in the future. They are also more likely to act violently and criminally, which may include abusing their own children. For instance, a study by a group of researchers revealed that women who had a history of sexual abuse were twice as likely to experience physical and/or sexual abuse as adults as non-abused, compared to females.

9.5.2. Risk and Protective Factors Related to Child Maltreatment

Children are not affected by CM predictably or consistently, just like they are by other types of trauma. Variability in both immediate and long-term results is caused by a number of interrelated factors, such as characteristics of the actual maltreatment experience (e.g., severity, chronicity), in addition to the child's traits (e.g., age, sex), as well as the child's family, relationships, and community environment. Some research shows that almost 25% of maltreated children show no long-term symptoms at all. This is probably due to the complex interaction between multiple risk and protective factors at any given point in a child's life.

Risk factors are those things that make someone more likely to act violently or become the victim of someone acting violently (USDHHS, 2001). Stated differently, a risk factor for childhood maltreatment (CM) is any attribute or situation that, when present for a particular child, increases the likelihood that the child will be abused. On the other hand, a protective factor lessens the chance of developing CM.

Risk and protective variables are dynamic and subject to change. Because individual and family-level factors were the most frequently looked at variables in research, researchers have long regarded family-level factors as the most influential in determining child exposure to maltreatment and related outcomes. A factor that increases the risk for CM at one life stage may or may not put the same child at risk at a later stage in development. But over the past few years, more data has emerged to highlight the critical roles that the community and larger environment also play in CM victimization and perpetration prediction.

Even though they cannot stop the harm that is done to them, certain traits of children have been shown time and time again to raise the likelihood of abuse; these traits include being younger than four years old and having special needs. Parental traits include ignorance of child development and parenting techniques; past child abuse; substance abuse and/or mental health problems; early age; lack of education; being a single parent; having many dependent children; having a low income; and having non-biological, temporary caregivers in the home (e.g., the mother's male partner), have also been linked to a higher chance of domestic abuse of children. Additional risk factors for the perpetration include inadequate and/or lack of social support networks; and additional types of domestic violence (e.g., intimate relationship violence, strained parent-child bonds, parenting pressures, communal violence, and concentrated neighborhood deprivation.

It is important to remember that, even though a history of CM may be a risk factor, it does not guarantee that someone will commit CM in the future. According to Thornberry, Knight, and Lovegrove (2012), more rigorous research studies produced contradictory findings, and the positive correlation between a history of CM and subsequent perpetration is primarily the consequence of methodologically flawed research designs. Safe, stable, and nurturing relationships have been found to moderate the relationship between intergenerational continuity in experiences of CM, according to methodologically sound research studies that do find such continuity. Despite their critical importance, protective factors have received far less attention in research than risk factors. Nonetheless, a child's positive relationship with at least one parent, strong perceived social support, and a family's socioeconomic standing above the poverty line have all been consistently linked to a decreased risk for CM.

9.5.3. Considerations for Nurses

Considering that childhood malnutrition (CM) is a major public health issue with detrimental effects on development, everyone who works with families must understand CM and how to prevent it. clinicians work in many different environments and perform a range of tasks (e.g., CM can be prevented and/or victims can be identified thanks to the special position that primary care, hospitals, schools, academic research institutions, patient and health advocacy, and community agencies hold. For instance, clinicians who work in pediatric, maternity, and neonatal intensive care units (NICUs) have the opportunity to mentor and watch primary caregivers as they provide care for their infants or children. Before the baby is sent home, NICU clinicians must make sure the parent is capable of providing competent care. Maternity clinicians frequently perform interventions to prevent abusive head trauma and promote safe sleep. When treating older infants and children admitted for treatment of injuries, ingestions, and acute or chronic conditions, clinicians working in the Emergency Department (ED) are in a critical position to assess for suspected maltreatment or identify the potential for maltreatment. In educational environments, clinicians can support educators and other staff members by offering prevention programs that are universal for child sexual abuse. When a student exhibits indications of possible abuse, school clinicians are best qualified to evaluate them. Clinicians must exercise extra caution because the symptoms and indicators of abuse can be mistaken for other medical issues.

Laws requiring mandatory reporting also apply to clinicians in each of these settings. Laws in each of the 50 states mandate that certain professionals report suspected child maltreatment (CM) to child protective services, law enforcement, or a "hotline" phone number. In addition to other professionals like doctors, psychologists, educators, and law enforcement officers, this frequently includes nurses. Though it's vital to remember that laws do differ from state to state, mandatory reporting statutes typically demand that a report be filed whenever there is "reasonable cause" to think that a child has been abused or exposed to circumstances that could lead to abuse. The decision to launch an investigation is ultimately up to child protective service agencies, but reports—like those from nurses, for example—are frequently what initiate this process. It is crucial to remember that reporting obligations take precedence over obligations to maintain professional secrecy. In actuality, neglecting to file a report may result in civil or criminal fines, as well as complaints of malpractice and professional ethics. When reports are made in good faith and without malice, all states offer criminal and civil immunity from liability.

Studies show that many cases of abuse remain unreported by professionals, even in spite of mandatory reporting laws. According to research, several factors can affect reporting, such as the severity of the situation as perceived, ignorance of the proper reporting procedures, fear of misinterpreting cultural customs, or worries about exacerbating the situation or severing a therapeutic relationship. It's critical to never assume that a report has already been made and to always submit one when requested to the proper authority. A validated CPS report has the potential to stop future occurrences of more severe and potentially fatal CM. Unsubstantiated CPS reports may also prevent CM due to the support and additional services that families may receive as a result. For instance, the majority of states (72.5%) send cases that are both substantiated and unsubstantiated to community agencies to receive services.

9.5.4. The Importance of Prevention in Child Maltreatment

Since CM is a serious public health issue, prevention strategies must be multifaceted. Preventive measures should focus on risk and protective variables at the individual, interpersonal, group, and societal levels, as well as other levels of the social ecology. Depending on the target of interest, prevention programs frequently fall into one of three categories on a continuum: indicated, selected, or universal prevention. Coordinating resources throughout this whole continuum is one of the strategies included in a comprehensive system of care aimed at improving outcomes for families and children. The following lists the various forms of prevention, each followed by a brief synopsis and a program example that is supported by data proving its efficacy. In many of these initiatives, clinicians serve as the main practitioners of prevention (Figure 9.3).

Child abuse is rated thirteenth on a list of community issues.

There were six times more people who had no concerns at all than there were people who were concerned about the problem of child abuse.

Child abuse is rated less concerning than transport, traffic, and roads.

Community concern about child abuse has not changed since 2003.

71% of respondents did not recall seeing or hearing any advertising or news related to child abuse or the protection of children in the past 12 months.

Figure 9.3. *Findings from a study on child abuse and child protection in Australia.*

Source: Tucci, J., & Mitchell, J., (2022). Still unseen and ignored: Tracking community knowledge and attitudes about child abuse and child protection in Australia. Front. Psychol., 13, 860212. doi: 10.3389/fpsyg.2022.860212.

9.5.4.1. Universal Prevention Programs

Programs for universal prevention are offered to all members of the public and frequently seek to inform them about the nature and potential consequences of childhood malformations (CM) before they happen. Public service announcements that promote positive parenting, school-based initiatives to prevent child sexual abuse, and hospital-based abusive head trauma (AHT) treatments are a few examples of universal approaches. Maternity clinicians in many hospitals perform AHT prevention interventions with all mothers and babies before they are sent home. Most of these educational programs require clinicians to ask parents to watch a brief videotape and read a brief booklet that addresses the risks of violently shaking an infant and offers strategies for handling crying. Period of Purple Crying is one such program that seeks to recognize that while baby cries can be upsetting, there are other solutions available besides simply shaking the child. Participating mothers reported learning more about AHT and infant crying, and they were more likely to have discussed the need of walking away from frustration and the risks associated with shaking your baby. There are presently randomized clinical trials for this and other AHT programs funded by the CDC. The goal of this study is to offer more thorough details regarding how these programs affect the prevalence of AHT in the population. To support safe, stable, and nurturing relationships and environments (SSNRs) for all children, states and communities can take into consideration the framework of primary prevention strategies for all forms of maltreatment provided by another CDC initiative, Essentials for Childhood.

9.5.4.2. Selected Prevention Programs

Individuals who have been classified as at-risk or who possess one or more risk factors linked to chronic muscle disease (e.g., poverty, substance abuse by parents, and young age of parents). Services for neighborhoods or communities with a high incidence of risk may also be the focus of certain programs. Behaviorally-based parent training programs, home visit programs that educate and support expectant and new mothers, parent-child centers that offer comprehensive educational and parent support to economically disadvantaged children and their parents, and education programs in high schools that target teenage parents are a few examples of specific preventive initiatives. Programs for home visits have been implemented extensively and are endorsed by numerous associations, such as the American Academy of Pediatrics. The Nurse-Family Partnership is an instance of a program of this kind. It is an evidence-based preventive intervention that usually enrolls first-time, low-income mothers. NFP home visits can last until the child turns two and always start during pregnancy. NFP home visitors are registered clinicians who work with participating families to address various issues, such as promoting healthy behaviors (e.g., diet); lowering harmful habits (e.g., alcohol, tobacco, and other drug use); identifying symptoms of illness in children; and establishing secure homes. Extensive research on NFP indicates that the program is successful in preventing CM in first-time, low-income mothers, and that the effects last over time. When compared to women in the comparison group, the NFP program has also been demonstrated to lower the number of subsequent pregnancies, welfare utilization, and criminal activity among women who took part in the home visiting program.

9.5.4.3. Indicated Prevention Activities

The focus of recommended preventive initiatives is on families who have already experienced abuse. These initiatives aim to lessen the harmful effects of abuse and stop it from happening again. Programs for indicated prevention could include mental health services for abused children and their families, as well as intensive family preservation services that put a licensed mental health counselor at the families' disposal. One type of conjoint child and parent psychotherapy approach for children and youth experiencing emotional distress related to traumatic life events is trauma-focused cognitive behavioral therapy (TF-CBT). TF-CBT is intended to prevent and lessen emotional distress that follows maltreatment, even though it is not specifically meant to prevent maltreatment. Numerous randomized controlled trials have shown that TF-CBT reduces internalizing (e.g., anxiety) more effectively than supportive therapies and nondirective play therapy, with effects that are sustained over time. (e.g., anxiety, depression) and externalizing (e.g., symptoms such as conduct issues, sexualized behaviors, in kids who have had CM.

The majority of empirical support has gone toward cognitive behavioral strategies for treating CM victims, which reduce psychological and behavioral symptomatology. These techniques usually focus on the way the child thinks, feels, and behaves in response to the CM. It is crucial to first ensure that the child or adolescent is safe from any potential harm in the future from the offender and from unsupportive or nonbelieving family members who may impede the victim's ability to achieve adaptive psychosocial outcomes. Notable programs include Triple P, which offers primary, selected, and indicated prevention programming components covering the prevention continuum. The five intervention levels in this system, which was created as a population-level parenting and family support system, are all focused on improving parental competence and preventing or altering dysfunctional parenting techniques.

The initial phase comprises a communications campaign that will make use of various resources (e.g., radio spots, newspaper articles, and public service announcements) to teach locals the fundamentals of positive parenting. The approaches taken by Levels 2 through 5 are not universal, and they represent an increase in the level of support provided to parents who might require more specialized, one-on-one help. This system of parenting interventions, though not specifically intended as a CM prevention program, was found in a recent South Carolina study to have reduced substantiated abuse cases by 28%, child out-of-home placements by 44%, and hospitalizations and ER visits for child injuries by 35%.

It is evident that CM is a serious public health issue with potential long-term harm to people, families, and society. It's crucial to remember, though, that child abuse is avoidable. A multifaceted strategy that supports secure, stable, and nurturing relationships and environments for all children and families is crucial to the prevention of CM. As primary preventive practitioners, clinicians play a crucial role in fostering safe, stable, and nurturing relationships and environments with all the families they interact with. Clinicians are also essential in identifying possible victims and helping CM victims receive treatment and/or referrals. Nursing professionals are at the forefront of the fight to attain the goal of a healthier population, as research indicates that this movement starts in childhood (Figure 9.4).

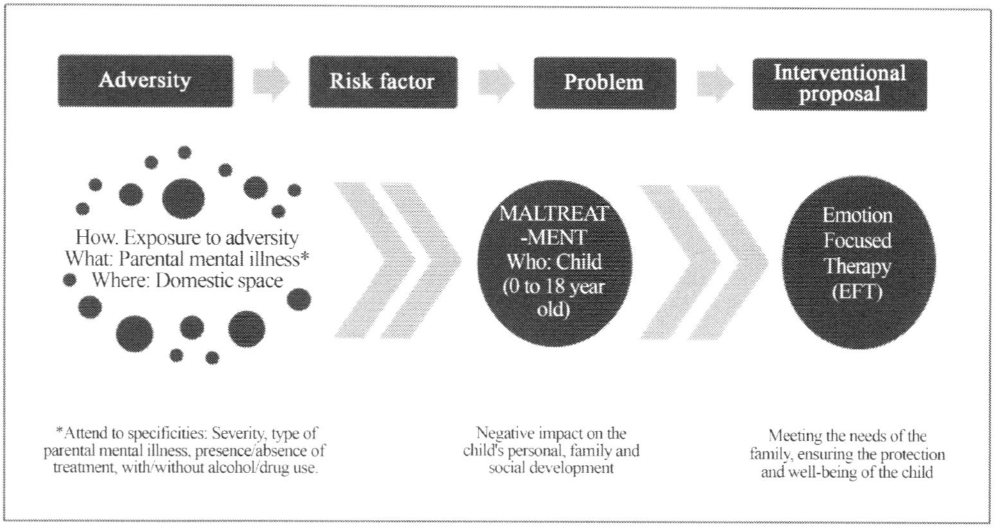

Figure 9.4. *Addressing maltreatment.*

Source: Lopes, A. I., Leal, J., & Sani, A. I., (2021). Parental mental health problems and the risk of child maltreatment: The potential role of psychotherapy. Societies, 11(3), 108. https://doi.org/10.3390/soc11030108.

A Closer Look

Osteogenesis Imperfecta

Osteogenesis imperfecta (OI) is an uncommon genetic connective tissue disease characterized by easily fractured, brittle bones. Collagen is a major component of connective tissue, and OI results from abnormal or reduced production of this protein due to a genetic defect. OI comes in four varieties, each with unique symptoms and intensities.

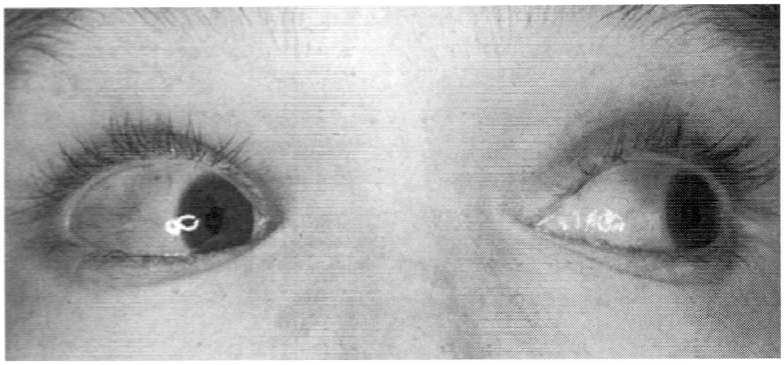

Source: By Herbert, L., Fred, M. D., & Hendrik, A., van Dijk – http://cnx.org/contents/_on798ZB@3/Images-of-Memorable-Cases-Case, CC BY-SA 3.0, https://commons.wikimedia.org/w/index.php?curid=11893313.

Infants with the most common type of Osteogenesis Imperfecta, known as type I, are born normally but may experience fractures in the following years. The frequency of fractures typically decreases after puberty. A bluish tint in the sclerae of the eyes may be present due to their thinness, allowing pigmentation to show. Hearing loss may result from abnormalities in the inner ear bones and pressure on the auditory nerve due to skull canal deformities. Double-jointedness, brittle teeth, and thin skin are common in type I. Type II, the most severe form, often leads to stillbirth or fractures at birth with a high likelihood of severe disability and low chance of survival to adulthood. Type III presents similar symptoms to type I but more severe. Type IV, while moderately severe, is also similar to type I with normal sclerae.

OI has no known cure; instead, management focuses on building bone mass, reducing symptoms, and avoiding fractures. Some patients have found success with bisphosphonate medication treatment, and deformities may be prevented or corrected surgically by inserting metal rods into specific bones.

Summary

- Traumatic injury is a term which refers to physical injuries of sudden onset and severity which require immediate medical attention. The insult may cause systemic shock called "shock trauma", and may require immediate resuscitation and interventions to save life and limb.
- In early infancy, emotional abuse may blunt emotional expressiveness and decrease interest in the environment. Emotional abuse commonly results in failure to thrive and is often misdiagnosed as intellectual disability or physical illness. Delayed development of social and language skills may be a sign of inadequate parental stimulation and interaction.
- Childhood injuries resulting from falls are typically solitary and occur on the forehead, chin, or mouth or extensor surfaces of the extremities, particularly elbows, knees, forearms, and shins. Bruises on the buttocks and the back of the legs are extremely rare from falls.
- Prevention of maltreatment should be a part of every well-child office visit through education of parents, caregivers, and children and identification of risk factors. At-risk families should be referred to appropriate community services. Parents who were victims of maltreatment are at increased risk of abusing their own children.
- Child maltreatment (CM) is a significant public health problem, affecting hundreds of millions of children globally. CM has been linked to a variety of short- and long-term health consequences, including poor physical and mental health, changes to brain architecture and development, altered biological factors, reduced cognitive ability and educational achievement, and impaired psychosocial functioning.

References

1. Barnes, J. E., Noll, J. G., Putnam, F. W., & Trickett, P. K. (2009). Sexual and physical revictimization among victims of severe childhood sexual abuse. *Child Abuse and Neglect, 33*, 412–420.
2. Barr, R. G., Rivara, F. P., Barr, M., Cummings, P., Taylor, J., Lengua, L. J., & Meredith-Benitz, E. (2009). Effectiveness of educational materials designed to change knowledge and behaviors regarding crying and shaken-baby syndrome in mothers of newborns: A randomized controlled trial. *Pediatrics, 123*, 972–980.
3. Berlin, L. J., Appleyard, K., & Dodge, K. A. (2011). Intergenerational continuity in child maltreatment: Mediating mechanisms and implications for prevention. *Child Development, 82*, 162–176.
4. Bolger, K. E., & Patterson, C. J. (2001). Children's internalizing problems and perceptions of control as functions of multiple types of maltreatment. *Development and Psychopathology, 13*, 913–940.
5. Briere, J., & Jordan, C.E. (2009). The relationship between childhood maltreatment, moderating variables, and adult psychological difficulties in women: An overview. *Trauma, Violence, and Abuse: A Review Journal, 10*, 375–388.
6. Centers for Disease Control & Prevention. (2013a). Child maltreatment: Risk and protective factors. Retrieved from www.cdc.gov/ViolencePrevention/childmaltreatment/riskprotectivefactors.html (accessed on 17 May 2024).

7. Centers for Disease Control & Prevention. (2013b). Steps to create safe, stable, and nurturing relationships. Retrieved from www.cdc.gov/violenceprevention/childmaltreatment/essentials/ (accessed on 17 May 2024).

8. Child Welfare Information Gateway. (2003). Decision-making in unsubstantiated child protective services cases: Synthesis of recent research. Washington, DC: United States Department of Health & Human Services. Retrieved from www.childwelfare.gov/pubs/focus/decisionmaking/decisionmaking.pdf. (accessed on 17 May 2024).

9. Cicchetti, D., & Toth, S. L. (2005). Child maltreatment. *Annual Review of Clinical Psychology, 1*, 409–438.

10. Cohen, J. A., Mannarino, A. P., & Iyengar, S. (2011). Community treatment of posttraumatic stress disorder for children exposed to intimate partner violence. *Archives of Pediatrics & Adolescent Medicine, 165*, 16–21.

11. Conger, R. D., Schofield, T. J., Neppl, T. K., & Merrick, M. T. (2013). Disrupting intergenerational continuity in harsh and abusive parenting: The importance of a nurturing relationship with a romantic partner. *Journal of Adolescent Health, 53*, S11–S17.

12. Coulton, C. J, Crampton, D. S., Irwin, M., Spilsbury, J. C., & Korbin, J. E. (2007). How neighborhoods influence child maltreatment: A review of the literature and alternative pathways. *Child Abuse and Neglect, 31*, 1117–1142.

13. Dallam, S. J. (2001). The long-term medical consequences of childhood maltreatment. In K. Franey, R. Geffner, & R. Falconer (Eds.), *The cost of child maltreatment: Who pays? We all do* (pp. 1–14). San Diego, CA: Family Violence & Sexual Assault Institute.

14. Deblinger, E., Mannarino, A. P., Cohen, J. A., & Steer, R. A. (2006). A multisite, randomized controlled trial for children with sexual abuse-related PTSD symptoms: Examining predictors of treatment response. *Journal of the American Academy of Child and Adolescent Psychiatry, 45*, 1474–1484.

15. Department of Health and Human Services (DHHS). (2001). Administration on children, youth, and families. *Understanding the effects of maltreatment on early brain development.* Washington, DC: Government Printing Office.

16. DePrince, A. P., Weinzierl, K. M., & Combs, M. D. (2009). Executive function performance and trauma exposure in a community sample of children. *Child Abuse and Neglect, 33*, 353–361.

17. Dias, M. S., Smith, K., GeGuehery, K., Mazur, P., Li, V., & Shaffer, M. L. (2005). Preventing abusive head trauma among infants and young children: A hospital-based parent education program. *Pediatrics, 115*(4), e470–e477.

18. Eckenrode, J., Ganzel, B., Henderson, C. R. J., Smith, E., Olds, D. L., Powers, J., ... Sidora, K. (2000). Preventing child abuse and neglect with a program of nurse home visitation: The limiting effects of domestic violence. *JAMA: The Journal of the American Medical Association, 284*(11), 1385–1391.

19. Everson, M. D., Hunter, W. M., Runyon, D. K., Edelsohn, G. A., & Coulter, M. L. (1991). Maternal support following disclosure of incest. In S. Chess & M. E. Hertzig (Eds.), *Annual Progress in Child Psychiatry and Child Development, 1990* (pp. 292–306). Philadelphia, PA: Brunner/Mazel.

20. Felitti, V. J., Anda, R. F., Nordenberg, D., Williamson, D. F., Spitz, A. M., Edwards, V., ... Marks, J. S. (1998). Relationship of childhood abuse and household dysfunction to many of the leading causes of death in adults. *American Journal of Preventive Medicine, 14*, 245–258.

21. Finkelhor, D., Turner, H. A., Shattuck, A., & Hamby, S. L. (2013). Violence, crime, and abuse exposure in a national sample of children and youth: An update. *JAMA Pediatrics, 167*(7).

22. Finkelhor, D., Turner, H., Ormrod, R., Hamby, S., & Kracke, K. (2009). Children's exposure to violence: A comprehensive national survey. *Juvenile Justice Bulletin*. US Department of Justice, Office of Justice Programs, Office of Juvenile Justice and Delinquency Prevention, Washington, DC.

23. Fluke, J. D., Shusterman, G. R., Hollinshead, D., & Yuan, Y. T. (2005). Rereporting and recurrence of child maltreatment: Findings from NCANDS. Washington, DC: U.S. Department of Health and Human Services, Office of the Assistant Secretary for Planning and Evaluation.

24. Fortson, B. L., & Mercy, J. (2012). Violence against children. In J. M. Rippe (Ed.), *Encyclopedia of Lifestyle Medicine and Health* (pp. 2818–2829). Thousand Oaks, CA: Sage.

Chapter

10

IMMUNIZATION, INFECTIOUS DISEASES, AND MANAGING ILL-NESS

Contents

Unit Introduction 314
10.1. Importance of Childhood Immunization 316
10.2 Integrated Management of New-born and Childhood Illness (IMNCI) 319
10.3. Childhood Illnesses 322
10.4. Nutritional Management 323
10.5. Care for a Sick Child 333
Summary 341
References 341

Unit Introduction

One of the best public health strategies for preventing infectious diseases and shielding individuals, groups, and populations from disease, disability, and death is vaccination. By administering vaccines, one can develop immunity without actually contracting the disease because the immune system is primed to identify and fight particular pathogens. Immunization campaigns have played a significant role in lowering the global burden of infectious diseases and in the control, eradication, and even total eradication of numerous deadly pathogens. Throughout history, vaccination campaigns have been essential in the fight against infectious diseases. Among the historic successes is the complete eradication of smallpox, which was made possible by an international immunization drive spearheaded by the World Health Organization (WHO). In a similar vein, extensive immunization campaigns have significantly decreased the prevalence of illnesses like rubella, polio, measles, diphtheria, and pertussis.

High vaccination rates within populations are necessary for immunization programs to be successful; this is referred to as "herd immunity" or "community immunity." A protective barrier that stops the pathogen from spreading is created when a sizable portion of the population is vaccinated against a specific disease. This protects those who cannot get vaccinations, such as young children, the elderly, or people with specific medical conditions. On the other hand, the risk of outbreaks and the resurgence of diseases that can be prevented by vaccination rises when vaccination rates fall, as has been shown in recent years by measles outbreaks around the globe. These outbreaks can be caused by vaccine hesitancy, false information, or restricted access to vaccines. Immunization campaigns have major positive social and economic effects in addition to preventing disease and death. Vaccination helps to lower healthcare costs, increase societal resilience, and improve productivity by lessening the burden of infectious diseases. Additionally, immunization campaigns can maximize the effectiveness and cost-effectiveness of other critical health interventions by acting as platforms for the delivery of deworming, vitamin supplements, and maternal and child health services.

Even with the amazing advancements made possible by vaccination, there are still issues with maintaining high vaccination rates around the world and providing fair access to vaccines. In low- and middle-income nations, where logistical, financial, and infrastructural obstacles may impede vaccine delivery and uptake, disparities in vaccine access are still present. Furthermore, mistrust and misinformation-based vaccine hesitancy pose a serious threat to public health initiatives by eroding vaccine confidence and jeopardizing community immunity. Concerted efforts are required to strengthen immunization systems, improve vaccine access and delivery, improve public awareness and education, and combat vaccine misinformation to address these issues and maintain progress in the fight against infectious diseases. We can continue to harness the power of vaccines to protect the health and well-being of people and communities around the world by making immunization a top priority, funding vaccine research and development, and encouraging cooperation between governments, healthcare providers, communities, and international partners.

Orientation and Directional Terms

Term	Definition	Illustration
Infectious diseases	Infectious diseases are illnesses caused by harmful organisms that enter the body from outside sources, such as bacteria, viruses, fungi, or parasites.	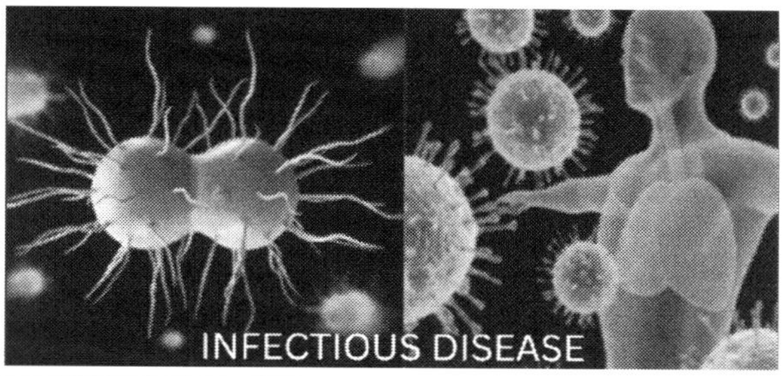
Bacteria	Bacteria are ubiquitous, mostly free-living organisms often consisting of one biological cell.	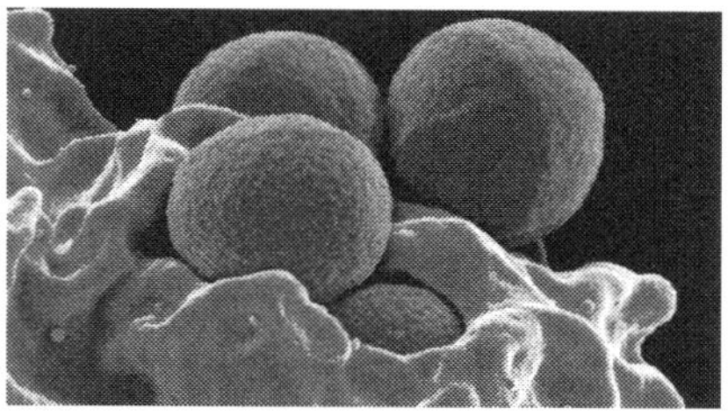
Healthcare infrastructure	Healthcare infrastructure refers to the facilities, systems, and services that are essential for maintaining public health and well-being.	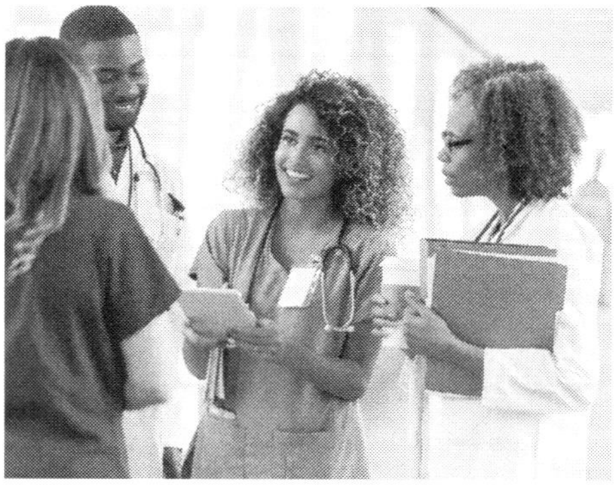
Influenza	influenza, is an infection of the nose, throat and lungs, which are part of the respiratory system.	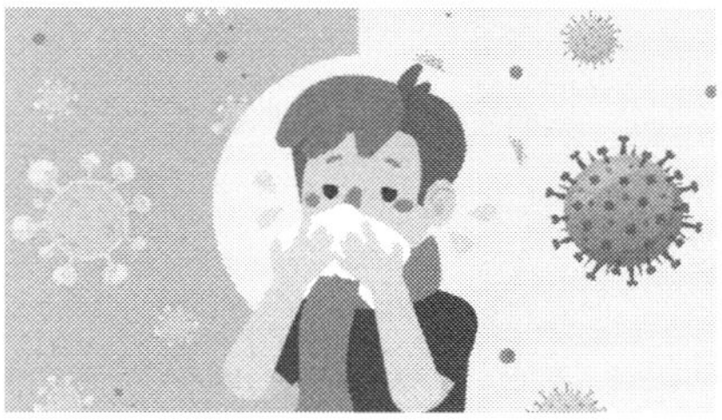
Diagnosis	Diagnosis, the process of determining the nature of a disease or disorder and distinguishing it from other possible conditions.	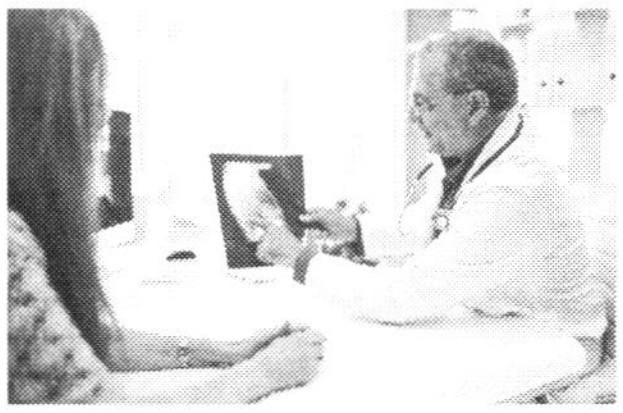

10.1. Importance of Childhood Immunization

A vital component of public health, childhood vaccinations are essential for preserving the health and welfare of children everywhere. Immunization campaigns aim to strengthen children's immune systems' capacity to identify and combat particular pathogens, thereby shielding them from dangerous and possibly fatal infectious diseases. The value of childhood vaccinations cannot be emphasized because they serve the larger objectives of disease prevention, public health, and public safety in addition to shielding individual children from disease and disability.

The prevention of vaccine-preventable diseases, which pose serious risks to children's health and can result in serious complications, long-term disabilities, and even death, is one of the main advantages of childhood vaccination. Measles, polio, diphtheria, pertussis, and tetanus are just a few of the illnesses that vaccinations have helped to lower in frequency, preventing millions of cases and saving countless lives annually. Vaccines lessen a child's vulnerability to infection and slow the spread of disease within communities by immunizing them against these pathogens.

Furthermore, childhood vaccination supports the idea of "herd immunity," also known as "community immunity," which holds that populations with high vaccination rates form a barrier that prevents the spread of infectious agents. A large percentage of the population being vaccinated lowers the general prevalence of disease in the community, protecting vulnerable people who might not be able to get vaccinations because of age, medical conditions, or other factors. Protecting infants who are too young to receive a full vaccination and people with weakened immune systems who may be more susceptible to serious illness are two reasons why herd immunity is crucial. Immunizations against disease and injury in children also have significant positive social and economic effects. Immunization programs help to lower healthcare costs, increase societal resilience, and improve productivity by lessening the burden of diseases that can be prevented by vaccination. In addition to saving lives, vaccines ease the burden on healthcare systems by lowering the need for hospital stays, medical services, and intensive care interventions related to diseases that can be prevented by vaccination. Additionally, immunization campaigns can maximize the effectiveness and cost-effectiveness of other critical health interventions by acting as platforms for the delivery of deworming, vitamin supplements, and maternal and child health services.

Notwithstanding the indisputable advantages of childhood vaccination, there are still obstacles in the way of maintaining high vaccination rates around the world and providing fair access to vaccines. In low- and middle-income nations, where logistical, financial, and infrastructural obstacles may impede vaccine delivery and uptake, disparities in vaccine access are still present. Furthermore, vaccine hesitancy jeopardizes community immunity and undermines vaccine confidence. It is driven by misinformation, mistrust, and complacency and poses a serious threat to public health initiatives. Concerted efforts are required to strengthen immunization systems, improve vaccine access and delivery, improve public awareness and education, and combat vaccine misinformation to address these issues and maintain progress in the fight against infectious diseases.

We can continue to use vaccines to safeguard children's health and wellbeing around the globe by emphasizing childhood immunization as a cornerstone of public health, funding vaccine research and development, and encouraging cooperation between governments, healthcare providers, communities, and international partners.

10.1.1. Common Childhood Infectious Diseases

Common childhood infectious diseases are a group of illnesses that mainly affect babies, toddlers, and early children and are brought on by bacteria, viruses, parasites, or fungi. These illnesses can spread quickly through daycare centers, schools, and communities because they are frequently very contagious. While immunization and good hygiene can prevent many infectious childhood diseases, these illnesses nevertheless pose a serious threat to global public health.

Some of the most common childhood infectious diseases include:

1. **Chickenpox (Varicella):** It is caused by the varicella-zoster virus and is characterized by an itchy rash, fever, and fatigue. It is highly contagious and spreads through respiratory droplets or direct contact with the rash. Vaccination has greatly reduced the incidence of chickenpox in many countries.
2. **Measles:** It is a highly contagious viral infection that causes fever, cough, runny nose, and a characteristic red rash. Complications of measles can be severe and include pneumonia, encephalitis, and death. Vaccination with the measles-mumps-rubella (MMR) vaccine is highly effective in preventing measles.
3. **Mumps:** It is a viral infection that causes swelling of the salivary glands, leading to fever, headache, muscle aches, and fatigue. Complications of mumps can include inflammation of the testicles or ovaries, deafness, and meningitis. Vaccination with the MMR vaccine protects against mumps.
4. **Rubella (German Measles):** It is a viral infection that causes a mild rash and fever. However, rubella infection during pregnancy can lead to congenital rubella syndrome, which can cause birth defects such as deafness, blindness, and heart defects. The MMR vaccine provides immunity against rubella.
5. **Whooping Cough (Pertussis):** It is a bacterial infection of the respiratory tract that causes severe coughing fits, often followed by a "whooping" sound when the child inhales. Complications of pertussis can be especially severe in infants, including pneumonia, seizures, and brain damage. Vaccination with the DTaP vaccine (diphtheria, tetanus, and pertussis) is crucial for preventing whooping cough.
6. **Rotavirus Infection:** It is a highly contagious virus that causes severe diarrhea and vomiting, leading to dehydration and sometimes death, particularly in infants and young children. Vaccination with the rotavirus vaccine has significantly reduced the burden of rotavirus gastroenteritis.
7. **Hand, Foot, and Mouth Disease (HFMD):** It is a viral illness caused by several different viruses, including enteroviruses. It is characterized by fever, sore throat, and a rash on the hands, feet, and mouth. HFMD is common in young children and typically resolves on its own without treatment.
8. **Scarlet Fever:** It is a bacterial infection caused by group A Streptococcus bacteria. It is characterized by a red rash, sore throat, fever, and a "strawberry tongue." Antibiotics are usually prescribed to treat scarlet fever and prevent complications such as rheumatic fever.

9. **Conjunctivitis (Pink Eye):** It is an inflammation of the conjunctiva, the thin membrane that covers the white part of the eye and lines the inside of the eyelid. It can be caused by bacteria, viruses, or allergies and is highly contagious, especially in childcare settings.
10. **Respiratory Syncytial Virus (RSV) Infection:** It is a common respiratory virus that causes cold-like symptoms, such as coughing, wheezing, and difficulty breathing. RSV infections are most severe in infants, particularly those born prematurely or with underlying health conditions.

The prevention and control of these infectious diseases in children include immunization, hand washing and other good hygiene habits, staying at home when sick, and avoiding close contact with sick people. Furthermore, controlling these infections and averting complications depend on early diagnosis and treatment.

10.1.2. Vaccination Schedules and Coverage

The timing and frequency of vaccinations differ based on factors like country-specific regulations, healthcare infrastructure, and epidemiological factors. Despite these variations, there are overarching principles and guidelines that serve as a foundation for vaccination programs internationally.

1. **Childhood Vaccination Schedule:** In many countries, childhood vaccination schedules begin shortly after birth and continue through adolescence. Common childhood vaccines include those against diseases such as measles, mumps, rubella, diphtheria, tetanus, pertussis, polio, hepatitis B, Haemophilus influenzae type b (Hib), rotavirus, pneumococcus, and varicella (chickenpox). Vaccines are typically administered in multiple doses at specific ages to ensure optimal immune response and long-lasting protection.
2. **Recommended Vaccines for Adolescents:** Adolescents may receive additional vaccines to protect against diseases such as meningococcal meningitis, human papillomavirus (HPV) infections (which can lead to cervical cancer and other cancers), and influenza (flu). Vaccination against HPV is particularly important for preventing certain types of cancer later in life.
3. **Adult Vaccination Schedule:** Adults may require booster doses or catch-up vaccinations to maintain immunity against certain diseases, such as tetanus, diphtheria, pertussis, and influenza. Additionally, adults may be advised to receive vaccines against diseases like pneumococcus, shingles (herpes zoster), and hepatitis A and B, depending on individual risk factors and health status.
4. **Travel Vaccinations:** Individuals traveling to certain regions may need additional vaccinations to protect against diseases prevalent in those areas. These may include vaccines against yellow fever, typhoid fever, cholera, Japanese encephalitis, and rabies, among others. Travelers should consult with healthcare providers or travel medicine specialists well in advance of their trip to determine which vaccines are recommended or required.
5. **Special Populations:** Certain populations, such as pregnant women, healthcare workers, and individuals with chronic medical conditions or

immunocompromising conditions, may have specific vaccination recommendations tailored to their needs. For example, pregnant women are advised to receive the influenza vaccine and the Tdap vaccine (tetanus, diphtheria, and pertussis) during each pregnancy to protect both themselves and their infants.

6. **Vaccination Coverage:** It refers to the proportion of the population that has received recommended vaccines within a specified time frame. High vaccination coverage rates are essential for achieving herd immunity and preventing outbreaks of vaccine-preventable diseases. Monitoring vaccination coverage allows public health authorities to assess the effectiveness of immunization programs, identify areas of low coverage, and implement targeted interventions to improve vaccine uptake.

Public education campaigns, healthcare provider training, outreach programs, and legislation aiming at enhancing vaccine accessibility and affordability are some of the measures used to raise vaccination coverage rates. Public health organizations regularly gather and assess vaccination coverage data to guide vaccination programs and assess advancements made toward disease control and elimination objectives.

10.2 Integrated Management of New-born and Childhood Illness (IMNCI)

Approximately 9 million children in developing nations pass away before turning five each year, with many of them doing so in their first year of life. With over 321,000 under-five deaths annually, Ethiopia has one of the highest rates of under-five mortality worldwide. Malnutrition, pneumonia, diarrhoea, malaria, measles, and other five diseases account for more than 70% of these child fatalities, and these illnesses frequently coexist.

At least three out of every four children who visit medical facilities do so for treatment of these diseases. Given that children typically present with multiple conditions, an integrated approach was deemed necessary to manage the child holistically, which involves considering all of the child's issues, including major childhood illnesses, in the assessment and treatment of illness. The Integrated Management of Newborn and Childhood Illness (IMNCI) strategy was created as a result of this.

IMNCI is a comprehensive strategy for child health that emphasizes the overall well-being of the child. The main goal of IMNCI is to decrease mortality, sickness, and disabilities, while also fostering better growth and development in children under five years old. This approach encompasses preventive and treatment measures that are carried out by families, communities, and healthcare facilities.

The IMNCI strategy includes three main components:

- Improving case management skills of healthcare staff.
- Improving the health systems.
- Improving family and community health practices.

In health facilities, the IMNCI strategy:

- promotes the accurate identification of childhood illnesses in out-patient settings
- ensures appropriate combined treatment of all major illnesses
- strengthens the counselling of caregivers

- Speeds up the referral of severely ill children.

In the home setting, IMNCI:

- promotes appropriate care-seeking behaviors
- helps to improve nutrition and preventative care, and
- Supports the correct implementation of prescribed care.

This module's integrated case management process will assist you in promptly taking into account every symptom a child exhibits and ensuring you don't miss anything. You'll discover how to assess a child's level of illness and whether they require an immediate referral. Additionally, you will learn how to manage a child's illness and advise caregivers to take care of a child at home for those infants and kids who don't require an urgent referral. ..

10.2.1 The IMNCI Strategy

The Integrated Management of Childhood Illnesses (IMNCI) approach combines all available interventions for disease prevention, early identification and treatment of childhood illnesses, and encouraging healthy behaviors in the home and community. The plan ensures a comprehensive approach to child health by combining better nutrition and immunization practices with improved management of newborn and childhood illnesses.

Healthcare professionals at all levels, from community health workers to facility-based clinicians, are trained in a systematic method of diagnosing, categorizing, and treating common childhood illnesses as part of IMNCI. In addition to medical management, this training teaches caregivers communication and counseling techniques and emphasizes the value of prompt health-seeking behavior.

In order to avoid complications and guarantee recovery, IMNCI places a strong emphasis on the necessity of early and accurate diagnosis, appropriate and timely treatment, and ongoing follow-up. It encourages the use of a standardized treatment plan, which makes it easier for medical professionals to make decisions and guarantees consistency in the provision of care. Furthermore, the approach promotes family and community involvement in the care process, acknowledging their critical role in preserving child health and averting disease.

Preventive measures like encouraging breastfeeding, making sure one is eating enough, giving vaccinations, and keeping one's hands and mouth clean are also part of the plan. With a focus on these areas, IMNCI aims to significantly lower the death rate for children under five by treating and preventing illnesses.

The overall goal of the IMNCI strategy is to create a sustainable impact on child health outcomes in settings with limited resources by combining treatment and prevention, involving multiple stakeholders, and taking a holistic and integrated approach to child health.

The overall goal of the IMNCI strategy is to create a sustainable impact on child health outcomes in settings with limited resources by combining treatment and prevention, involving multiple stakeholders, and taking a holistic and integrated approach to child health.

10.2.2 Importance and Objectives of the IMNCI Strategy

An Integrated Management of Newborn and Childhood Illness strategy is crucial because it allows for a standardized and consistent approach to address the primary causes of morbidity and mortality in children under five, which account for over 90% of the mortality in this age group in Ethiopia. The following are the estimated leading causes of death for children under five: pneumonia (28%), neonatal issues (25%), malaria (20%), diarrhea (20%), measles (4%), AIDS (1%), and other causes (2%), as illustrated in Figure 10.1 below. Figure 10.1 also shows that malnutrition is linked to approximately 60% of deaths in children under five.

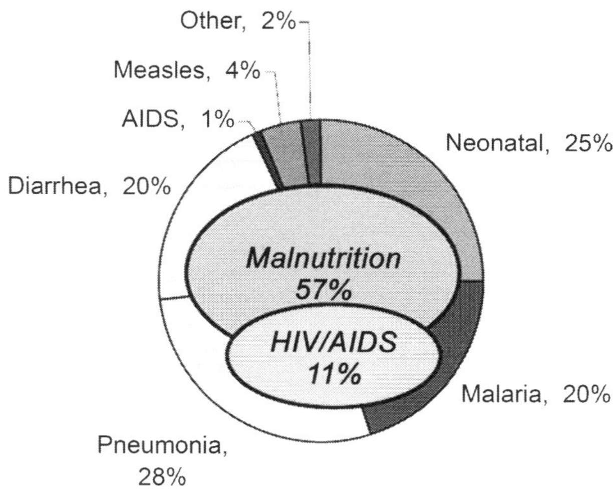

Figure 10.1. Major causes of under-five mortality in Ethiopia.

Source: *Child Health in Ethiopia, Background Document for the National Child Survival Conference, April 2004*, Family Health Department, Ministry of Health.

The objectives of the IMNCI strategy are:

- to reduce mortality and morbidity associated with the major causes of disease in children less than five years of age, and
- To contribute to the healthy growth and development of children.

Integrated case management of the most prevalent childhood issues, with an emphasis on the leading causes of death, forms the basis of the IMNCI strategy. The clinical guidelines are intended to help with the management of sick children up to the age of five. These include techniques for identifying symptoms of serious illness, evaluating a child's diet, immunization history, and breastfeeding habits, instructing parents on how to care for their child at home, offering guidance to parents on how to address feeding issues, and advising parents on when to bring their child back to a medical facility. ..

IMNCI has the following advantages:

- Promotes the accurate identification of childhood illnesses in out-patient settings
- Ensures appropriate combined treatment of all major childhood illnesses

- Strengthens the counselling of mothers or caregivers
- Strengthens the provision of preventive services
- Speeds up the referral of severely ill children
- Aims to improve the quality of care of sick children at the referral level.

10.2.3 The IMNCI Assessment

Instead of arriving at a diagnosis when evaluating a sick child, a combination of individual signs leads to one or more classifications. The action-oriented illness categories known as IMNCI classifications allow a medical professional to decide whether a child needs to be immediately referred to a health center, whether the child can be treated at the health post (e.g. using ORS, an oral antibiotic, an antimalarial, etc.), or whether the kid can be raised safely at home.

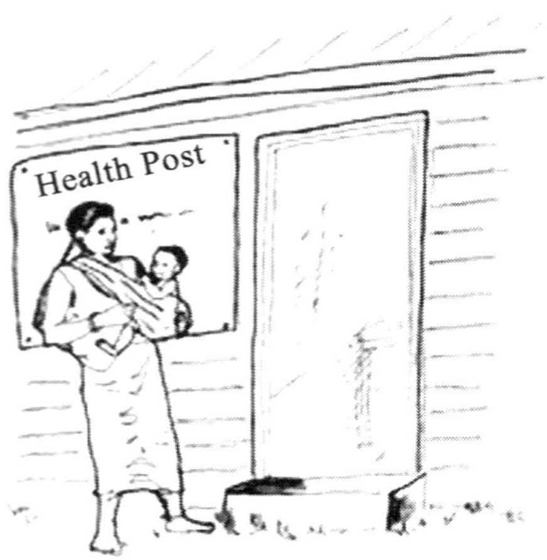

Figure 10.2. A mother and child arrive at the health post.

Source:- https://www.open.edu/openlearncreate/mod/oucontent/view.php?id=245&printable=1

The guidelines for Integrated Management of Neonatal and Childhood Illness (IMNCI) outline the proper care for children who visit your health post for illness treatment or follow-up appointments. These guidelines include procedures for assessing general danger signs, identifying bacterial infections in infants, detecting common illnesses, malnutrition, and anemia, and checking for other health concerns. Along with treatment recommendations, the guidelines also cover preventive measures to help maintain overall health.

10.3. Childhood Illnesses

Every child should have access to top-notch healthcare. To ensure your child is receiving the best care possible, it is crucial for parents to be informed about the most recent treatment guidelines. The American Academy of Pediatrics (AAP) provides a list of some of the most prevalent childhood illnesses along with recommended treatments. The therapies covered here are supported by best practices and scientific data. Your child's pediatrician may have different recommendations for your child for a variety of reasons, particularly if your child has a chronic illness or allergy. Any treatment modifications will be discussed with you by your pediatrician. Please contact your pediatrician with any questions you may have about providing your child with the best care possible.

10.4. Nutritional Management

Health workers should follow the counseling advice. A mother's card with pictures of the advice can be helpful for the mother to take home as a reminder.

10.4.1. Supporting Breastfeeding

Breastfeeding is most important for protecting infants from illness and for their recovery from illness.

- Exclusive breastfeeding is recommended from birth until 6 months of age.
- Continued breastfeeding, with adequate complementary foods, is recommended from 6 months to ≥ 2 years.

Health workers treating sick young children have the responsibility to encourage mothers to breastfeed and to help them overcome any difficulties.

10.4.2. Assessing a Breastfeed

Take a breastfeeding history by asking about the infant's feeding and behavior. Observe the mother while breastfeeding to decide whether she needs help. Observe:

How the infant is attached to the breast. Signs of good attachment are:

- Areola visible above the infant's mouth;
- Mouth wide open;
- Lower lip turned out;
- Infant's chin touching the breast;
- How the mother holds her infant;
- Should be held close to the mother;
- Should face the breast;
- The body should be in a straight line with the head;
- The whole body should be supported.

10.4.3. Overcoming Difficulties

10.4.3.1. 'Not Enough Milk'

Almost all mothers can produce enough breast milk for one or even two infants; however, sometimes an infant is not getting enough breast milk (Figure 10.3). The signs are:

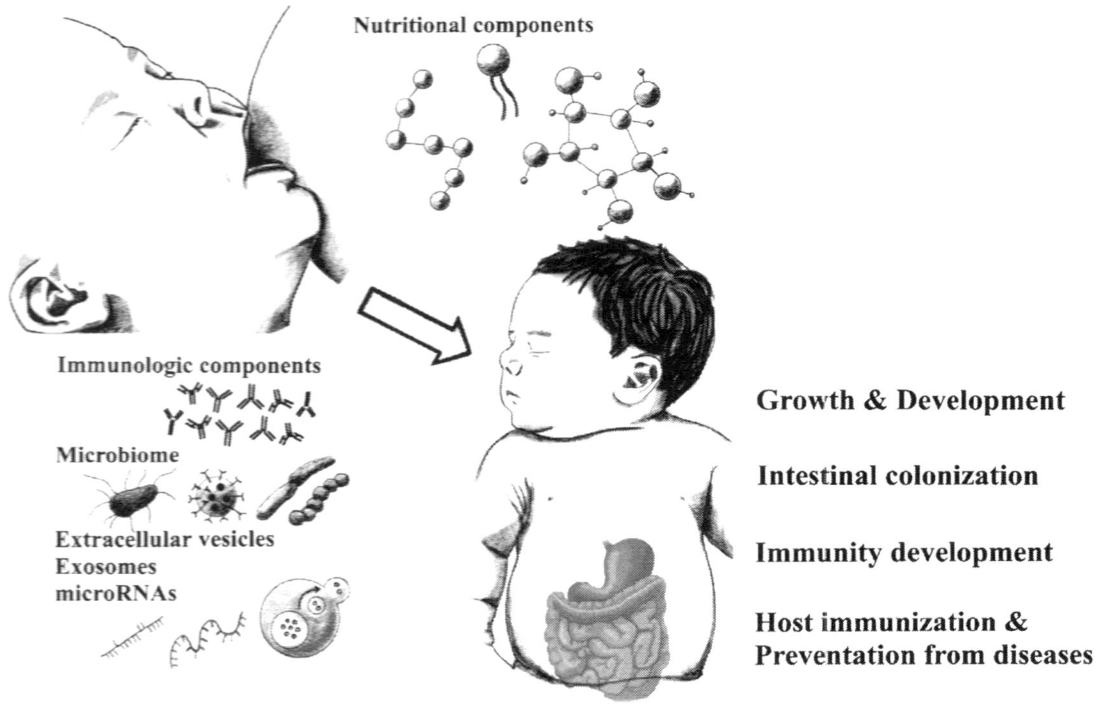

Figure 10.3. *Breastfeeding is an important aspect of motherhood.*

Source: *Yi, D. Y., & Kim, S. Y., (2021). Human breast milk composition and function in human health: From nutritional components to microbiome and microRNAs. Nutrients, 13(9), 3094. https://doi.org/10.3390/nu13093094.*

- Poor weight gain (< 500 g/month or < 125 g/week or infant weighing less than the birth weight after 2 weeks).
- Passing a small amount of concentrated urine (less than six times a day, yellow and strong-smelling).

Common reasons why an infant may not be getting enough breast milk are:

- **Poor Breastfeeding Practices:** Poor attachment (very common cause), delayed start of breastfeeding, feeding at fixed times, no night feeds, short feeds, use of bottles, pacifiers, other foods and other fluids.
- **Psychological Factors in the Mother:** Lack of confidence, worry, stress, depression, dislike of breastfeeding, rejection of infant, tiredness.
- **Mother's Physical Condition:** Chronic illness (e.g., TB, severe anemiaor rheumatic heart disease), contraceptive pill, diuretics, pregnancy, severe malnutrition, alcohol, smoking, retained piece of the placenta (rare).
- **Infant's Condition:** Illness or congenital anomaly (such as cleft palate or congenital heart disease) that interferes with feeding.

A mother whose breast milk supply is reduced will have to increase it, while a mother who has stopped breastfeeding may need to relactate.

Help a mother to breastfeed again by:

- Keeping the infant close to her and not giving him or her to other carers.
- Ensuring plenty of skin-to-skin contact between the mother and the infant at all times.
- Offering the infant her breast whenever the infant is willing to suckle.
- Helping the infant to take the breast by expressing breast milk into the infant's mouth, and positioning the infant so that he or she can easily attach to the breast.
- Avoiding the use of bottles, teats and pacifiers. If necessary, express the breast milk and give it by a cup. If this cannot be done, artificial feeds may be needed until an adequate milk supply is established.

10.4.3.2. How to Increase the Milk Supply?

The main way to increase or restart the supply of breast milk is for the infant to suckle often to stimulate the breast.

Give other feeds from a cup while waiting for breast milk to come. Do not use bottles or pacifiers. Reduce the other milk by 30–60 ml per day as the mother's breast milk starts to increase. Monitor the infant's weight gain.

10.4.3.3. Refusal or Reluctance to Breastfeed

The main reasons why an infant might refuse to breastfeed are:

- The infant is ill, in pain or sedated.
- If the infant is able to suckle, encourage the mother to breastfeed more often. If the infant is very ill, the mother may need to express breast milk and feed by cup or gastric tube until the infant can breastfeed again.
- If the infant is in hospital, arrange for the mother to stay with the infant to breastfeed.
- Help the mother to find a way to hold her infant without pressing on a painful place.
- Explain to the mother how to clear a blocked nose. Suggest short feeds, more often than usual, for a few days.
- A sore mouth may be due to Candida infection (thrush) or teething. Treat the infection with nystatin (100 000 U/ml) suspension. Give 1–2 ml dropped into the mouth four times a day for 7 days. If this is not available, apply 1% gentian violet solution. Encourage the mother of a teething infant to be patient and keep offering the breast.
- If the mother is on regular sedation, reduce the dose or try a less sedating alternative.
- There is difficulty with the breastfeeding technique
- Help the mother with her technique: ensure that the infant is positioned and attached well without pressing on the infant's head or shaking the breast.
- Advise her not to use a feeding bottle or pacifier: if necessary, use a cup.
- Treat engorgement by removing milk from the breast; otherwise, mastitis or an abscess may develop. If the infant is not able to suckle, help the mother to express her milk.
- Help reduce oversupply. If an infant is poorly attached and suckles ineffectively, the infant may breastfeed more frequently or for a longer time, stimulating the breast so that more

milk is produced than required. Oversupply may also occur if a mother tries to make her infant feed from both breasts at each feed, when this is not necessary.

- A change has upset the infant.
- Changes such as separation from the mother, a new carer, illness of the mother, a change in the family routine or the mother's smell (due to a different soap, food or menstruation) can upset the infant and cause refusal to breastfeed.

10.4.3.4. Low-Birth-Weight and Sick Infants

Infants with a birth weight < 2.5 kg need breast milk even more than larger infants; often, however, they cannot breastfeed immediately after birth, especially if they are very small.

For the first few days, an infant may not be able to take oral feeds and may have to be fed IV. Initiate early feeding with small oral feeds even on day 1 or as soon as the infant can tolerate enteral feeds.

Very low-birth-weight infants (< 1.5 kg) may have to be fed by naso- or orogastric tube during the first days of life. Preferably give the mother's expressed breast milk. The mother can let the infant suck on her cleaned finger while being tube fed. This may stimulate the infant's digestive tract and help weight gain.

Low-birth-weight infants at ≥ 32 weeks' gestational age can start suckling on the breast. Let the mother put her infant to the breast as soon as the infant is well enough. Continue giving expressed breast milk by cup or tube to make sure that the infant gets all the nutrition needed. Infants at ≥ 34–36 weeks' gestational age can usually take all that they need directly from the breast.

10.4.3.5. Infants Who Cannot Breastfeed

Non-breastfed infants should receive either:

- Expressed breast milk (preferably from their own mothers) or donor human milk where safe and affordable milk-banking facilities are available
- Formula milk prepared with clean water according to instructions or, if possible, ready-made liquid formula
- If the above are not available, consider animal milk. Dilute cow's milk by adding 50 ml of water to 100 ml of milk, then add 10 g of sugar, with an approved micronutrient supplement. If possible, do not use for premature infants.

Expressed breast milk is the best choice, in the following amounts:

- Infants ≥ 2.0 kg: Give 150 ml/kg daily, divided into eight feeds at 3-h intervals.
- Infants < 2.0 kg: for detailed guidance for low-birth-weight infants.
- If the child is too weak to suck but can swallow, feeding can be done with a cup. Feed by naso- or orogastric tube if the child is lethargic or severely anorexic or unable to swallow.

10.4.4. Nutritional Management of Sick Children

The principles for feeding sick infants and young children are:

- Continue breastfeeding.
- Do not withhold food.
- Give frequent, small feeds, every 2–3 h.
- Coax, encourage, and be patient.
- Feed by nasogastric tube if the child is severely anorexic.
- Promote catch-up growth after the appetite returns.

The food provided should be:

- Palatable (to the child);
- Easily eaten (soft or liquid consistency);
- Easily digested;
- Nutritious: rich in energy and nutrients.

The fundamental tenet of nutritional management is to include enough foods that provide energy and high-quality proteins in the diet. Foods high in oil or fat are advised; fat can make up as much as 30–40% of the total calories. To attain a high energy intake, frequent feedings are also required. Give multivitamins and mineral supplements to children who are ill. It is best to encourage the child to eat frequently in relatively small amounts. Young children may not eat enough if they are forced to compete with their siblings for food or if they are left to fend for themselves. A clogged nose, accompanied by thick or dry mucus, can make eating difficult. To help loosen mucus, insert saline drops into the nose using a moistened wick.

A small percentage of kids who go several days without eating (because, e.g., a nasogastric tube to be fed due to respiratory distress in severe pneumonia or impaired consciousness in meningitis. Giving frequent small volumes and making sure the tube is in the stomach before each feed will help lower the risk of aspiration. During convalescence, feeding should be increased to make up for any lost weight to support the child's nutritional management while they are in the hospital. When a child's appetite increases, it's critical that the mother or other caregiver feeds them more often than usual—at least one extra meal per day.

10.4.5. Fluid Management

The total daily fluid requirement of a child is calculated from the following formula: 100 ml/kg for the first 10 kg, then 50 ml/kg for the next 10 kg, thereafter 25 ml/kg for each subsequent kg. For example, an 8-kg infant receives 8 x 100 ml = 800 ml per day, a 15 kg child (10 x 100) + (5 x 50) = 1250 ml per day (Table 10.1).

Table 10.1. *Complementary Feeding Practices*

Breast-fed infants:

- Practice exclusive breastfeeding from birth to 6 months of age, and introduce complementary foods at 6 months of age while continuing to breastfeed
- Continue frequent, on-demand breastfeeding until 2 years of age or beyond
- Practice responsive feeding, applying the principles of psycho-social care
- Practice good hygiene and proper food handling
- Start feeding small amounts of complementary foods at 6 months of age and increase the quantity as the child gets older, while maintaining frequent breastfeeding
- Gradually increase food consistency and variety as the infant gets older, adapting to the infant's requirements and abilities
- Increase the number of times that the child is fed complementary foods as they get older
- Feed a variety of foods to ensure that nutrient needs are met
- Use fortified complementary foods or vitamin-mineral supplements for the infant as required
- Increase fluid intake during illness, including more frequent breastfeeding and encourage child to eat soft, varied, appetizing, favorite foods. Following illness, give more food than usual and encourage the child to eat more

Non-breastfed infants:

- Ensure energy needs are met: 600kcal per day at 6-8 months of age, 700 kcal per day at 9-11 months of age, and 900 kcal per day at 12-23 months of age
- Gradually increase food consistency and variety as the infant gets older, adapting to the infant's requirements and abilities
- For the average healthy infant, meals should be provided 4-5 times per day, with additional nutritious snacks offered 1-2 times per day, as desired
- Feed a variety of foods to ensure that nutrient needs are met
- As needed, use fortified foods or vitamin-mineral supplements (preferably mixed with or fed with food) that contain iron (8-10 mg/d at 6-12 months, 5-7 mg/d at 12-24 months)
- Non-breastfed infants and young children need at least 400-600 mL/d of extra fluids (in addition to the 200-700 mL/d of water that is estimated to come from milk and other foods) in a temperate climate, and 800-1200 mL/d in a hot climate. Plain, clean (boiled, if necessary) water should be offered several times per day to ensure that the infant's thirst is satisfied
- Practice good hygiene and proper food handling
- Practice responsive feeding, applying the principle of psycho-social care
- Increase fluid intake during illness and encourage the child to eat soft, varied, appetizing, favorite foods. After illness, give food more often than usual and encourage child to eat more

Source: *Harrison, L., Padhani, Z., Salam, R., Oh, C., Rahim, K., Maqsood, M., Ali, A., Charbonneau, K., Keats, E. C., Lassi, Z. S., et al., (2023). Dietary strategies for complementary feeding between 6 and 24 months of age: The evidence. Nutrients, 15(13), 3041. https://doi.org/10.3390/nu15133041.*

10.4.5.1. Monitoring Fluid Intake

When caring for very ill children, keep in mind that they may not have had any oral fluid intake in a while. It is preferable to administer fluids orally (via the mouth or a nasogastric tube). If intravenous fluids are required, close monitoring of the infusion is necessary due to the potential risk of fluid overload, which can result in heart failure or cerebral edema. The IV route should only be used to treat severe dehydration, septic shock, administer IV antibiotics, and treat children for whom oral fluids are contraindicated (such as those with intestinal perforations or other surgical abdominal problems) if close monitoring of the IV fluid infusion is not possible. Half-normal saline plus 5% or 10% glucose are examples of potential IV maintenance fluids. Giving 5% glucose on its own should not be done since it can cause hyponatraemia.

10.4.6. Management of Fever

The temperatures given in these guidelines are rectal temperatures, unless otherwise stated. Oral and axillary temperatures are lower by approximately 0.5 °C and 0.8 °C, respectively.

Fever is not an indication for antibiotic treatment and may help the immune defense against infection. High fever (> 39 °C or > 102.2 °F) can have harmful effects, such as:

- Reducing the appetite;
- Making the child irritable;
- Precipitating convulsions in some children aged 6 months to 5 years;
- Increasing oxygen consumption (e.g., in a child with very severe pneumonia, heart failure or meningitis).

All children with fever should be examined for signs and symptoms that indicate the underlying cause of the fever, and should be treated accordingly.

10.4.6.1. Antipyretic Treatment

1. **Paracetamol:** Treatment with oral paracetamol should be restricted to children aged ≥ 2 months who have a fever of ≥ 39 °C (≥ 102.2 °F) and are uncomfortable or distressed because of the high fever. Children who are alert and active are unlikely to benefit from paracetamol.

- Paracetamol dose is 15 mg/kg every 6 h.

2. **Ibuprofen:** The effectiveness in lowering temperature and the safety of ibuprofen and acetaminophen are comparable, except that ibuprofen, like any NSAID, can cause gastritis and is slightly more expensive.

- Ibuprofen dose is 10 mg/kg every 6–8 h.

3. **Other Agents:** Because aspirin has been associated with Reye syndrome, a rare but dangerous disorder affecting the liver and brain, it is not advised to use aspirin as a first-line antipyretic. Children suffering from dengue fever, chickenpox, or other hemorrhagic illnesses should not be given aspirin. Due to their toxicity and lack of effectiveness, other agents (dipyrone, phenylbutazone) are not advised.

10.4.7. Pain Control

Correct use of analgesics will relieve pain in most children with pain due to medical illness, when given as follows:

- Give analgesics in two steps according to whether the pain is mild or moderate-to-severe.
- Give analgesics regularly ('by the clock'), so that the child does not have to experience recurrence of severe pain to obtain another dose of analgesic.
- Administer by the most appropriate, simplest, most effective and least painful route, by mouth when possible (IM treatment can be painful and, if shock is present, can delay the effect).
- Tailor the dose for each child, because children have different dose requirements for the same effect, and progressively titrate the dose to ensure adequate pain relief.

Use the following drugs for effective pain control:

1. **Mild Pain:** Such as headaches, post-traumatic pain and pain due to spasticity. Give paracetamol or ibuprofen to children > 3 months who can take oral medication. For infants < 3 months of age, use only paracetamol.

- paracetamol at 10–15 mg/kg every 4–6 h;
- ibuprofen at 5–10 mg/kg every 6–8 h.

Moderate-to-severe pain and pain that does not respond to the above treatment: strong opioids:

- Give morphine orally or IV every 4–6 h or by continuous IV infusion.
- If morphine does not adequately relieve pain, then switch to alternative opioids, such as fentanyl or hydromorphone.

2. **Adjuvant Medicines:** Adjuvant therapy does not appear to be effective in treating chronic pain or certain types of pain in children, such as neuropathic pain, bone pain, or pain related to muscle spasms. Drugs that are frequently used include corticosteroids (like dexamethasone) for pain caused by an inflammatory swelling pressing on a nerve, diazepam for muscle spasm, and carbamazepine for neuralgic pain.

10.4.7.1. Pain Control for Procedures

1. **Local Anesthetics:** For painful lesions in the skin or mucosa or during painful procedures (lidocaine infiltration at 1–2%).

- Lidocaine: apply (with gloves) on a gauze pad to painful mouth ulcers before feeds; acts within 2–5 min.
- Tetracaine, adrenaline and cocaine: apply to a gauze pad and place over open wounds; particularly useful during suturing.

10.4.8. Management of Anemia

1. **Non-Severe Anemia:** Young children (aged < 6 years) are anaemic if their Hb is < 9.3 g/dl (approximately equivalent to an EVF of < 27%). If anemia is present, begin treatment, unless the child has severe acute malnutrition.

Give (home) treatment with iron (daily iron-folate tablet or dose of iron syrup) for 14 days. Ask the parent to return with the child in 14 days. Treat for 3 months when possible, as it takes 2–4 weeks to correct anemia and 1–3 months to build up iron stores.

If the child is ≥ 1 year and has not received mebendazole in the previous 6 months, give one dose of mebendazole (500 mg) for possible hookworm or whipworm infestation.

Advise the mother about good feeding practices.

2. **Severe Anaemia:** Give a blood transfusion as soon as possible to:

- All children with an EVF of ≤ 12% or Hb of ≤ 4 g/dl
- Less severely anemic children (EVF, 13–18%; Hb, 4–6 g/dl) with any of the following clinical features:
- Clinically detectable dehydration

- Shock
- Impaired consciousness
- Heart failure
- Deep, labored breathing
- Very high malaria parasitemia (> 10% of red cells with parasites).
- If packed cells are available, give 10 ml/kg over 3–4 h in preference to whole blood. If not available, give fresh whole blood (20 ml/kg) over 3–4 h.
- Check the respiratory rate and pulse rate every 15 min. If either rises or there is other evidence of heart failure, such as basal lung crepitations, enlarged liver or raised jugular venous pressure, transfuse more slowly. If there is any evidence of fluid overload due to the blood transfusion, give IV furosemide at 1–2 mg/kg, up to a maximum total of 20 mg.
- After the transfusion, if the Hb remains as low as before, repeat the transfusion.
- In children with severe acute malnutrition, fluid overload is a common and serious complication. Give packed cells when available or whole blood at 10 ml/kg (rather than 20 ml/kg), and do not repeat transfusion based on the Hb level, or within 4 days of transfusion.

10.4.8.1. Blood Transfusion: Storage of Blood

Use blood that has undergone screening to rule out infections that could spread during transfusion. Blood that is past its expiration date or has been left out of the refrigerator for longer than two hours should not be used. Hypothermia, particularly in small infants, can result from large-volume, fast transfusion of blood stored at 4 °C at a rate greater than 15 ml/kg per hour.

10.4.8.2. Problems in Blood Transfusion

Blood can be the medium through which infections (e.g., HIV, hepatitis B and C, syphilis, and malaria). As a result, check as many of these infections as you can on donors. Give blood transfusions only when absolutely necessary to reduce the risk.

1. **Indications for Blood Transfusion:** There are five general indications for blood transfusion:
   - Acute blood loss, when 20–30% of the total blood volume has been lost, and bleeding is continuing.
   - Severe anemia.
   - Septic shock (if IV fluids are insufficient to maintain adequate circulation; transfusion to be given in addition to antibiotic therapy).
   - Whole fresh blood is required to provide plasma and platelets for clotting factors if specific blood components are not available.
   - Exchange transfusion in neonates with severe jaundice.
2. **Giving a Blood Transfusion:** Before transfusion, check that:
   - The blood is the correct group, and the patient's name and number are on both the label and the form (in an emergency, reduce the risk for incompatibility or transfusion reactions by cross-matching group-specific blood or giving O-negative blood if available)
   - The blood transfusion bag has no leaks
   - The blood pack has not been out of the refrigerator for more than 2 h, the plasma is not pink or has large clots, and the red cells do not look purple or black

- The child has no signs of heart failure. If present, give 1 mg/kg of furosemide IV at the start of the transfusion to children whose circulating blood volume is normal. Do not inject into the blood pack.

Make baseline recordings of the child's temperature, respiratory rate and pulse rate.

The volume of whole blood transfused should initially be 20 ml/kg, given over 3–4 h.

i. During Transfusion:

- If available, use an infusion device to control the rate of transfusion.
- Check that the blood is flowing at the correct speed.
- Look for signs of a transfusion reaction, particularly carefully in the first 15 min of transfusion.
- Record the child's general appearance, temperature, pulse and respiratory rate every 30 min.
- Record the times the transfusion was started and ended, the volume of blood transfused and any reactions.

ii. After Transfusion:

- Reassess the child. If more blood is needed, a similar quantity should be transfused and the dose of furosemide (if given) repeated.

10.4.8.3. Transfusion Reactions

If a transfusion reaction occurs, first check the blood pack labels and the patient's identity. If there is any discrepancy, stop the transfusion immediately and notify the blood bank.

Ø **Mild reaction:** Due to mild hypersensitivity. Signs and symptoms:

- Itchy rash.

Ø **Management:**

- Slow the transfusion.
- Give chlorphenamine at 0.1 mg/kg IM, if available.
- Continue the transfusion at the normal rate if there is no progression of symptoms after 30 min.
- If the symptoms persist, treat as a moderately severe reaction.

Ø **Moderately Severe Reaction:** Due to moderate hypersensitivity, non-hemolytic reactions, pyrogens or bacterial contamination. Signs and symptoms:

- Severe itchy rash (urticaria).
- Flushing.
- Fever > 38 °C (> 100.4 °F) (Note: Fever may have been present before the transfusion.).
- Rigor.
- Restlessness.
- Raised heart rate.

Ø **Management:** Stop the transfusion, and remove the IV line but not the cannula. Set up a new infusion with normal saline.

- Give 200 mg hydrocortisone IV or 0.25 mg/kg chlorphenamine IM, if available.
- Give a bronchodilator if wheezing.
- Send the following to the blood bank: the blood-giving set that was used, a blood sample from another body site and urine samples collected over 24 h.
- If there is an improvement, restart the transfusion slowly with new blood and observe carefully.
- If there is no improvement in

15 min, treat as a life-threatening reaction, and report to the doctor in charge and to the blood bank.

Ø **Life-Threatening Reaction:** Due to hemolysis, bacterial contamination and septic shock, fluid overload or anaphylaxis. Signs and symptoms:

- Fever > 38 °C (> 100.4 °F) (Note: Fever may have been present before the transfusion.);
- Rigor;
- Restlessness;
- Raised heart rate;
- Fast breathing;
- Black or dark-red urine (hemoglobinuria);
- Unexplained bleeding;
- Confusion;
- Collapse.

Note that in an unconscious child, uncontrolled bleeding or shock may be the only signs of a life-threatening reaction.

Ø **Management:** Stop the transfusion, take out the IV line, but keep in the cannula. Set up an IV infusion with normal saline.

- Maintain airway and give oxygen.
- Give adrenaline 0.15 ml of 1:1000 solution IM.
- Treat shock.
- Give 200 mg hydrocortisone IV or chlorphenamine 0.1 mg/kg IM, if available.
- Give a bronchodilator, if there is wheezing.
- Report to the doctor in charge and to the blood laboratory as soon as possible.
- Maintain renal blood flow with IV furosemide at 1 mg/kg.
- Give antibiotics as for septicemia.

10.5. Care for a Sick Child

It can be distressing and stressful to have a sick child. While you're wondering if it's time to call the doctor, your child might be struggling to feel comfortable and cope with pain. There are various things you can do to make sure your sick child is comfortable and making progress toward recovery if they are at home.

10.5.1. Making a Sick Child Comfortable

1. **Provide Emotional Support:** Being sick is uncomfortable and your child may be worried or upset because of how he or she feels. Giving your child some extra attention and care may help. For example, you can:

- Sit with your child.
- Read your child a book.
- Sing to your child.
- Hold your child's hand.
- Hold your baby in your arms.

2. **Elevate Your Child or Baby's Head:** A cough can get worse if your child is lying flat on his or her back. To keep your child's head elevated, try putting a book or towel under the mattress of your baby's crib or under the legs at the head of the crib or bed (Figure 10.4).
   - • You can also give your child an extra pillow or use a wedge pillow to help your child stay upright.

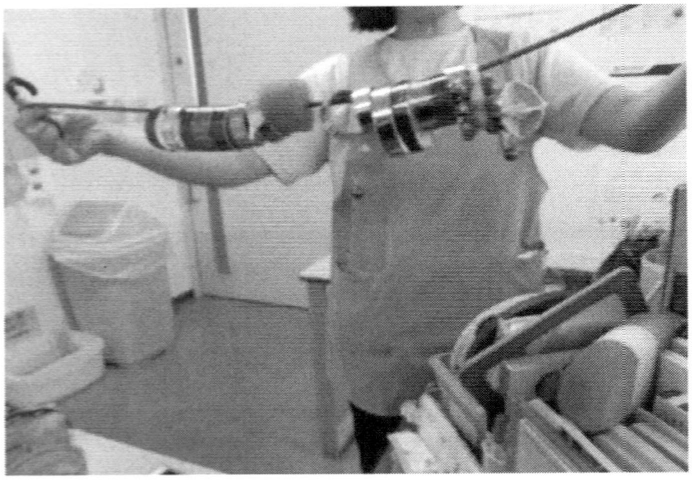

Figure 10.4. *Caring for sick children: This toy consists of a cord, hooks, and various materials with holes, such as rings made from glittering tapes of different colors and bells, threaded onto the cord. For children in bed, the cord is hooked at the bedrail, and rings are slid toward the opposite side at a signal from HPS, such as "Here they go! Choo!," so that they enjoy the movements and sounds of rings that move while rotating and changes of color.*

Source: *Kihara, N., & Yamamoto, T., (2018). Developmental support for sick children through play in Japan's ECEC system: A comparison with hospital play specialists. Children, 5(10), 133. https://doi.org/10.3390/children5100133.*

3. **Turn on a Humidifier:** Dry air can make a cough or sore throat feel worse. Try using a humidifier or cool-mist vaporizer to keep the air in your child's room moist. This can help to reduce coughing, congestion, and discomfort.
   - Make sure to change the water in your humidifier frequently.
   - Wash the humidifier according to the manufacturer's instructions to prevent mold from growing in it.
4. **Provide a Quiet Environment:** Keep your home as quiet and peaceful as possible to make it easier for your child to rest. Stimulation from television or computers prevents

sleep and your child needs as much rest as possible, so you may consider removing devices from your child's bedroom or at least limiting your child's use of devices.

5. **Keep Your Home at a Comfortable Temperature:** Your child may feel hot or cold depending on the illness, so adjusting the temperature in your home may help your child to feel more comfortable. It may be helpful to keep your home between 65° and 70°, but you can also adjust this temperature if your child is too hot or too cold.

10.5.2. Feeding a Sick Child

1. **Give Your Child Plenty of Clear Liquids:** Dehydration can make matters worse when your child is sick. Prevent dehydration in your child by making sure your child drinks fluids frequently. Offer your child:
   - Water;
   - Ice pops;
   - Ginger ale;
   - Diluted fruit juice;
   - Electrolyte-enhanced beverages.
2. **Provide Foods That are Easy to Digest:** Give your child nutritious foods that won't upset their stomach. Choice of food might depend on your child's symptoms. Good options include:
   - Salty crackers;
   - Bananas;
   - Applesauce;
   - Toast;
   - Cooked cereals;
   - Mashed potatoes.
3. **Give Your Child Chicken Soup:** Although it will not cure your child, warm chicken soup helps relieve cold and flu symptoms by making mucus thinner and acting as an anti-inflammatory. There are a number of recipes for making your own chicken soup, although many commercial varieties work well, too.

10.5.3. Treating a Sick Child at Home

1. **Give Your Child Plenty of Rest:** Encourage your child to sleep as often as he or she likes. Read your child a story or have your child listen to an audio book to make it easier to fall asleep. Your child needs as much rest as they can get.
2. **Use Over-the-Counter Medications with Caution:** If you decide to give medicine, try to stick to one product, such as acetaminophen or ibuprofen, rather than alternating medications or giving combinations of medications. Ask your doctor or pharmacist about which medicines might be appropriate for your child.
   - Do not give ibuprofen to a child under 6 months old.
   - Do not give cough and cold medicines to a child under 4 years old, and preferably not until at least 8 years old. These medicines have the potential to cause life-threatening side effects and have not been shown to be very effective either.
   - Do not give infants, children, or teenagers acetylsalicylic acid (aspirin) because this can cause a rare but serious illness called Reye's syndrome.
3. **Encourage Your Child to Gargle with Warm Salt Water:** Add ¼ teaspoon

of regular table salt to 8 ounces of lukewarm water. Have your child gargle and spit out the salty water when finished. Gargling with salt water can help relieve throat pain.

- • For younger children or for nasal congestion, you can also use salt water (saline) nasal drops or sprays. You can make a saline spray yourself or buy some at the pharmacy. For infants, you can use a bulb syringe to suction the nose after using the drops.

4. **Keep Your Home Free of Irritants:** Avoid smoking around your child and avoid wearing especially strong perfumes. Postpone activities like painting or cleaning. The fumes can irritate your child's throat and lungs and make their illness worse.
5. **Air Out Your Child's Room:** Periodically open the windows in your child's room to keep the air fresh. Do this when the child is in the bathroom so they don't get cold. Give your child extra blankets as necessary.

10.5.4. Seeing a Doctor

1. **Determine Whether Your Child has the Flu:** Take symptoms of an infection with the influenza virus seriously. It is a potentially dangerous illness that often develops suddenly. Contact your child's doctor if you think your child may have the flu, especially if your child is under age 2 or has medical problems such as asthma. Symptoms of the flu include:
    - High fever and/or chills;
    - Cough;
    - Sore throat;
    - Runny nose;
    - Body or muscle aches;
    - Headache;
    - Tiredness and/or weakness;
    - Diarrhea and/or vomiting.
2. **Take Your Child's Temperature:** Check to see if your child has chills, a flushed appearance, is sweating, or feels very warm to the touch if you do not have a thermometer.
3. **Ask Your Child if he or She Has Any Pain:** Ask your child how much pain he or she is in and where the pain is located. You may also want to apply gentle pressure to the spot your child is complaining about to get an idea of how severe it is.
4. **Watch for Signs of Serious Illness:** Pay careful attention to signs that indicate your child needs to be seen by a medical professional immediately. These include:
    - Fever in a child under three months old;
    - Severe headache or a stiff neck;
    - Changes in breathing patterns, especially any trouble breathing;
    - Changes in skin color, such as looking very pale, reddish, or bluish;
    - Child refuses to drink fluids or stops urinating;
    - No tears when crying;
    - Severe or persistent vomiting;
    - Child is difficult waking up or is unresponsive;
    - Child is unusually quiet and inactive;
    - Signs of extreme irritability or pain;

- Pain or pressure in the chest or stomach;
- Sudden or prolonged dizziness;
- Confusion;
- Flu-like symptoms improve but then get worse.

5. **Visit Your Local Pharmacist:** Talk to your local pharmacist if you are not sure whether your child needs to be seen by a doctor. She or he can help determine if your child's symptoms require medical attention and can offer advice on medications if they are needed.
   - You can also call your doctor's office, as there is almost always someone available to help you decide what to do and to provide home care advice.

10.5.5. Reducing the Spread of Illness in Childcare

There is always a risk of infection transmission when kids are around each other. This is particularly true for young children, as they frequently touch other kids or handle toys after wiping their noses or rubbing their eyes with their hands. The virus spreads from one child's nose or eyes to another through hands or toys, and so on, until the youngest child touches his own nose or rubs his own eyes. Additionally, during the first few years of life, children are more prone to illness as their bodies develop immunity to infections.

Due to staffing levels or space constraints, many childcare centers are unable to provide adequate care for a sick child; however, in other centers, the child can be kept comfortable and given time to rest when necessary in a different part of the room where they have already exposed the other kids. An ill child who is being excluded should wait to be picked up in a place where they are not in contact with people who have not yet been exposed to their infection. To keep the child under close supervision and stop the illness from spreading throughout the facility, it is usually best for the child to remain in one location. In certain programs, a staff member who is qualified to care for sick children and who is familiar with the child may look after them in a designated area where no one else will see them. When a child needs to rest, there might be a spot where they can lie down and still be seen by a staff member if their condition only requires minimal care and doesn't require exclusion. For kids with minor ailments who can't participate in regular daycare or who require more attention than the staff can give, some communities have created special sick child care centers.

It's possible that some infections will still spread throughout the child care facility despite all of these preventative efforts. A child is contagious for many of these infections for up to a day before they show symptoms. Make sure to frequently wash your hands and your child's hands. You never know when a virus or bacteria is being passed from one child to another. Your child may occasionally get sick at daycare and have to be sent home. To ensure that someone can pick him up, you will need to have a plan. Thankfully, some illnesses—like ear infections—are not communicable. There's no need to keep your sick child apart from the other kids in these situations. You can schedule most medications to be administered exclusively at home. If your child needs medication during the day, make sure the facility has trained staff members who can administer medication and that there are clear procedures in place. Find out how they make sure the right medication is being given to the right child at the right time, via the right route, in the right dose, and record each dosage.

10.5.6. Measures to Promote Good Hygiene in Childcare

To reduce the risk of disease in child care settings as well as schools, the facility should meet certain criteria that promote good hygiene.

- Are there sinks in every room, and are there separate sinks for preparing food and washing hands? Is food handled in areas separate from the toilets and diaper-changing tables?
- Are the toilets and sinks clean and readily available for the children and staff? Are disposable paper towels used so each child will use only his own towel and not share with others?
- Are toys that infants and toddlers put in their mouths sanitized before others can play with them?
- Are all doors and cabinet handles, drinking fountains, and all surfaces in the toileting and diapering areas cleaned and disinfected at the end of every day?
- Are all changing tables and any potty chairs cleaned and disinfected after each use?
- Are staff and other children fully immunized, especially against the flu?
- Is food brought in from home properly stored? Is food prepared on site properly handled?
- Is breast milk labeled and stored correctly?
- Are children and their caregivers or teachers instructed to wash their hands throughout the day, including:
- When they arrive at the facility
- Before and after handling food, feeding a child, or eating
- After using the toilet, changing a diaper, or helping a child use the bathroom (Following a diaper change, the caregiver's and child's hands should be washed and the diaper-changing surfaces should be disinfected.)
- After helping a child wipe his nose or mouth or tending to a cut or sore
- After playing in sandboxes
- Before and after playing in water that is used by other children
- Before and after staff members give medicine to a child
- After handling wastebaskets or garbage
- After handling a pet or other animal
- Make sure your own child understands good hygiene and the importance of hand washing after using the toilet and before and after eating.
- Is health consultation available to deal with outbreaks or to review policies?
-

A Closer Look

Immunization

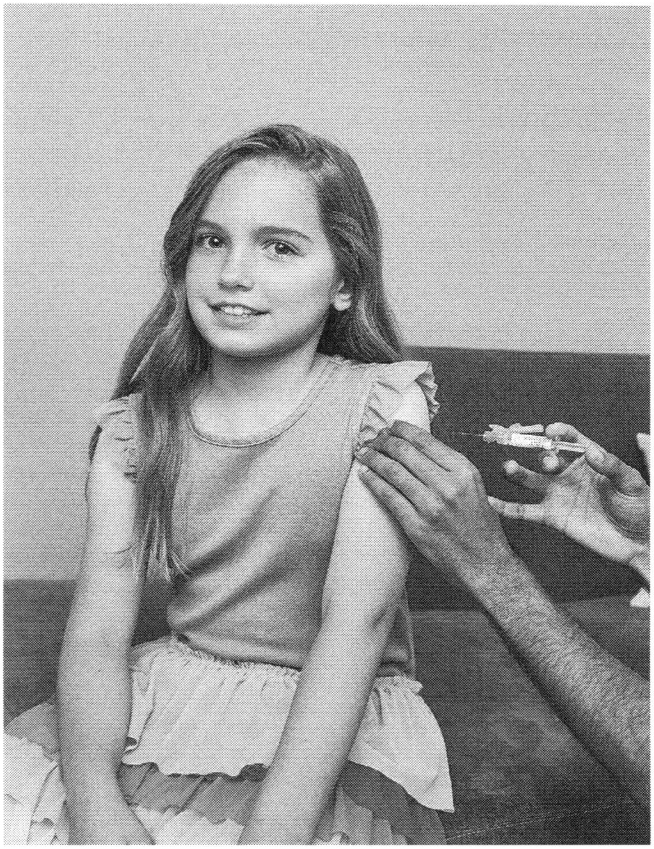

Source: By SELF Magazine – Young girl about to receive a vaccine in her upper arm, CC BY 2.0, https://commons.wikimedia.org/w/index.php?curid=81631650.

One of the best ways to guard against infectious diseases for yourself, your kids, and future generations is through immunization. Put differently, immunization contributes to the eradication of diseases that have the potential to proliferate in the future.

In addition to taking care of your own family, you are also safeguarding the weaker members of your community by making sure you and your family adhere to the National Immunization Program Schedule established by the Australian Government. A disease can spread less widely and fewer people will become infected the more vaccines people receive. Immunizations prevent fatalities. Even in the 1950s, diseases like whooping cough (pertussis), diphtheria, and tetanus caused thousands of deaths in children each year. Fortunately, large-scale immunization campaigns that were started in the 1960s and 1970s and are still going strong today have made it extremely rare for anyone in Australia to pass away from these infectious diseases.

Every vaccination functions in the same way. The vaccination boosts immunity to an infection before it affects you by utilizing your body's immune system. Stated differently, it is akin to having a disease infection but not exhibiting any symptoms. Following vaccination, your body fights off infections to prevent you from contracting the illness, or it may only give you a mild case. In contrast to alternative immunization strategies (like homeopathy), vaccinations have undergone extensive testing to confirm their efficacy and safety in preventing infectious diseases.

Summary

- The Integrated Management of Childhood Illness (IMCI) is an integrated approach to child health that focuses on the well-being of the whole child.
- The tactile (touch) health check involves gently rubbing your hand on the child's back, shoulder, or head as you greet him or her.
- Mild illness is common among children. Most children will not need to be excluded from their usual source of care for mild illnesses.
- The child should be removed from direct contact with other children and should be cared for in an area where the toys, equipment, and surfaces will not be used by other children or adults until after the ill child leaves and after the surfaces and toys have been cleaned and disinfected.
- The child should be encouraged to eat relatively small amounts frequently. If young children are left to feed themselves or have to compete with siblings for food, they may not get enough to eat.

References

1. McIntyre J. Management of fever in children. Arc Dis Child. 2011;96:1173–1174.
2. Neto G. Fever in the young infant. In: Moyer VA, Eliott EJ, Gilbert R, Klassen T, Logan S, et al., editors. Evidence-based pediatrics and child health. 2nd ed. BMJ Books/Blackwell publishing; 2004. pp. 257–66.
3. Yeung K, Duclos P, Nelson E, Hutubessy R. An update of the global burden of pertussis in children younger than 5 years: a modelling study. *Lancet Infect Dis.* 2017;**17**(9):974–980.
4. Crowcroft N, Stein C, Duclos P, Birmingham M. How best to estimate the global burden of pertussis? *Lancet Infect Dis.* 2003;**3**(7):413–418.
5. Legesse E, Dechasa W. An assessment of child immunization coverage and its determinants in Sinana District, Southeast Ethiopia. *BMC Pediatr.* 2015;**15**(1):31.
6. Lakew Y, Bekele A, Biadgilign S. Factors influencing full immunization coverage among 12–23 months of age children in Ethiopia: evidence from the national demographic and health survey in 2011. *BMC Public Health.* 2015;**15**(1):728.

INDEX

A

Abdominal 54, 55, 56, 65, 70, 71
Abortion 9, 16
Abruptio placentae 131
Adolescence 181, 183, 192, 222, 223, 225
Adolescent health 183
Adolescents 2, 17, 34, 183, 207
Adrenal cortisol 51
Adrenocorticosteroids 69
Adverse childhood experiences (ACEs) 216
Advocacy 242, 245, 269
Allergy 323
American Congress of Obstetricians and Gynecologists (ACOG) 131
Analytic epidemiology 258
Anemia 9
Anesthesia 130, 131, 132, 133, 134
Anganwadi Workers (AWWs) 84
Antibiotic therapy 331
Antifungal medication 158
Anxiety 284, 287, 292, 293, 298, 302, 306
Asparagus 191
Auditory Brain Stem Response (ABR) 169
Auscultatory 60
Avoidance 133, 138

B

Bacterial infection 317
Bacterial sinusitis 195
Ballottement 57
Bladder irritation 67
Blood pressure 48, 61, 62, 64, 78
Bloodstream 89, 103
Blood volume expansion 62
Bluish skin 155
Braxton Hicks 56
Braxton Hicks contractions 127
Bronchiolitis 194
Brussels sprouts 190, 191

C

Cantaloupe 192
Carbon dioxide 65, 66
Cardiotocography 135
Cardiovascular system 224
Cardiovascular System 60
Catecholamines 122
Cauliflower 192
Cells crystallizing 58
Cervix development 91
Chest transillumination 166
Chickenpox 90, 317
Chickpeas 191
Child health 2, 4, 5, 7, 8, 9, 10, 11, 13, 16, 17, 19, 22, 34, 40, 41, 42
Childhood diseases 196
Childhood immunization 316

Childhood vaccination 316, 318
Child maltreatment 284, 286, 287, 288, 289, 299, 300, 301, 304, 307, 309, 310, 311
Child protection agency 14
Chloasma 68
Chorioamnionitis 131
Chronic bronchitis 194
Chronic infections 9
Citrus fruits 192
Cognitive development 213, 227, 234
Cognitive development milestones 176
Communication 10, 15, 16, 17, 35
Community-based clinics 247
Community health nurse 244, 245
Community immunity 314, 316
Community organizations 210
Comprehensive strategy 203
Congenital adrenal hyperplasia (CAH) 167
Conservation 177
Continuous positive airway pressure (CPAP) 163
Convulsions 137
Corpus luteum 48, 74
Cost containment 7
Criminal Behavior 200
Critical Congenital Heart Disease (CCHD) 168, 169
Cultural taboos 9
Cyprus 98

D

Depression 287
Dexamethasone 51
Diaphragm elevation 65
Diarrhea 9, 158
Digital health technologies 222
Diphtheria 314, 316, 317, 318, 319, 340
Disaster management 220, 221
Disease 214, 215, 216, 219, 220, 221, 222, 226
Disease Control and Prevention (CDC) 137, 213, 248, 252
Disease surveillance 219
Disequilibrium 92, 94
Diuretics 324
Droplet nuclei 254
Dyslipidemia 184
Dystocia 128, 135, 137, 141
Dysuria 67

E

Eclampsia 124, 131, 137
Economic power 2
Edematous 57
Emergency preparedness 220
Epidemiology 219
Epistaxis 65
Estrogen 48, 54, 56, 58, 59, 60, 65, 66, 69, 70, 72, 73, 74, 75
Estrogen stimulation 56
Etiologic 253, 257, 260
Eustachian tubes 65
Every Woman, Every Child (EWEC) 247
Expected Date of Delivery (EDD) 82
Exploitation 284, 286, 289, 300
External fetal monitoring (EFM) 135

F

Family planning 9
Fatigue 52
Fetal demise 131
Fetal movements 52, 57
Fetal waste products 67
Fetus's growth and development 48, 75
Financial assistance 202
Fluid intake 86
Foodborne pathogens 187
Fortified cereals 191, 192

G

Gastric cancer 185
Gastrointestinal discomforts 93
Gestational 153, 154, 158, 164, 165, 166, 170, 171
Gestational Age 153, 170
Gestational hypertension 131
Glomerular filtration rate (GFR) 67
Glucose 51, 67, 68, 75
Glucose intolerance 184
Glucose tolerance test 51
Glucosuria during pregnancy 68

Gravidity 50
Gray mucoid discharge 58
Growth hormone 51
Growth retardation 9
Guarantee consistency 17
Gum hypertrophy 70
Gynecological disorders 287
Gynecology 129, 142, 148

H

Habitual spontaneous abortion 93
Hand hygiene 219
Handicapped children 9
Haphazard assessment 93
Healthcare 2, 5, 7, 8, 9, 10, 11, 14, 15, 16, 17, 18, 19, 21, 22, 30, 31, 33, 34, 35, 36, 39, 40, 43
Healthcare paradigm 244
Healthcare quality 9
Healthcare services 2, 7, 8, 10
Health Management Information System (HMIS) 85
Health promotion 10, 11, 19, 22
Healthy lifestyle 210, 215, 225
Heart rhythm 192
Hemodilution 62
Hemoglobin concentration 129
Heterosexual marriages 14
High-quality healthcare 174
Hirsutism 70
Homocystinuria 167
Hormone 125, 129, 130, 144
Hpertrophy 54, 55, 57, 59, 60, 67
Human chorionic gonadotropin (hCG) 48
Human Immunodeficiency Virus (HIV) 82
Human papillomavirus (HPV) 21
Hygiene 247
Hyperemia 65, 67
Hyperemia appear 65
Hyperpigmentation 68
Hyperplasia 54, 57, 58, 59, 67, 75
Hypertension 56, 68
Hypertensive disorders 217
Hypotensive syndrome 61, 62
Hypothesis 93
Hypothyroidism 167

I

Immature circulation 152
Immigration 181
Immune function 213, 227
Immunity 255, 257
Immunizations 210, 215, 217
Immunocompromising 319
Immunological response 191
Infants 157, 165, 166, 169
Infection prevention 150
Infections 155, 156, 157, 158, 167
Infectious diseases 215, 219, 314, 316, 317, 318, 339, 340
Inferior vena cava 62
Inflammatory response 65
Influence 2, 6, 11, 33, 37, 41
Influenza 318, 319, 336
Insecticide-treated mosquito nets (ITNs) 247
Insulin tolerance test 51
Integrated Management of Childhood Illness (IMCI) 195
Integrated Management of Newborn and Childhood Illness (IMNCI) 319
Integumentary system 68
Intermittent mandatory ventilation (IMV) 163
Intervillous spaces 56
Intraosseous 165
Intrauterine device (IUD) 129
Intrauterine pressure catheter (IUPC) 136
Intravenous fluids 328

J

Jaundice 156

L

Lactation 60
Language development 214
Last Menstrual Period (LMP) 82
Lentils 191
Ligaments 48, 55, 65, 74
Local anesthesias 96

Long-acting reversible contraception (LARC) 129
Lysosomal 168

M

Macronutrients 181, 182
Malnutrition 9, 180, 181, 200, 217, 218, 226
Maltreatment 284, 286, 287, 289, 291, 292, 294, 296, 298, 299, 300, 303, 305
Maternal and child health (MCH) 4, 246
Maternal arterial pressure 56
Maternal health 2, 9, 29, 41, 42, 43, 246, 247, 248, 252
Mean arterial pressure (MAP) 61
Measles-mumps-rubella (MMR) 317
Medical supervision 61
Medical Termination of Pregnancy (MTP) 83
Mental Health 8, 21
Mental health management 214
Metabolic rate 65, 66, 70
Metabolism 183
Metyrapone 51
Milestones 176, 177, 178, 179
Mineralocorticoids 51
Ministry of Women and Child Development (MoW-CD) 85
Misinformation 314, 316
Morbidity 241, 247, 252, 253, 267, 270, 275
Mucous plug 58
Multifaceted strategy 284, 288, 307
Muscle contraction 192
Musculoskeletal 48, 53
Mushrooms 192
Mysterious 213

N

Naloxone 165
Narcotic pain medications 194
National Institutes of Health (NIH) 191
Neglected tropical diseases (NTDs) 247
Neonatal 8, 10, 16, 26, 29, 45
Neonatal lungs 163
Neonatal morbidity 10
Neonatal resuscitation 158, 159, 160, 161
Neonatal technology 8
Nervous system 192
Newborn 150, 152, 153, 154, 155, 156, 158, 159, 160, 161, 163, 168, 169, 171, 172
Newborn death 90
Non-communicable diseases (NCDs) 287
Normal hemoglobin 62
Normal phenomenon 52
Nuckolls 93
Nullipara's cervix 57
Numerous clinicians 244
Nutrition 2, 7, 30, 84, 86, 87, 118, 213, 218, 227

O

Obesity 287
Optimal operation 182
Oral rehydration therapy (ORT) 247
Otoacoustic Emissions (OAE) 169
Oxytocin 125

P

Painless Braxton 56
Pain management 10, 15
Pancreatic insulin 51
Papanicolaou 57
Patient education 215
Patricia Benner 19
Peak inspiratory pressure (PIP) 163
Pediatrician 182, 193, 194
Perineum 59
Perspiration 67
Pharmaceutical 242
Pharmaceutical regulation 222
Phenomenon 126
Phenylketonuria 167
Physical skills 181
Physiologic 48, 52, 68, 71
Physiological alterations 158
Physiological changes 79, 81
Physiological functions 48
Playgroups 216
Pleural effusion 166

Pneumonia 217, 235, 317, 319, 321, 327, 329
Pneumothorax 165
point of maximal intensity (PMI) 60
Positive end-expiratory pressure (PEEP) 163
Positive pressure ventilation (PPV) 161, 163
Postpartum 51, 59, 65, 70, 74
Postpartum hemorrhage 96
Postpartum infections 96
Postpartum process 2
Post-term pregnancy 131
Post-traumatic stress disorder (PTSD) 200, 201
Posttraumatic stress disorder (PTSD) 138
Potassium regulates 192
Potatoes 190, 192
Preeclampsia 90, 91, 131
Pregnancy 2, 4, 6, 7, 8, 9, 10, 11, 17, 19, 21, 23, 24, 26, 28, 29, 30, 33, 34, 37, 38, 39, 40, 41, 42, 43, 45, 47, 48, 50, 51, 52, 53, 57, 60, 61, 64, 65, 66, 67, 70, 73, 78
Premature atrial contractions 61
Prenatal care 79, 81, 88, 97, 99, 100, 119
Primigravida 50
Progesterone 91, 116
Promote healthy growth 180, 183
Promoting maternal 2, 5
Promotion 11, 20
Properly disinfected 187
Prophylactic medication 219
Prosperous 7
Protects health 185
Proteinuria 68
Psychological 92, 93, 94, 96, 97, 98
Psychological distress 287
Psychological health 183, 200
Psychomotor 180
Psychosocial factors 122
Psychosocial repercussions 184
Public health 2, 4, 5, 41
Public Health Security 242
Public Health Service 22
Puerperal sepsis 9
Puerperium 11
Pulmonary function 65
Pulse oximetry 168, 169

R

Rapid assessment 162
Rapid breathing 156
Rapid Plasma Reagin (RPR) 82
Red blood cells (RBCs) 62
Regional anesthetics 134
Relaxation reduce 133
Renal function 67
Renal plasma flow (RPF) 67
Respiratory 9
Respiratory Syncytial Virus (RSV) 318
Resuscitation 150, 158, 159, 161, 165, 166
Retinol activity equivalents (RAE) 191
Risk assessment 220

S

School health 9
Self-Help Groups (SHGs) 84
Sexual abuse 284, 289, 290
Sexually transmitted infections (STIs) 140, 218
Sexual violence 286
Smoking 287
Social inequality 288
Social services 9
Sociocultural practices 9
Socioeconomic 252, 257, 258, 273
Spinach 191, 192
Spiritual dimension 214
Squamocolumnar junction 57
Stimulus 94, 97
Strawberries 192
Strengthening healthcare systems 218
Stretch marks 69
Striae gravidarum 59, 69
Surveillance 213, 219
Sustainable Development Goals (SDGs) 4, 247
Sweat gland activity 66
Syndromic surveillance 219

T

Thermal care 150
Thoracic 60, 65
Tocodynamometer 136
Tomatoes 192
Toxemia 96
Transmission 253, 254, 255, 257, 260
Tuberculosis 9, 33, 34, 241, 254
Tympanic membranes 65

U

Umbilicus 54, 71
Unintended pregnancy 287
Universal health coverage (UHC) 221
Unscarred cervix 57
Ureters lengthen 67
Urine production 67
Uterine blood flow 56
Uterine enlargement 54, 55
Uterine isthmus 56
Uterus 54

V

Vaccination 215, 219
Vagina 125, 127, 132, 133
Varicella 317, 318
Vegetarian 189
Venereal Disease Research Laboratory (VDRL) 82
Ventilation efficacy 163
Village Health and Nutrition Day (VHND) 84
Volume expansion 165

W

Weight-to-height relationship (BMI) 184
Workforce planning 222
World Health Organization (WHO) 5

Y

Youth Media Campaign Longitudinal Survey (YM-CLS) 213

FSC
www.fsc.org
MIX
Papier | Fördert gute Waldnutzung
FSC® C083411

Kolibri 360 GmbH
Ferdinand-Jühlke-Straße 7
99095 Erfurt, Deutschland
produktsicherheit@kolibri360.de